Birth, Bonding and Baby Behaviour

Carmen Power

Birth, Bonding and Baby Behaviour

Understanding the Links Between Childbirth Experience and Early Infant Behaviour

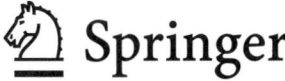

Dr. Carmen Power
Independent Researcher/Consultant/Educator
Bristol, Somerset, UK

ISBN 978-3-032-05844-7   ISBN 978-3-032-05845-4 (eBook)
https://doi.org/10.1007/978-3-032-05845-4

© The Editor(s) (if applicable) and The Author(s), under exclusive license to Springer Nature Switzerland AG 2025

This work is subject to copyright. All rights are solely and exclusively licensed by the Publisher, whether the whole or part of the material is concerned, specifically the rights of translation, reprinting, reuse of illustrations, recitation, broadcasting, reproduction on microfilms or in any other physical way, and transmission or information storage and retrieval, electronic adaptation, computer software, or by similar or dissimilar methodology now known or hereafter developed.

The use of general descriptive names, registered names, trademarks, service marks, etc. in this publication does not imply, even in the absence of a specific statement, that such names are exempt from the relevant protective laws and regulations and therefore free for general use.

The publisher, the authors and the editors are safe to assume that the advice and information in this book are believed to be true and accurate at the date of publication. Neither the publisher nor the authors or the editors give a warranty, expressed or implied, with respect to the material contained herein or for any errors or omissions that may have been made. The publisher remains neutral with regard to jurisdictional claims in published maps and institutional affiliations.

This Springer imprint is published by the registered company Springer Nature Switzerland AG
The registered company address is: Gewerbestrasse 11, 6330 Cham, Switzerland

If disposing of this product, please recycle the paper.

This book is dedicated to Jasmine and Sophie Power, and to the next generation of young people thinking about or planning to have a baby.

Foreword

Birth is the beginning of life. It starts with the journey of a baby—a unique human being—into the outside world, and the phenomenal adaptation of the baby's anatomy, physiology and psychology required for adjustment to life beyond the womb. For the woman, it is a metamorphosis into motherhood. The experiences of both the baby and the mother during this critical and highly sensitive period—labour, giving birth and being born—will make all the difference, not only to the beginning of life but to all of life. The impact of care during this time will have a profound and enduring effect. Birth should be a time full of potential for the future: for health, wellbeing and happiness. Care during this time can contribute to a start in life where this potential may be realised; a lack of care may reduce it. For the woman, a positive experience is of vital importance to her and to her ability to mother her child. And let's not forget the father or the other parent, who is also making a profound adaptation and is critical to the baby's future.

Birth is a time when those bonds that tie us to one another, that enable us to provide the adjustment and commitment needed for mothering or parenting, when perhaps recovering from physical trauma, usually exhausted, may be strengthened or weakened. Secure attachments and strong, enduring relationships form a vital foundation for both short and long term health and happiness. The development of this bond, between mother, baby, father and family, is reciprocal. How the mother feels, how the baby feels—expressed at this time only through behaviour—and the father's experience will affect their interactions.

Over many years as a midwife, I have worked with women and babies where the baby, unsettled, fussy, screaming, kicking away, has brought to the exhausted parents a feeling that they are being rejected. I learned from the midwives of the 1960s that some babies are 'born with a headache'. Clearly distressed, a baby with a headache needed to be soothed and calmed. I have worked with women and babies where a gentle birth has altered the Apgar score because there was no crying, only a wide-eyed gazing. It is simply easier to love a baby who is easily cuddled and consoled.

The formation of attachments around birth and the health of mother and baby are supported by a highly intricate interplay of physiology and psychology. This delicate balance may be easily disturbed by fear, anxiety, complications, interventions, threats, poverty, ethnicity, inequalities or ill health. If we are to provide care aimed at thriving rather than just surviving, an understanding of the profound importance of the mother's and baby's experience, as well as the physiological and psychological basis of the bonds that tie us to one another, is vital.

Yet I have seen, in my work as a midwife over the years, and in many parts of the world, that there is a blind spot, a denial even, to the importance of our support for the development of strong, enduring bonds. This intricate interplay between physiology and psychology is often overlooked when making decisions about interventions. Babies are still separated from their mothers. Routines override relationships, quiet and recovery. Overstretched, under-resourced, poorly led services lead to neglect of mothers and babies, and moral distress and emotional trauma to staff. Rather than knowing joy and achievement and delight in their baby, too many women are being physically and psychologically traumatised. Since the 1980s, we have known about the capabilities of newborns and how their behaviour communicates their needs. Yet this is seldom spoken about. There is still a silence around the baby's voice.

This is why, when I read 'Birth, Bonding and Baby Behaviour', I was filled with a sense of excitement, optimism and relief. After years of working with disparate, scattered resources in journals and lectures, here is a book that has brought them all together. It builds on our knowledge, based on sound research, exploring the impact of care during labour, birth and early life on the experience of the baby and the mother, and the relationship between them. As far as I know, nobody has done this before. In well over 40 years of experience as a midwife, in hands-on practice and management, then as professor doing academic work and developing practice, organisations and policy at national and international levels, I have become acutely aware of this blind spot and denial of a need that is fundamental if we are to support health and wellbeing around this vital time of life.

Birth, Bonding and Baby Behaviour helps us see into the blind spot. In conducting a deep exploration fired by curiosity arising from her own very different experiences of giving birth, Carmen has gone to the centre of what is important. When I first heard her speak at a conference in London some years ago, I realised that Carmen's research was going to fill a missing piece in our work to humanise childbirth. Now, brought together in the pages of this book are three in-depth studies about childbirth and baby behaviour, an up-to-date account of the literature and an understanding of our modern-day context. The methodology is rigorous yet infused with a clear humanity. Here, at last, is a resource—a book that turns our attention, shines a light on a higher aim: to support, through our care, health, happiness and wellbeing in both the short and long term. Dr Carmen Power aims to bring to a wider audience an exploration of how the experience of childbirth potentially affects us all. Here is a deeply humane scientist who has asked profound questions, and rather than shy away from their complexity, has embraced them with continuing curiosity.

Drawing from robust research and personal insight, Carmen explores the profound interconnections between birth, bonding and baby behaviour. She illuminates the experience of the baby, so often absent from our understanding, and brings the voices of mothers and midwives to the forefront. Through mixed-methods research, she builds a compelling case for care that honours the mother's and baby's intertwined physiology and psychology. She describes her work as joining the dots or putting missing pieces into a puzzle. This work shows us that the baby's behaviour is a meaningful expression—that how a baby is received into the world matters deeply. It also reminds us that love and connection between mother and baby are supported or undermined by the nature of the care they receive.

Birth, Bonding and Baby Behaviour is a vital resource for policymakers, midwives, health visitors, doctors and doulas. It will be of interest to women about to give birth, or thinking about it, to help inform their choices. Above all, the book sets our sights on a higher level of thinking about how we provide care while also addressing detailed concerns. If we take this higher level of thinking into practice, we will help give babies a better start in life. This is of importance to us all.

Visiting Professor in the Department Lesley Page
of Women & Children's Health,
Faculty of Life Science & Medicine
King's College London
London, UK
2025

Acknowledgements

There are many remarkable individuals without whom this book could not have been written. First and foremost, my heartfelt gratitude goes to all the mothers, midwives, health visitors and doulas who participated in the original research, sharing their experiences, perceptions and beliefs about birth, bonding and baby behaviour so honestly, openly and in such great depth. I hope I have managed to capture some of your profound insights and words of wisdom.

I would like to thank my initial research collaborators, Professors Amy Brown and Claire Williams, for showing me the ropes and guiding me through the process. Huge thanks to Spoorthy Deepak, whose graphic wizardry helped bring some of the dry numerical data to life. And a big thank you to everyone who reviewed chapters and made valuable contributions, including Grégoire Capron, Lucy Power, midwives Rebecca Johnson and Julika Johanna Hudson, obstetric sonographers Jane Chippett and Amie Whittard, and Kim Thomas—CEO of the Birth Trauma Association and author of the national Birth Trauma Inquiry report. I'm also grateful to Professor Susan Ayers for introducing me to Kim and, through her extensive and inspiring work on birth trauma, for encouraging us all to see childbirth from a more holistic, psychological perspective rather than a purely physical or medical one.

I am enormously grateful to my lovely editor, Marie-Elia Come-Garry, who enthusiastically embraced the initial idea, allowed great flexibility as the book developed and provided helpful feedback and encouragement throughout the writing process. I'd also like to thank Pinky Sathishkumar and the rest of the production team at Springer Nature, who kept the book on track in a friendly, efficient and supportive manner. Additionally, I appreciate their patience at the end, when I kept on wanting to revise 'just one more thing'.

Profound gratitude to my dear friend, colleague and mentor, midwifery professor Lesley Page, who readily agreed to write the foreword—for her support throughout this project and for meticulously reviewing and providing invaluable feedback on the entire book, which dramatically improved it by helping me turn its focus further towards its audience. I feel very privileged to have you on board and am thrilled to be involved in some of your projects too.

To friends and family—particularly my inspiring parents, who passed on all their writerly tips and a whole lot more; and my late 'bonus father', Professor Sir John Hills, who provided so much guidance, enthusiasm and support throughout this research, greatly influencing the direction the writing took by advocating for an awareness of the impacts of health and wealth inequalities on outcomes for mothers and babies. Also to the very special people who have constantly cheered me on and never fail to lift my spirits: Jeany, Judy, Inga, Annie, and of course, my wonderful children—the initial inspiration for this research. Thank you all for your unwavering belief.

Finally, and from the bottom of my heart, I am grateful to Mike, who gave me the space to focus and write, even on high days and holidays when we were supposed to be relaxing and having fun together, but the mounting pressure of a looming book deadline constantly drove me back to my desk. I can't ever thank you enough for your unerring faith, kindness, patience and jovial good humour—all of which helped me to just keep on writing.

About the Book

The *Birth, Bonding and Baby Behaviour* book is an introduction to the physical and psychological impacts of childbirth on mother and baby. It demonstrates how the birth experience can affect parents' mental health, parent-infant bonding and baby behaviour, and have a ripple effect on infant development and the baby's future physical and mental health.

The book has been written as a resource for health professionals seeking to understand more about the physiological and psychological needs of parents and babies during childbirth, how they can contribute to positive outcomes for mother and baby, and how best to support the whole family through this pivotal, life-changing transition. This aim encompasses all families, regardless of ethnicity, disability, gender, neurodiversity or any other factors that may require particular care during the early stages of the birthing and parenting journey. In writing about it here, I hope to bring this vital research to the desks of influential policymakers as well as to the health professional's coffee table and the midwifery student's rucksack.

I would like this to be a book that practising midwives, doulas, health visitors, obstetricians, neonatologists, paediatricians and students in all these fields will be drawn to pick up and read a few pages of at a time, whenever they find a spare moment amid their busy lives. If you are one of these people, whose work is essential to positive outcomes for mother and baby, the wider family and the society in which we live, I hope it inspires you and increases your resolve to practise holistically and humanely—that is, to always remember that in every birthing situation there is the long-term physical and emotional wellbeing of at least two people at stake. Therefore, the mother's and baby's human rights need to be upheld at every point of the process. Giving birth to a live baby is the very least that parents should be able to expect in the twenty-first century. Bringing babies into the world who can grow up happily and healthily in a society that cares for their wellbeing and welfare from the outset must become our ultimate ambition.

Carmen Power

Endorsements

Commentary 1

"A difficult birth can have a profound psychological effect on mothers, many of whom report finding it hard to bond with their baby. But what effect does the birth itself have on the baby? This is the under-researched topic Carmen Power explores in her fascinating book. Using survey and interview data from both mothers and health professionals, Power explores the interplay between the type of birth, the mother's psychological state and the baby's behaviour, such as its ability to settle. Her research demonstrates how birth can influence the mental wellbeing of both mother and baby and highlights the importance of making sure that mothers feel safe and well looked after during birth. Its valuable insights make it a must-read for midwives, health visitors and anyone who works with pregnant women and new mothers."

(*Dr Kim Thomas, CEO of the Birth Trauma Association and author of the 2024 National Birth Trauma Inquiry*)

Commentary 2

"This book powerfully details why childbirth matters when it comes to infant mental health and why we need to respect and protect the mother-infant pair from the start. Drawing on her own research and experience, Dr Carmen Power makes the strong argument that infant behaviour is closely linked to childbirth practices and experiences, effortlessly weaving in decades of evidence from a variety of disciplines. A must-read for professionals, policymakers and parents alike."

(*Dr Julika Hudson Community Midwife, Infant Mental Health Team, Dublin*)

Contents

1 **An Introduction to Early Infant Behaviour in the Context of Childbirth**......................... 1
   1.1 A Brief History of Maternity and Neonatal Care Practices and Beliefs 2
   1.2 Infant Mental Health 7
   1.3 The Possibility of Long-Term Physiological Changes Taking Place During Childbirth................ 9
   1.4 Joining the Dots 10
   1.5 Motivation for This Research................... 12
   1.6 How the Studies Were Carried Out 14
   1.7 Outline of Chapters 16
   References.. 16

2 **A Brief Introduction to Infant Temperament and Parent-Infant Bonding** 21
   2.1 Infant Temperament: What Is It and Why Does It Matter? 21
   2.2 Where It All Began: The Origins of Infant Temperament Research 22
   2.3 Neonatal Behavioural Assessment Scale 24
   2.4 Why Is It Important to Protect Infant Temperament Development? 25
   2.5 Parent-Infant Bonding and Its Relationship to Infant Behaviour and Temperament........... 26
   References.. 31

3 **How Is Childbirth Related to Bonding and Baby Behaviour?** *Physical Factors That Might Influence the Course of Childbirth and Infant Outcomes* 35
   3.1 Birth Mode: How the Type of Birth Can Affect Mother and Baby 36
   3.2 Birthplace..................................... 46
   3.3 Induction of Labour and Its Potential Impacts on Mother and Baby........................... 47
   3.4 Pain Relief and Its Relationship to Obstetric Interventions and Infant Outcomes 52

	3.5	Alternatives to Using Medical Pain Relief During Childbirth 56
	3.6	Why Is It Essential to Reduce Pain and Distress During Labour? 59
	3.7	Labour Positions 59
	3.8	Conclusion: Where Does This Leave Us Now? 61
	References 62	
4	**Psychological Impacts of Childbirth on Mother and Baby** 73	
	4.1	Introduction to the Psychology of Childbirth 73
	4.2	The Psychology of Pregnancy 75
	4.3	The Psychology of Childbirth 76
	4.4	Postnatal Mental Health 80
	References 91	
5	**Maternity Care Providers' Perceptions of Childbirth and Baby Behaviour** 101	
	5.1	Introduction to the Study 101
	5.2	What the Interviews Uncovered About Birth, Bonding and Baby Behaviour 102
		5.2.1 The Baby's Response to Childbirth 103
		5.2.2 The Mother's Response to Childbirth 108
		5.2.3 Chapter Summary, Conclusions and New Insights 118
	References 120	
6	**Mothers' Childbirth Experiences and Perceptions of Their Baby's Behaviour** 123	
	6.1	Introduction to Mothers' Perceptions of Childbirth and Baby Behaviour 123
	6.2	Outline of Childbirth Experiences and Baby Behaviour 124
	6.3	What the Mothers Said About Their Birth Experience and Their Baby's Behaviour 126
		6.3.1 Physical Birth Experience 127
		6.3.2 Psychological Birth Experience 139
	References 151	
7	**Physical and Psychological Experiences of Childbirth and Baby Behaviour** 157	
	7.1	Introduction to the Survey 157
	7.2	How the Survey Was Carried Out 159
	7.3	The Findings: Relationships Between Childbirth Experiences and Baby Behaviour 163
	7.4	Maternal Personality, Postnatal Mood and Current Mental State (Anxious/Relaxed) 200
	7.5	Summary of the Survey Findings So Far 202
	References 202	

8	**Physical and Psychological Experiences of Childbirth and Baby Behaviour** 207
	8.1 Introduction 207
	8.2 Perinatal Factors Predicting 24-Hour Baby Outcomes 208
	8.3 Perinatal Factors Predicting Mother and Baby Scale Outcomes (0–6 Months) 210
	8.4 Summary of the Birth and Perinatal Factors Predicting Mother and Baby Outcomes 216
	8.5 What Does This Study Show Us, and Where Do We Go from Here? 220
	8.6 Summary 222
	References 222
9	**Joining the Dots:** *What Does This All Mean for the Future of Maternity Care?* 225
	9.1 Placing the Findings in the Context of Other Research 225
	9.2 New Insights into Childbirth Experiences and Baby Behaviour 228
	9.3 Conclusion 237
	References 239

About the Author

Carmen Power is a writer, researcher, educator and consultant specialising in the interconnected fields of childbirth, perinatal mental health, parent-infant bonding, baby behaviour and infant development. She is an active member of the World Association of Infant Mental Health and has served on the committee of the Society for Reproductive and Infant Psychology for several years. She holds a PhD in Public Health, which focused on childbirth experiences and baby behaviour, viewed from both health professionals' and mothers' perspectives.

With a background in Psychology and Education, she is also a trained doula, hypnobirthing practitioner and early years specialist. She is currently involved in several international collaborations, including Investigating Maternal Perinatal Stress and Adverse Outcomes in the Offspring with *TREASURE*, a European Cooperation in Science and Technology (COST Action), and ongoing projects around Humanising Childbirth and the Polarisation of Maternity Care with Oxford University medical sociologist, Professor Sue Ziebland, and leading midwifery professors, Lesley Page (CBE) and Soo Downe.

In addition to her academic work, she provides consultancy, research, analysis and report writing on childbirth, parent-infant bonding and infant social-emotional development for various charities, including the Parent Infant Foundation, the Royal Foundation and the Birth Trauma Association. She regularly presents at international conferences on midwifery, reproductive health and infant psychology, and teaches Psychology, Education and Public Health to students at universities across the UK.

List of Figures

Fig. 5.1	The baby's response to childbirth	104
Fig. 5.2	The mother's response to childbirth	109
Fig. 6.1	Type of birth and baby behaviour	125
Fig. 6.2	Overall birth experience and baby behaviour	126
Fig. 6.3	Did the birth affect your baby?	126
Fig. 6.4	An overview of birth mothers' experiences and their baby's behaviour	128
Fig. 7.1	Relationship between 24-Hour Baby and early infant behavioural style	164
Fig. 7.2	Relationship between 24-Hour Baby and maternal confidence	165
Fig. 7.3	24-Hour Baby according to birthplace	167
Fig. 7.4	Baby behaviour (0–6 months) according to birthplace	168
Fig. 7.5	Maternal confidence according to birthplace	168
Fig. 7.6	24-Hour Baby after tear or episiotomy	169
Fig. 7.7	Baby behaviour (0–6 months) after tear or episiotomy	170
Fig. 7.8	Maternal confidence after tear or episiotomy	171
Fig. 7.9	24-Hour Baby according to the start of labour method	171
Fig. 7.10	Baby behaviour (0–6 months) according to start of labour	172
Fig. 7.11	Maternal confidence according to start of labour	173
Fig. 7.12	Labour interventions and 24-Hour Baby	174
Fig. 7.13	Labour interventions and Baby Behaviour (0–6 months)	175
Fig. 7.14	Labour interventions and maternal confidence	176
Fig. 7.15	24-Hour Baby according to birth mode	178
Fig. 7.16	Baby behaviour (0–6 months) according to mode of birth	178
Fig. 7.17	Maternal confidence according to mode of birth	179
Fig. 7.18	Pain Ratings, Pain Relief and Baby Behaviour	181
Fig. 7.19	Baby distress signals and 24-Hour Baby	182
Fig. 7.20	Baby distress signals and baby behaviour (0–6 months)	183
Fig. 7.21	Baby distress signals and maternal confidence	183
Fig. 7.22	Gentle birth and 24-Hour Baby	184
Fig. 7.23	Baby behaviour (0–6 months) following a gentle/non-gentle birth	185

Fig. 7.24	Maternal confidence following a gentle/non-gentle birth	186
Fig. 7.25	24-Hour Baby following to skin to skin	186
Fig. 7.26	Baby behaviour (0–6 months) following skin to skin	187
Fig. 7.27	Maternal confidence following skin to skin	188
Fig. 7.28	24-Hour Baby according to first feed	189
Fig. 7.29	Baby behaviour (0–6 months) according to first feed	189
Fig. 7.30	Maternal confidence according to first feed	190
Fig. 7.31	24-Hour Baby according to current feeding method	190
Fig. 7.32	Baby behaviour (0–6 months) according to current feeding method	191
Fig. 7.33	Maternal confidence according to current feeding method	191
Fig. 7.34	Subjective pregnancy states and baby behaviour	193
Fig. 7.35	Birth emotions and baby behaviour	194
Fig. 7.36	Subjective postnatal states and baby behaviour	195
Fig. 7.37	Overall perceptions of childbirth and baby behaviour	197
Fig. 7.38	Birth emotions according to birth mode	198
Fig. 7.39	Subjective postnatal states according to birth mode	199
Fig. 7.40	Perceptions of childbirth according to birth mode	199
Fig. 7.41	Maternal personality, mental health and baby behaviour	201
Fig. 7.42	Summary of physical and psychological factors relating to baby behaviour	202
Fig. 8.1	Predictors of Cry-Fuss 24-Hour Baby	209
Fig. 8.2	Predictors of alert-content 24-Hour Baby	210
Fig. 8.3	Predictors of Positive Baby Behaviour	211
Fig. 8.4	Predictors of Neutral Behaviour (0–6 months)	212
Fig. 8.5	Predictors of negative baby behaviours (0–6 months)	213
Fig. 8.6	Predictors of global confidence (during the first 6 months)	215
Fig. 8.7	Predictors of Lack of confidence in caretaking and breastfeeding (0–6 months)	216
Fig. 8.8	Correlations and predictors of baby behaviour	218
Fig. 8.9	Mother-infant bonding predicts the ongoing mother-child relationship	219
Fig. 9.1	Factors that most contribute to baby behaviour during the first 6 months	227

List of Table

Table 7.1   Mother and Baby Scales (MABS) 162

An Introduction to Early Infant Behaviour in the Context of Childbirth

The *Birth, Bonding and Baby Behaviour* book is based on three studies from a PhD in Public Health, examining mothers' and health professionals' experiences and perceptions of childbirth and its relationship to bonding, baby behaviour and the development of infant temperament. The studies were carried out in collaboration with PhD supervisors, Professors Amy Brown and Claire Williams. While we have published each of these studies as a scientific paper in peer-reviewed journals [77–79], this book aims to bring them to a broader audience (beyond academic researchers)—to reach practising clinicians working in maternity or neonatal care. After setting the scene within the context of modern and historical childbirth practices, the book explores how the experience of childbirth potentially affects us all. In other words, it affects everyone who is born, not just those who give birth or who are supporting another person to give birth (e.g. partners, family members, midwives, doctors and doulas). The book investigates the potential short- and long-term impacts of childbirth experience on the infant's future physical and psychological health. It discusses how the way birth is managed, including both maternity and neonatal care, could be improved to make childbirth a happier, safer, more fulfilling and empowering experience for parents, babies and midwives. A positive childbirth experience, as outlined by the World Health Organization's intrapartum guidelines [96], should leave the mother with confidence and self-efficacy in her new role [68], benefitting not only herself but also her baby, partner and wider family.

The *Birth, Bonding and Baby Behaviour* book presents the relevant connections between childbirth experience and infant behaviour. It examines in detail the particular and very personal horrors of a traumatic birth experience, alongside looking at what happens when birth goes well and the mother feels content with—or even euphoric about—her birth experience. The book explores how parent-infant bonding and a newborn baby's physiological wellbeing and behaviour might benefit from a more "humane" birth than is common in many overrun and under-resourced maternity care settings today—in other words, one that provides personalised, respectful and compassionate care that responds to the mother and baby's physiological, psychological and emotional as well as medical needs. This should occur without any *unnecessary* medicalisation (where intervention is not either required or requested by the mother) and be based on respecting and honouring parents' informed choices and personalised preferences, their cultural and socioeconomic background and their current life situation [68, 70].

*For ease of use, the terms "mother", "woman", "she" and "her" are used throughout to incorporate all individuals who give birth to a baby, including those who are gender-neutral or diverse. These terms therefore denote intentions of inclusivity throughout the book. To easily distinguish the baby from the person who gives birth to them (and because I would really rather not refer to any baby as "it"), when the baby's gender is unknown, I use the male terms "he/him/his" to encompass all babies. The baby's caregivers are referred to here as their "parents"—although the use of this term incorporates all people responsible for caring intimately for the baby after childbirth, including adoptive or step-parents.

1.1 A Brief History of Maternity and Neonatal Care Practices and Beliefs

Childbirth has undergone significant changes, not just since the Industrial Revolution, as is sometimes claimed [60, 91]. Even since the early days of "Call the Midwife", where midwives rode on bicycles in pairs to attend homebirths in some of the poorest parts of London, childbirth practices have altered almost beyond recognition. Some of these changes are positive, such as the availability of pain relief and having modern technology readily available for an expedited birth if needed. Others, however, are less so and could even be damaging when used as blanket interventions or without the appropriate scientific evidence to support their effectiveness or safety. Certain changes have taken place and then been retracted, for example, the trend of separating mother and baby at birth, with the baby only being returned for brief 4 hourly breastfeeds. What is a widely accepted childbirth practice one day is often discounted and dismissed the next. This introduction to the subject of changing childbirth practices and their potential impact on mother and baby will cover a few key topics, some of which will be explored in more detail in Chaps. 3 and 4 and later in relation to the three studies presented in Chaps. 5, 6, 7 and 8.

Mother-Baby Separation, Interventions and Birth Trauma
If there is one major way in which the medicalisation of childbirth has been responsible for interrupting parent-infant bonding, attachment and consequently healthy infant development and long-term wellbeing, it is probably the practice of separating mother and baby post-birth. Intuitively, we have always known that childbirth is a transformative milestone for mother and baby, who ideally should be cared for "as one" after the birth. There is an ever-increasing amount of research evidence emphasising the importance of not intruding on the mother and baby getting to know each other during these sensitive first few "golden" hours, providing there are no valid

medical reasons for their separation, and possibly even if there are (e.g. by replacing time in an incubator with parent-baby skin-to-skin care).

Modern technological advances in maternity and neonatal healthcare have led to many life-saving gains as well as some potential issues. One problem that has appeared alongside the medicalisation of childbirth is the idea that we can treat the mother and baby as two separate entities, the minute the birth itself is over. Although the mother and newborn baby's instinctive need to remain together after childbirth has been known since time immemorial, the evolution of medically based maternity care has meant that these intrinsic needs can sometimes be overlooked in the haste of the moment. Another critical issue is the misguided concept that only the physical safety (and thus physical care) of mother and baby is essential and, therefore, attention to emotional care is unnecessary.

Sometimes a mother or baby may need medical attention during or immediately after childbirth. However, it is often possible to treat them together, as is often done in Nordic countries, who recognise the significance of this sensitive time for parent-infant bonding [50, 54]. What affects the mother will undoubtedly affect the baby. When this precious time for parents and babies to bond gets thwarted, infant development may suffer, with potentially long-term impacts on the child. A Japanese study reveals that a lack of bonding during infancy (i.e. during the first 2 years) increases the likelihood of 5-year-old children exhibiting "difficult" and "asocial" behaviours, with this effect being particularly pronounced in male babies [51]. However, although an extensive study investigating over 1000 women has shown us that separation of mother and baby post-birth provokes the highest number of "extreme distress" hotspots, interpersonal difficulties and post-traumatic stress symptoms [14], the mother's physiological and psychological wellbeing is currently not given enough focus in busy maternity wards.

Bringing this complex topic of maternal distress to public attention, the UK government cross-party Birth Trauma Inquiry established that a general lack of care and compassion, accentuated by a severe midwifery shortage after years of austerity and the COVID-19 pandemic, has led to many women being traumatised by their birth and postnatal care experiences [92]. As the author of this report has observed, many traumatised women also mention challenging, unsettled baby behaviour, often asking whether this is normal. However, as the inquiry did not ask specific questions about infant outcomes, it is difficult to know just how many babies are affected by birth trauma. Out of 1,300 responses to the public inquiry, approximately 200 mothers talked about how the birth experience had disturbed early mother-baby bonding, sometimes due to pain and immobility after a traumatic birth, and sometimes due to the sheer horror of their unsupported birth experiences—but this is a topic for another book!

Examining birth trauma from another perspective, health professionals (including midwives and obstetricians) who witness traumatic childbirth—even where there is no blame attached—often suffer complex emotions linked to secondary trauma such as guilt, shame and remorse. This may affect their short- and long-term psychosocial health and wellbeing, leading to psychological burnout, stress or depression—mental states that are not conducive to safer practice [85, 86]. Traumatic childbirth experiences from both perspectives—mothers' and health professionals'—are reinforced by our risk-averse safety culture, where "defensive medicine" is practised, and women and babies are subjected to multiple "unnecessary interventions" [96]. This self-perpetuating situation is caused by hospitals' and health professionals' ever-increasing fear of litigation.

While historical customs vary worldwide, "confinement" (care with a focus on rest and assistance) was previously commonplace for the mother-infant pair. This practice was intended to promote successful breastfeeding, bonding and care of the newborn, but has been in decline since the early 1950s, with possible negative impacts on the mother's physical and mental health, as well as the baby's overall wellbeing and ability to thrive [35]. It has been suggested that changes in practice have come about in response to the emotionally supportive care that midwives once provided being gradually eroded by hierarchical systems dominated by men. This has meant the focus in maternity care became more efficiency- and productivity-based, with technology- and task-orientated care now the norm for both doctors and midwives, resulting in more (often unconsented) interventions as midwives attempt to fulfil the extensive medical criteria demanded by current maternity care systems [95].

In many Western countries, the ancient tradition of keeping mother and baby together after childbirth was replaced with them being instantly and automatically separated for medical checks and infection control [12]. With the medicalisation of childbirth, and until relatively recent times, mothers were often whisked straight off for a bath or stitches while their baby was briskly wiped down with a rough towel, hung upside down by their feet until they cried, placed naked on a set of cold metal weighing scales and then carted off to the nursery and lain alone in a tiny cot, far away from everything the newborn baby instinctively wants and needs to survive: love, warmth and food—ideally from their parents [93]. This routine separation of the mother and baby after childbirth had some serious unintended consequences for mother-baby relationships and infant care. Original research comparing nursery care (where mother and baby are separated) with rooming-in (where mother and baby are kept together) showed that removing newborn infants from their mothers resulted in less frequent breastfeeding and consequently lower breastfeeding success rates as well as less sleep and more crying for the babies. Perhaps unsurprisingly, mothers whose babies were removed to the nursery also did not sleep any longer or better [52], no doubt because they were worrying about their babies.

All They Need Is Love
Since time immemorial, the baby's mother and everything she provides has been imperative to his survival [93]. Although it is possible to replace some of these essentials with modern replicas, for instance, replacing breast milk with bottle milk, we know from Harlow's [45] cruel monkey experiments that separating mothers and babies post-birth can cause profound disturbances, leading to bonding, attachment and developmental issues that could be long-lasting and extremely difficult to repair. How many thousands of babies have been inadvertently harmed

by these practices? In tandem with their newborn's instinctive needs and desires, mothers are highly attuned to their babies and can also become very distressed when their baby is distressed [46]. Therefore, promoting proximity is essential for both parties[39]. Sadly, while it now seems obvious that a human baby is born with basic human needs and rights that require proximity and close contact with another human being, and preferably one who loves them and can feed them, science had to prove this—that the newborn baby needs love and intimate proximity to their mother—before our healthcare systems were willing to contemplate "rooming-in" policies. These days, it could almost appear that keeping mother and baby together after childbirth was a modern innovation rather than an instinctive ancient practice.

The Seeing and Hearing Newborn
Along similar lines, until quite recently (only a matter of decades), we still believed the human baby was incapable of seeing or hearing anything much during (or for some time after) pregnancy and childbirth. Yet scientists have discovered that the foetus can hear and respond to sounds inside and outside the womb from just 16 gestational weeks [59]. This ability to listen is thought to be in preparation for language acquisition. Experimenters have even compared the cries of French and German newborn infants and discovered they are different, remarkably reflecting their mothers' voice contours and intonations from the moment of birth [47]. By 19 weeks, the foetus may "dance" to music from inside the amniotic sac, stretching and exercising its limbs in response to sounds in a way that positively influences their future behaviour [33], neurodevelopment and temperament [7]. And it was a complete revelation when scientists discovered that newborn babies recognise their parents' voices as soon as they are born while showing a preference for their biological mother's voice as she is likely to be the one who they heard most often while still inside the womb [58].

When it comes to sight, rather than still being blind at the moment of birth as previously assumed, research over the past couple of decades has clearly shown that the newborn infant does in fact see, if not very far to begin with, and can even integrate visual stimuli with other sensory input [40]. As demonstrated by Nugent et al. [69], a newborn baby will typically turn their head to locate and follow a nearby sound, such as a tinkling bell and a moving colourful shape, like a red ball. In fact, it is not just bright colours that newborn babies see. They can notice and pay attention to any moving object [32]. The human infant is also programmed to socially engage in mutual gazing with "closely connected" others from birth, and these skills are vital for their survival and attachment [43]. Interestingly, newborns are also perfectly happy to stare at a non-human primate's face, such as a monkey [31], perhaps illustrating that, as a race, we are even more similar to monkeys than we previously thought! Andrew Meltzoff [62] demonstrated in his experiments on infants' imitations of facial expressions that newborn babies can perceive another human face and are programmed to socially interact with their fellow humans from birth.

So, when does human consciousness begin? Due to our inability to remember our earliest days or ask newborns how they feel, this is a challenging question to answer; hence the early assumption that newborn babies do not think or feel until they are old enough to express themselves in a way we can understand. Recently, however, through functional magnetic resonance imaging (fMRI brain scans), scientists have been able to show that the human subjective experience (i.e. how we think and feel) might begin when still in the womb—where thalamocortical connectivity (transferring sensory messages to the brain) is established from as young as 26 gestational weeks [41].

"It's Just Wind"
To continue with this list of "scientific" follies, with new evidence constantly disproving the old, newborn babies were believed to smile only when releasing "wind". According to this old "wisdom", they also cried only to expand their lungs and breathed only once their umbilical cord was clamped and cut immediately after being born. Until quite recently in fact, babies were not believed capable of half the things we now know they can do, think and feel. However, the research evidence has accumulated, showing that babies are intelligent mini scientists, conducting their own physical and social experiments as soon as they can grasp and drop, performing complex analyses of cause and effect. For example, "If I drop this spoon, it makes a sound as it hits the floor and (bonus) my parent comes running to pick it up for me". Directly contradicting Piaget's [71] previously influential assumptions of complete egocentricity during the "pre-operational" stage (2–7 years), even very young infants can put themselves in another's shoes and imagine other human experiences to their own [42].

This relatively newly discovered infant intelligence involves acknowledging the newborn baby's innate social and emotional intelligence, as well as their ability to experience distress, although tragically and similar to sight and hearing, scientists did not used to believe babies were capable of experiencing any emotions. Thankfully, multiple studies over the past three decades have shown this to be untrue. Indeed, newborn babies experience extreme distress when separated from their mother during the early moments, hours or days after being born [20]. And even very young infants respond and react to their mother's distress [36]. Well, why *wouldn't* they? Babies are programmed to think, feel and relate to others from birth, and scientists are finally beginning to understand *how* they think and feel. For example, babies gaze for longer at unexpected or impossible events (e.g. a toy car passing through a wall) than at more predictable and physically feasible ones (such as the same toy car riding on the ground). And babies as young as 5 months old have expectations about what is going to happen [10]. In the words of Gopnik [42], babies and young children can no longer be viewed merely as "defective adults".

1.2   Infant Mental Health

Infant mental health is an increasing concern as incidences of poor developmental mental health in our children and young people seem to be rising year on year. This is happening even in Nordic countries, which have set a shining example to the rest of the world for many years by providing extensive support for parents, babies and families during the first few years after childbirth and beyond. In 2024, the World Association for Infant Mental Health (WAIMH) held their World Congress in Finland—one of the world's most progressive countries in terms of caring for its most vulnerable citizens. This event brings together leading clinicians and researchers in infant mental health from around the world, and I was fortunate enough to be able to attend and listen to many fascinating talks. Professor Mette Skovgaard Vaever of Copenhagen University, Denmark, drew attention to the fact that, even though parenting is a much more equal affair across Scandinavia—where both parents are given lengthy paid leave during the first year after childbirth (a total of 12 months between them), and where children are rated as the happiest in the world—perinatal and infant mental health issues do still exist. In Denmark, figures have risen to 8% of children receiving at least one psychiatric diagnosis by the age of ten, and this figure is almost doubled for children growing up in at-risk families. These families need to be given appropriate support and early interventions if the Danes are to maintain their happy, healthy society, as mental health issues that begin in infancy may have lifelong consequences for the child who is left untreated or not given the necessary caregiving (Professor Skovgaard Vaever, live at WAIMH World Congress, June 2024).

Meanwhile, Professor Astrid Berg from Cape Town discussed how babies are born with an acute awareness of their surroundings and the people around them. They possess feelings, even if they cannot yet articulate them in adult language. Therefore, providing good physical and emotional care for both the baby and the parents must begin as early as possible (i.e. during pregnancy). She questioned how we can best support parents and babies safely during times of uncertainty and world disasters, emphasising that it all begins in the womb. Nurturing parents and babies throughout pregnancy, childbirth and the postnatal period will set the child on the path to a life of sound physical and mental health.

Understanding Pain and Distress in the Newborn
According to Professor Campbell (live at WAIMH World Congress, June 2024), hospitalised infants can and *do* experience pain, distress and trauma. However, doctors and other staff are often either unaware of this or fail to consider it, perhaps because they are "too busy fixing the body to think about potential damage to the mind". He explained how the primary focus in maternity and neonatal care has always been on the baby's *physical* wellbeing and development, including motor skills, feeding and sleeping. And yet, the baby "arrives in the world programmed to be ready for engagement with people, seeking connection". When aided and supported, even very young infants can "retain hope in the face of persistent medical trauma and hospitalisation". Infants who have lost hope exhibit this by behaving in

a "depressed" way—by being withdrawn or distressed. Therefore, it is vital to protect the sick infant from fear and engage them in joy and play (Professor Campbell, live at WAIMH World Congress, June 2024).

Until the late 1980s to early 1990s, we lacked scientific evidence that the newborn infant could experience pain, despite their indignant screams while being dried with a rough towel, placed abruptly onto cold metal scales or having the post-birth heel prick. As the saying goes, how often does the "scientific truth" of one day become an obsolete untruth the next? Because premature babies are frequently not yet strong enough to cry after they are born, for a long time, they were believed to be even less capable of experiencing pain than full-term infants. A pair of Italian researchers, Giovanna Axia and Sabrina Bonichini [8], in their studies assessing infants' stress responses to vaccinations, showed that, in fact, the opposite is true—pain-related distress is even stronger in *younger* infants, such as premature babies, possibly due to their immature nervous systems, which make it more difficult for them to regulate their emotional responses to pain.

For generations of premature babies, painful and repetitive operations, including skin breaking procedures such as lumbar punctures and inserting feeding tubes down the baby's throat or nostrils to initiate tube feeding, were often carried out after birth without any analgesia or even a parent present to hold and soothe the baby [4, 75]. Thankfully, since research on neonatal pain has progressed, procedures performed on newborn babies are more likely to occur with a low dose of analgesia, as recommended initially by Pokela [73], facilitating the treatment by diminishing the baby's pain. However, analgesics should not be given repeatedly due to their impact on respiratory depression when used in excess [61]. Alternatively, a topical anaesthesia [64] or skin-to-skin contact with a parent and a small sucrose tablet to suck on are safer methods for soothing neonatal pain and distress during painful procedures [19]. Despite these discoveries around neonatal pain and distress, we still often underestimate the impact that childbirth complications and interventions may have on the newborn, affecting their neurobiological wellbeing and behaviour post-birth [27].

The Neonatal Facial Coding System (NFCS), developed by researchers Grunau and Craig [44], was a breakthrough for previous sceptics of newborn pain and pain-related distress. It was developed to help health professionals assess the expressions of newborn infants in their care while enabling researchers to better understand a newborn baby's behavioural and emotional state in response to external stimuli, such as pain, stress or pleasure, by reading and coding the tiny movements and configurations of their facial muscles. For example, an eye squeeze, furrowing around the brow, nose and mouth areas or tongue protrusion may signify pain, stress or discomfort, whereas an open mouth indicates the baby's relaxation or pleasure [22]. Alongside rating the newborn baby's heart rate and crying time, the Neonatal Facial Coding System and similar measures of neonatal pain have made it possible to study the impacts of various obstetric interventions, as well as harsh environmental factors such as loud noise or bright lights in a ward of highly sensitive premature infants. Scientists studying these things have made strong recommendations regarding necessary adjustments to environmental settings, alongside the vital (yet still undervalued) role of parents in non-pharmacological pain relief methods during operations, including touch, holding and soothing [11, 18].

A sparsity of research evidence around the possible impacts of childbirth on the baby presents a serious question: could the infant's birth and early postnatal experiences—if they are negative and the appropriate care and support are not in place—count as adverse childhood experiences (ACEs)? Are we over-flooding the sensory experiences of newborns as they are being born? If this is true, then it is possible that babies who have negative birth experiences, if not given the sensitive care they need to aid their recovery from birth trauma, might be more susceptible to all the future mental health issues linked to ACEs—such as depression, anxiety and severe headaches [5]. Potentially, a lack of appropriate care could also affect whether or to what degree they trust in their caregivers and how securely or insecurely they are attached. Insecurely attached infants, including those with avoidant, ambivalent or disorganised attachment, are more likely to struggle with emotional regulation, affecting them during childhood and into adolescence [21]. ACE research suggests that a lack of trust in caregivers during infancy and childhood may lead to more challenging romantic relationships in adulthood [65] and increased stress in their future parenting [89]. In becoming adults with children themselves, parents with their own ACEs may lack the ability and resilience to cope with and care sensitively for their offspring, perpetuating a negative cycle of suboptimal care within families.

Research has shown that increases in the mother's stress response to her baby's distress predict harsher parenting during toddlerhood, and this reaction negatively impacts both the mother's and baby's stress physiology over time, creating a self-perpetuating negative cycle of distress [80]. One thing that seems certain is—if we want to promote healthy relationships and healthy happy people within our society—it is time to provide trauma-informed maternity and neonatal care [66] and to put babies' psychosocial wellbeing and their social and emotional development firmly on the agenda (Professor Mette Skovgaard Væver, live at WAIMH World Congress, June 2024).

1.3 The Possibility of Long-Term Physiological Changes Taking Place During Childbirth

There are several interesting concepts on which more research evidence is emerging every day, enlightening our awareness of the unborn foetus' and newborn infant's sensitivity to internal and external stimuli. One of these is *foetal programming*, which takes place in the womb via the mother's physical, emotional, hormonal and mental state [13, 25, 26]. An Italian researcher named Piontelli [72] was one of the first people to propose an "interplay" between the previously dichotomous nature and nurture argument, suggesting that what happens in the womb might "have a profound emotional effect on the child", especially if this is reinforced by their postnatal experiences. We now know that when mothers are stressed or depressed during pregnancy, their child is more likely to have difficult temperament traits such as negative affectivity, meaning the tendency to experience negative emotions [57, 63], although these traits are less likely to play out in a sensitive and supportive postnatal environment [56].

While foetal programming is still a relatively new concept, there is increasing evidence about the potential negative impacts of epigenetic changes on the baby's genome. "Genome" refers to the entire set of DNA instructions found in each cell's nucleus, containing all the information needed for the infant to learn, develop and function in the world [67]. These are long-lasting or possibly permanent changes to the foetus or infant that may occur during pregnancy or postnatally in response to their environment. Upon observing increased crying, fussing and other "unsettled" behaviours following obstetric interventions, a few prominent scientists have speculated about a potentially permanent dysregulation of the baby's hypothalamic-pituitary-adrenal (HPA) axis [23, 24, 34]. The HPA axis is one of the body's physiological systems linked to stress regulation and is responsible for the baby's stress response. Despite this earlier research, however, there has been very little focus to date on the possible impacts of complications and interventions during childbirth on the baby's genome.

Disruption of the infant microbiome is another issue that scientists are fast discovering more about. Like the genome, this could also be affected by the mother's health and the birth experience. With these new discoveries and speculative theories fast emerging, it doesn't seem so far-fetched to wonder whether the birth experience might affect the newborn baby's physical and mental health as well as the mother's, although research on this is still limited. Perhaps the main issue with "outdated professional attitudes" is that newborn babies cannot speak, and preterm neonates are even less able to mount a strong vocal or behavioural response [4, p. 177]. But, if we listen carefully, the newborn baby tries very hard to express themselves. In addition to their cries, whimpers and screams, we can pick up on their subtle cues and what their facial expressions, grimaces, bodily movements and behaviour are trying to tell us about their birth and early postnatal experiences [15].

1.4 Joining the Dots

The *Birth, Bonding and Baby Behaviour* book investigates numerous physiological and psychological factors that could influence the newborn baby's physiological wellbeing and consequently their early behaviour and developing temperament. It seeks to highlight and unify different fields of research evidence in order to "join the dots" between a mother's experience of the perinatal period (from pregnancy and childbirth to the early postnatal days with her baby, including bonding and attachment), mother and infant mental health and the baby's temperament and behaviour. Increasingly, rigorous scientific evidence is showing how the mother's physical ("objective") and psychological ("subjective") birth experiences are linked to her mental health in the postnatal period. If the birth is experienced as particularly negative or traumatic, this may lead to the distressing symptoms of post-traumatic stress disorder [9, 97], with both direct and indirect impacts on the baby [57].

Furthermore, the birth experience may affect mother-infant bonding, especially if the mother is anxious, depressed or experiencing symptoms of post-traumatic stress [94]. The partner can step in to fill this gap in some instances, although they too may feel overwhelmed, distressed or depressed, and consequently in need of emotional support themselves [3, 6]. Experiencing such support should strengthen the partner and enable them to provide supportive care for the mother and baby [49]. In addition, a randomised controlled trial has shown that midwife-led counselling and similarly supportive interventions for the mother may help lessen symptoms of distress, reducing the risk of developing PTSD [87]. Otherwise, the consequences of a negative birth and postnatal experience could have serious repercussions for the entire family [28–30].

Meanwhile, we might wonder how the newborn baby reacts to all this disruption. How do they respond to their own experience of being born and to their mother's physical and psychological experiences of birth, which are reflected in her physiology and hormonal state during and after childbirth? The mother releases beneficial hormones for herself and her baby, such as oxytocin, prolactin and prostaglandins during and after a positive experience, but is more likely to release an excess of stress hormones, such as cortisol, adrenaline and noradrenaline, during and after a negative, unsupported or traumatic birth (although a certain amount of these stress hormones are necessary during the final stages of labour and birth [16]). We know that the baby absorbs and reflects the mother's physiological state during pregnancy, birth and postnatally—via amniotic fluids pre- and during birth, as well as proximity and breast milk post-birth. Despite the risk of transferring stress hormones to the baby after a difficult birth experience, skin-to-skin care and breastfeeding may help the mother and baby release oxytocin, unwind, connect and recover after the birth [17].

The newborn also responds to their mother's *psychological* state after birth, and this influences the innately programmed and bidirectional parent-infant bonding processes that generally occur during this sensitive time [94]. We know that building a strong, secure relationship is an essential process for parents and babies and how bonding and attachment difficulties can have a devastating impact on the child's present and future wellbeing and development [1, 37, 38]. In this book, I aim to address some of the questions presented above by drawing on prior research evidence and presenting the three studies I conducted for my PhD, which explored this topic in depth [76].

The *Birth, Bonding and Baby Behaviour* book sets out to answer the following question:

Does the birth experience influence baby behaviour?

1.5 Motivation for This Research

I was initially motivated to carry out this research by the two very different births of my own children and their subsequent distinct natures and approaches to life. Both are now inspired and inspiring young adults whom I am very proud to call my daughters, though their beginnings could scarcely be more different. Like most (if not all) mothers, I could talk for hours about how my children were born, but I will try to keep this part brief, I promise. Although I remember every aspect of both my birth stories, as do most mothers, I'll therefore attempt to share only the most relevant parts with you.

My Own Birth Stories

My first birth experience was every expecting parent's nightmare: from the race along icy country lanes to a small cottage hospital with a midwife-led unit in the nearest town on a bitterly cold Christmas morning, to the ambulance transfer at midnight (still on Christmas day) to a large high-tech hospital, where the registrar had to be woken up to perform a rotational forceps delivery for our baby who had become completely stuck. After pushing against what felt like a brick wall for 2 hours under the instruction of a midwife who had turned off my music and told me firmly just to forget about my essential oils as they would definitely "not help", she finally called in the doctor, who diagnosed the situation as urgent and ordered an ambulance.

I lay for what seemed like an age outside the big hospital on a cold stretcher, covered only by a thin blanket and desperately clutching my tank of gas and air. We were locked out of the darkened building, and nobody appeared from within. The ambulance crew did not have the key. After a few frantic phone calls between the ambulance staff and the hospital, the side door we were parked outside finally opened, and I was brought inside to the warm and placed on a crisp white hospital bed in the middle of a room surrounded by machinery while we waited for the registrar to appear. By this time, my partner had managed to persuade himself that either I, the baby or both of us were going to die. The hospital staff—a smiling young midwife and a very nervous young doctor desperately clutching her board with shaking hands—were closely watching the baby's heartbeat on the monitor. Finally, a lovely Indian registrar with kind, quiet, empathic eyes came to perform the rotational forceps delivery, as the baby was in occiput posterior position (known as "back-to-back"), so first had to be turned before being pulled out. When he looked me in the eye and said, "We will work together now – you are going to push while I pull", I knew I was in safe hands. Meanwhile, despite all the surrounding commotion, the cheery, compassionate midwife, with bright blue smiling eyes I will never forget that looked straight down into mine, began a reassuring chant of "Cheeky baby!" before adding, "Your baby is fine in there, very comfy and cosy…no wonder they don't wanna come out!" I think it was those kind words coming from the midwife during my final moment of excruciating pain and panic that saved me from being traumatised by that birth.

1.5 Motivation for This Research

After the birth, the village doctor (who was also a sheep farmer) stomped into our cottage on an officious home visit, seemingly to reaffirm her opinion that we should never have attempted to have our baby in a midwife-led unit birth in the first place and that—as I had multiple stitches, was in acute pain and could hardly walk—my partner could get on with keeping the house clean. He was not overly impressed with this idea. However, he proved to be a diligent and doting father, dutifully looking after me and our new baby during the following days and weeks as we recovered from the physical and emotional impacts of the birth. As for our beautiful baby girl, who had been born screaming with a large bulbous red lump on the top of her head, she needed a lot of gentle care and attention, and we gave it to her, although it did not always seem to ease her crying or calm her unsettled temperament.

In contrast, the second birth involved a couple of quite painful yet blissfully fruitful hours in a birthing pool before the senior midwife, whose words and manner I will also never forget, gently urged me to, "Listen to your body. Just breathe your baby out". This time, the birth was a joyful and empowering experience, and I had a smiling and contented baby to show for it. Almost immediately, I felt like a happy, confident mother. After guiding me out of the pool by the hand and placing the baby over my stomach, the midwife massaged her back vigorously for a few quiet seconds. Finally, our second baby girl uttered a small cry and began to breathe. I was quite surprised that this baby had not been born screaming and suffering, as I had come to assume this was the way all babies were born. But no, seemingly not necessarily. Her head was smooth and unscathed—visual proof that she'd had a much easier time entering the world. When she smiled directly at her dad within a few hours of being born as he cradled her in his arms, looking down and speaking to her gently, we were abruptly informed by a passing nurse that it was just "wind". If this were the case, I wondered why our first baby had not also smiled after she was born. Instead, she had done a lot of what we playfully used to call "posh lips"—the pursed lips and tongue protrusions described as indications of pain in the Neonatal Facial Coding System described earlier [22]. But we didn't know that back then.

After the second baby was born and we'd had a couple of months of relatively easy parenting, filled with a deep sense of wonder, pride and complete euphoria about our new arrival, I began to question why I felt so differently to how I had after the first birth and why our baby seemed much calmer and easier to manage. At the time, I attributed this to the differences in midwifery and medical approaches, which appeared to have resulted in entirely different birth experiences. I concluded that their different physical birth experiences must have profoundly impacted my babies. I also realised that I may have experienced undiagnosed and, therefore, untreated postnatal depression after my firstborn, as every day felt like a challenging ordeal I had to endure. In contrast, this time, life felt busy yet good. A few months after the second birth, I began to research the subject of childbirth and its potential associations with infant behaviour and temperament. I couldn't find anything specific to determine whether there might be a connection and, if so, what the mechanisms behind this could be. I explored a range of related topics, from the potential benefits of continuity of care [81, 82] or having a doula [53, 55] to the drawbacks of guided or "forced" pushing techniques known as Valsalva [48], medication during childbirth [88] and routine episiotomies [74]. My passion for this under-researched area, exploring the possible effects of childbirth on infant wellbeing and temperament, grew with everything I read. I vowed to return to university to study it in more depth as soon as I had time and available funds. A mere 17 years later, I embarked on my PhD.

Later, I came across the aforementioned study by Douglas and Hill [34], which discussed crying and fussing behaviours in newborns and suggested that this could be due to a dysregulated HPA axis (the baby's delicate stress response system) during a challenging birth. In addition, Taylor et al. [90] considered how the mother's reaction to the birth might influence the baby's response. Then, in a moment of revelation, I encountered a meta-analysis by Professor Susan Ayers et al. [9] demonstrating how the *subjective* birth experience affected the mother's psychological outcomes and perceptions of birth trauma more than the objective physical experience. These three articles were pivotal in forming my theory about how childbirth might impact baby behaviour and developing temperament. The baby's stress response system could become dysregulated during a challenging birth experience, and perhaps the mother's too, making it difficult for her to support the baby's immature regulatory system postnatally, especially if she felt distressed or traumatised by the birth. However, if the mother perceived the birth positively, perhaps she would find it easier to soothe her baby, even after a challenging time.

1.6 How the Studies Were Carried Out

A mixed-method research programme was designed to answer my research question: *Does the birth experience influence baby behaviour?* This involved a combination of quantitative (measurable, objective, fixed and statistical) and qualitative (descriptive, subjective, interpretative and exploratory) methods, which together aimed to gather rich, diverse and in-depth data. Therefore, the research was based on a "pragmatist" paradigm, bringing together positivist (quantitative) and constructivist (qualitative) research methodologies to conduct a comprehensive scientific inquiry. Pragmatist methodology is frequently employed in public health research, providing a flexible framework for exploring research problems with the goal of enhancing healthcare services for patients. This action-orientated (leading to action or change) and patient-orientated (focused on patients' lived experiences) approach aims to strengthen the findings by actively involving individuals with lived experiences of the research problem. It seeks to gather diverse sources of information to find solutions to complex issues arising in our physical, psychological and social worlds. In other words, it investigates real-world problems by utilising multiple data sources to answer the research question [2].

The three studies presented here were set up and run simultaneously. As it was a part-time PhD, which took place alongside teaching work, this provided ample time for data collection. The quantitative survey, comprising approximately 150 detailed questions about childbirth experiences and infant behaviour, was initially completed by over 1000 mothers and ran from January 2014 to March 2017. The two sets of interviews were conducted with 40 health professionals, doulas and mothers, while the survey collected data. Here I will present the interviews first, as they are full of great insights and wisdom, before sharing the survey findings to enable a deeper scientific understanding of which birth and perinatal factors most impact mother and baby. The methods used for each study are outlined in more detail in the chapters where they are individually presented (Chaps. 5, 6, 7 and 8). If you have a strong preference for either quantitative (numerical, measurable) or qualitative (descriptive) data, please feel free to skip the other chapters and read only the summaries at the beginning and end of each chapter.

Reflexivity is a crucial aspect of all rigorous research, particularly when conducting qualitative, interpretative research on a topic that stems from a personal interest such as mine. The two interview studies of maternity care providers (including midwives, health visitors and doulas) and mothers with babies up to a year old provide an in-depth introduction to the topic as midwives and mothers share their personal insights and perspectives. These rich, in-depth studies offer the potential background workings to the quantitative findings and are therefore known as "mechanisms". When it came to listening to the mothers' birth stories, many snippets of which you will find in Chap. 6, I knew it would have been all too easy to say, "Me too, that happened to me", and to follow each remark or anecdote with a leading question. Thus, while engaging with these 40 inspiring women in their homes or cafes over a cuppa and cake and listening to their experiences and beliefs about childbirth and baby behaviour, I took determined care to maintain a constant awareness of myself as a scientist rather than as a mother who had also experienced some of the things they spoke about.

Perhaps because I had not only experienced a very challenging and potentially traumatising birth but had also experienced—in the words of the senior midwife who was there to catch my second baby—a "beautiful birth", I was able to listen to mothers' diverse stories, and those of the midwives, health visitors and doulas I interviewed, with a curious and open mind. The fact that I had experienced opposite ends of the spectrum in both childbirth experiences and baby behaviour meant I was able to offer some degree of recognition on every level, nodding in equal understanding at tales of sadness and disappointment or empowerment and joy. I like to think that this means the health professionals' and mothers' beliefs, perspectives and personal birth stories contained within this book come to you as they were presented to me—in a form as raw, open and honest as they were told [83, 84]. To help make sense of mothers' birth stories and the unique insights from both new and seasoned health professionals and doulas, I have organised the different elements or patterns I found in the data into themes. But I will explain this process in more detail when we arrive at those chapters. In the meantime, I hope you enjoy this book and find it helpful in practice.

1.7 Outline of Chapters

The next chapter (Chap. 2) introduces the concepts of baby behaviour, infant temperament and parent-infant bonding. Chapter 3 highlights the research around relevant physical factors linked to childbirth that could affect baby behaviour. There are very few studies that directly examine the potential associations between childbirth and baby behaviour and those that do tend to focus solely on physical aspects. Only when you examine each separate entity of the birth experience, such as interventions or pain relief, can you begin to uncover some of the mysteries behind birth, bonding and baby behaviour pathways. Chapter 3 weaves together a historical overview of prior evidence in multiple connected areas, delving into particular issues around childbirth that could influence infant wellbeing and behaviour, including medical interventions (from electronic foetal monitoring to Caesarean sections), neonatal pain and distress, pain relief medications used during labour and other perinatal factors that might influence infant temperament. It also explores physiological (and associated psychological) factors that may impact the baby, such as perinatal hormonal changes. Chapter 4 provides a more in-depth background to the psychological impacts of childbirth on mother and baby outcomes with a focus on perinatal mood disorders: how these are affected by pregnancy, birth and early postnatal experiences and how they in turn influence infant behaviour and development.

Chapter 5 presents the perceptions, beliefs and insights of 22 midwives, doulas and health visitors regarding childbirth and post-birth mother-infant wellbeing and behaviour. Chapter 6 presents 18 in-depth interviews with mothers of babies up to 12 months, asking mothers for their birth stories and to comment on their babies' behaviour. A survey of over 1000 mothers is presented in Chaps. 7 and 8. This substantial quantitative study investigates and discusses all the physical and psychological factors that appear to play a role in baby behavioural outcomes during the first 6 months of life. Drawing on all three studies, Chap. 9 brings the findings together and relates them to the broader literature on childbirth experiences, perinatal mental health, bonding and attachment and infant temperament and development. Finally, I offer a theoretical model based on my own and others' findings and ask: *How do we apply this evidence to current models of maternity and neonatal care? How can we make childbirth a better and more humane experience for all mothers and babies everywhere, regardless of their personal, cultural or socioeconomic background or where they happen to live?*

References

1. Abraham E, Feldman R. The neurobiology of human allomaternal care; implications for fathering, coparenting, and children's social development. Physiol Behav. 2018;193:25–34.
2. Allemang B, Sitter K, Dimitropoulos G. Pragmatism as a paradigm for patient-oriented research. Health Expect. 2022;25(1):38–47.
3. Álvarez-García P, García-Fernández R, Martín-Vázquez C, Calvo-Ayuso N, Quiroga-Sánchez E. Postpartum depression in fathers: a systematic review. J Clin Med. 2024;13(10):2949.
4. Anand KJS. Consensus statement for the prevention and management of pain in the newborn. Arch Pediatr Adolesc Med. 2001;155(2):173–80.

5. Anda R, Tietjen G, Schulman E, Felitti V, Croft J. Adverse childhood experiences and frequent headaches in adults. Headache. 2010;50(9):1473–81.
6. Ansari NS, Shah J, Dennis CL, Shah PS. Risk factors for postpartum depressive symptoms among fathers: a systematic review and meta-analysis. Acta Obstet Gynecol Scand. 2021;100(7):1186–99.
7. Antsaklis P, Antsaklis A. The assessment of fetal neurobehavior with four-dimensional ultrasound: the Kurjak antenatal neurodevelopmental test. Donald Sch J Ultrasound Obstet Gynecol. 2012;6(4):362–75.
8. Axia G, Bonichini S. Regulation of emotion after acute pain from 3 to 18 months: a longitudinal study. Early Dev Parenting. 1998;7(4):203–10.
9. Ayers S, Bond R, Bertullies S, Wijma K. The aetiology of post-traumatic stress following childbirth: a meta-analysis and theoretical framework. Psychol Med. 2016;46(6):1121–34.
10. Baillargeon R, Spelke ES, Wasserman S. Object permanence in five-month-old infants. Cognition. 1985;20(3):191–208.
11. Balice-Bourgois C, Zumstein-Shaha M, Vanoni F, Jaques C, Newman CJ, Simonetti GD. A systematic review of clinical practice guidelines for acute procedural pain on neonates. Clin J Pain. 2020;36(5):390–8.
12. Ball HL, Russell CK. Nighttime nurturing: an evolutionary perspective on breastfeeding and sleep. Oxford: Oxford University Press; 2012. p. 241–61.
13. Beijers R, Buitelaar JK, de Weerth C. Mechanisms underlying the effects of prenatal psychosocial stress on child outcomes: beyond the HPA axis. Eur Child Adolesc Psychiatry. 2014;23:943–56.
14. Blecker MK, Dähn D, Engel S, Schmiedgen S, Garthus-Niegel S, Knaevelsrud C, Schumacher S. Childbirth-related posttraumatic stress symptoms: exploring the predictive potential of intrapartum hotspots. J Psychosom Obstet Gynaecol. 2024;46(1):2469290.
15. Brazelton TB, Nugent JK. Neonatal behavioral assessment scale (no. 137). Cambridge: Cambridge University Press; 1995.
16. Buckley SJ. Executive summary of hormonal physiology of childbearing: evidence and implications for women, babies, and maternity care. J Perinat Educ. 2015;24(3):145–53.
17. Buckley S, Uvnäs-Moberg K. Nature and consequences of oxytocin and other neurohormones in the perinatal period. In: Downe S, Byrom S, editors. Squaring the circle: normal birth research, theory and practice in a technological age. London: Pinter and Martin; 2019. p. 19–31.
18. Campbell-Yeo M, Eriksson M, Benoit B. Assessment and management of pain in preterm infants: a practice update. Children. 2022;9(2):244.
19. Carter CS. Oxytocin pathways and the evolution of human behavior. Annu Rev Psychol. 2014;65:17–39.
20. Christensson K, Cabrera T, Christensson E, Uvnäs-Moberg K, Winberg J. Separation distress call in the human neonate in the absence of maternal body contact. Acta Paediatr. 1995;84(5):468–73.
21. Cooke JE, Kochendorfer LB, Stuart-Parrigon KL, Koehn AJ, Kerns KA. Parent–child attachment and children's experience and regulation of emotion: a meta-analytic review. Emotion. 2019;19(6):1103.
22. Craig KD, Whitfield MF, Grunau RV, Linton J, Hadjistavropoulos HD. Pain in the preterm neonate: behavioural and physiological indices. Pain. 1993;52(3):287–99.
23. Dahlen HG, Kennedy HP, Anderson CM, Bell AF, Clark A, Foureur M, Ohm JE, Shearman AM, Taylor JY, Wright ML, Downe S. The EPIIC hypothesis: intrapartum effects on the neonatal epigenome and consequent health outcomes. Med Hypotheses. 2013;80(5):656–62.
24. Dahlen HG, Downe S, Kennedy HP, Foureur M. Is society being reshaped on a microbiological and epigenetic level by the way women give birth? Midwifery. 2014;30(12):1149–51.
25. De Weerth C. Prenatal stress and the development of psychopathology: lifestyle behaviors as a fundamental part of the puzzle. Dev Psychopathol. 2018;30(3):1129–44.
26. De Weerth C, Buitelaar JK. Physiological stress reactivity in human pregnancy—a review. Neurosci Biobehav Rev. 2005;29(2):295–312.
27. De Weerth C, Buitelaar JK. Childbirth complications affect young infants' behavior. Eur Child Adolesc Psychiatry. 2007;16:379–88.

28. Delicate A, Ayers S. The impact of birth trauma on the couple relationship and related support requirements; a framework analysis of parents' perspectives. Midwifery. 2023;123:103732.
29. Delicate A, Ayers S, McMullen S. A systematic review and meta-synthesis of the impact of becoming parents on the couple relationship. Midwifery. 2018;61:88–96.
30. Delicate A, Ayers S, McMullen S. Health-care practitioners' assessment and observations of birth trauma in mothers and partners. J Reprod Infant Psychol. 2022;40(1):34–46.
31. Di Giorgio E, Leo I, Pascalis O, Simion F. Is the face-perception system human-specific at birth? Dev Psychol. 2012;48(4):1083.
32. Di Giorgio E, Lunghi M, Simion F, Vallortigara G. Visual cues of motion that trigger animacy perception at birth: the case of self-propulsion. Dev Sci. 2017;20(4):e12394.
33. DiPietro JA, Bornstein MH, Costigan KA, Pressman EK, Hahn CS, Painter K, et al. What does fetal movement predict about behavior during the first two years of life? Dev Psychobiol. 2002;40(4):358–71.
34. Douglas PS, Hill PS. A neurobiological model for cry-fuss problems in the first three to four months of life. Med Hypotheses. 2013;81(5):816–22.
35. Eberhard-Gran M, Garthus-Niegel S, Garthus-Niegel K, Eskild A. Postnatal care: a cross-cultural and historical perspective. Arch Womens Ment Health. 2010;13:459–66.
36. Enlow MB, Kitts RL, Blood E, Bizarro A, Hofmeister M, Wright RJ. Maternal posttraumatic stress symptoms and infant emotional reactivity and emotion regulation. Infant Behav Dev. 2011;34(4):487–503.
37. Feldman R. The adaptive human parental brain: implications for children's social development. Trends Neurosci. 2015;38(6):387–99.
38. Feldman R. The neurobiology of human attachments. Trends Cogn Sci. 2017;21(2):80–99.
39. Feldman R, Weller A, Leckman JF, Kuint J, Eidelman AI. The nature of the mother's tie to her infant: maternal bonding under conditions of proximity, separation, and potential loss. J Child Psychol Psychiatry Allied Discip. 1999;40(6):929–39.
40. Filippetti ML, Orioli G, Johnson MH, Farroni T. Newborn body perception: sensitivity to spatial congruency. Infancy. 2015;20(4):455–65.
41. Frohlich J, Bayne T, Crone JS, DallaVecchia A, Kirkeby-Hinrup A, Mediano PA, et al. Not with a "zap" but with a "beep": measuring the origins of perinatal experience: origins of perinatal experience. NeuroImage. 2023;273:120057.
42. Gopnik A. How babies think. Sci Am. 2010;303(1):76–81.
43. Green J, Staff, L., Bromley P, Jones L, Petty J. The implications of face masks for babies and families during the COVID-19 pandemic: a discussion paper. J Neonatal Nurs. 2021;27(1):21–5.
44. Grunau RV, Craig KD. Pain expression in neonates: facial action and cry. Pain. 1987;28(3):395–410.
45. Harlow HF. The nature of love. Am Psychol. 1958;13(12):673.
46. Hendrix CL, Stowe ZN, Newport DJ, Brennan PA. Physiological attunement in mother–infant dyads at clinical high risk: the influence of maternal depression and positive parenting. Dev Psychopathol. 2018;30(2):623–34.
47. Henriques J, Jauniaux E, de Maisieres AT, Gélat P. Sound before birth: foetal hearing and the auditory environment of the womb. In: Aural diversity. London: Routledge; 2022. p. 27–41.
48. Hollins Martin CJ. Effects of valsalva manoeuvre on maternal and fetal wellbeing. Br J Midwifery. 2009;17(5):279–85. https://doi.org/10.31234/osf.io/cy6g5.
49. Johansson M, Fenwick J, Premberg Å. A meta-synthesis of fathersx experiences of their partnerx s labour and the birth of their baby. Midwifery. 2015;31(1):9–18.
50. Johansson MW, Lilliesköld S, Jonas W, Thernström Blomqvist Y, Skiöld B, Linnér A. Early skin-to-skin contact and the risk of intraventricular haemorrhage and sepsis in preterm infants. Acta Paediatr. 2024;113(8):1796–802.
51. Kawasaki T, Noda Y, Hirano Y, Kawanami A, Sakurai K, Mori C, Shimizu E. The effects of mother-infant bonding on children's strengths and difficulties. Heliyon. 2025;11(3):e41727. https://doi.org/10.1016/j.heliyon.2025.e41727.
52. Keefe MR. The impact of infant rooming-in on maternal sleep at night. J Obstet Gynecol Neonatal Nurs. 1988;17(2):122–6.

References

53. Klaus MH, Kennell JH, Robertson SS, Sosa R. Effects of social support during parturition on maternal and infant morbidity. Br Med J (Clin Res Ed). 1986;293(6547):585–7.
54. Klemming S, Lilliesköld S, Westrup B. Mother-newborn couplet care from theory to practice to ensure zero separation for all newborns. Acta Paediatr. 2021;110(11):2951–7.
55. Kozhimannil KB, Vogelsang CA, Hardeman RR, Prasad S. Disrupting the pathways of social determinants of health: doula support during pregnancy and childbirth. J Am Board Fam Med. 2016;29(3):308–17.
56. Lahtela H, Flykt M, Nolvi S, Kataja EL, Eskola E, Tervahartiala K, et al. Mother–infant interaction and maternal postnatal psychological distress associate with child's social-emotional development during early childhood: a FinnBrain Birth Cohort Study. Child Psychiatry Hum Dev. 2024:1–16. https://doi.org/10.1007/s10578-024-01694-2.
57. Lahti-Pulkkinen M, Lähdepuro A, Lahti J, Girchenko P, Pyhälä R, Reynolds RM, et al. Maternal psychological distress and temperament traits in children from infancy to late childhood. JCPP Adv. 2024;4(3):e12242.
58. Lee GY, Kisilevsky BS. Fetuses respond to father's voice but prefer mother's voice after birth. Dev Psychobiol. 2014;56(1):1–11.
59. López-Teijón M, García-Faura Á, Prats-Galino A. Fetal facial expression in response to intravaginal music emission. Ultrasound. 2015;23(4):216–23.
60. Marland H, Rafferty AM, editors. Midwives, society and childbirth: debates and controversies in the modern period. London: Routledge; 2002.
61. McPherson C, Ortinau CM, Vesoulis Z. Practical approaches to sedation and analgesia in the newborn. J Perinatol. 2021;41(3):383–95.
62. Meltzoff AN. Elements of a developmental theory of imitation. In: The imitative mind: development, evolution, and brain bases. Cambridge: Cambridge University Press; 2002. p. 19–41.
63. Merced-Nieves FM, Lerman B, Colicino E, Enlow MB, Wright RO, Wright RJ. Maternal lifetime stress and psychological functioning in pregnancy is associated with preschoolers' temperament: exploring effect modification by race and ethnicity. Neurotoxicol Teratol. 2024;103:107355.
64. Miller NM, Fisk NM, Modi N, Glover V. Stress responses at birth: determinants of cord arterial cortisol and links with cortisol response in infancy. BJOG Int J Obstet Gynaecol. 2005;112(7):921–6.
65. Murphy A, Steele M, Dube SR, Bate J, Bonuck K, Meissner P, et al. Adverse childhood experiences (ACEs) questionnaire and adult attachment interview (AAI): implications for parent child relationships. Child Abuse Negl. 2014;38(2):224–33.
66. Murphy A, Steele H, Steele M, Allman B, Kastner T, Dube SR. The clinical adverse childhood experiences (ACEs) questionnaire: implications for trauma-informed behavioral healthcare. In: Integrated early childhood behavioral health in primary care: a guide to implementation and evaluation. Cham: Springer; 2016. p. 7–16.
67. National Human Genome Research Institute. Introduction to genomics. 2024. https://www.genome.gov/About-Genomics/Introduction-to-Genomics.
68. Newnham E, McKellar L, Pincombe J. Towards the humanisation of birth. A study of epidural analgesia & hospital birth culture. Cham: Palgrave Macmillan; 2018.
69. Nugent JK, Keefer CH, Minear S, Johnson LC, Blanchard Y. Understanding newborn behavior and early relationships: the Newborn Behavioral Observations (NBO) system handbook. Baltimore: Paul H Brookes Publishing; 2007.
70. Page L, Kitzinger C. From medicalisation to humanisation of birth and death. Midwifery Matters. 2021;168:13.
71. Piaget J. Piaget's theory of intelligence. Englewood Cliffs: Prentice Hall; 1978.
72. Piontelli A. From fetus to child, new library of psychoanalysis. London: Routledge; 1992.
73. Pokela ML. Pain relief can reduce hypoxemia in distressed neonates during routine treatment procedures. Pediatrics. 1994;93(3):379–83.
74. Polavarapu M, Odems DS, Banks S, Singh S. Role of obstetric violence and patient choice: factors associated with episiotomy. J Midwifery Womens Health. 2024;69:718–26. https://onlinelibrary.wiley.com/doi/pdfdirect/10.1111/jmwh.13655.
75. Porter FL, Grunau RE, Anand KJS. REVIEW ARTICLES:- long-term effects of pain in infants. J Dev Behav Pediatr. 1999;20(4):253–61.

76. Power C. The influence of maternal childbirth experience on early infant behavioural style. 2021. https://www.researchgate.net/publication/353039432_The_Influence_of_Maternal_Childbirth_Experience_on_Early_Infant_Behavioural_Style.
77. Power C, Williams C, Brown A. Does childbirth experience affect infant behaviour? Exploring the perceptions of maternity care providers. Midwifery. 2019;78:131–9.
78. Power C, Williams C, Brown A. Physical and psychological childbirth experiences and early infant temperament. Front Psychol. 2022;13:792392.
79. Power C, Williams C, Brown A. Does a mother's childbirth experience influence her perceptions of her baby's behaviour? A qualitative interview study. PLoS One. 2023;18(4):e0284183.
80. Ravindran N, Zhang X, Ku S. Within-person bidirectional associations between maternal cortisol reactivity and harsh parenting across infancy and toddlerhood. J Fam Psychol. 2024;38(6):911.
81. Sandall J, Soltani H, Gates S, Shennan A, Devane D. Midwife-led continuity models of care compared with other models of care for women during pregnancy, birth and early parenting. Cochrane Database Syst Rev. 2016;4(4):CD004667.
82. Sandall J, Turienzo CF, Devane D, Soltani H, Gillespie P, Gates S, et al. Midwife continuity of care models versus other models of care for childbearing women. Cochrane Database Syst Rev. 2024;4(4):CD004667.
83. Sandelowski M. Focus on research methods-whatever happened to qualitative description? Res Nurs Health. 2000;23(4):334–40.
84. Sandelowski M. What's in a name? Qualitative description revisited. Res Nurs Health. 2010;33(1):77–84.
85. Schrøder K, Larsen PV, Jørgensen JS, Hjelmborg JVB, Lamont RF, Hvidt NC. Psychosocial health and well-being among obstetricians and midwives involved in traumatic childbirth. Midwifery. 2016a;41:45–53.
86. Schrøder K, Jørgensen JS, Lamont RF, Hvidt NC. Blame and guilt–a mixed methods study of obstetricians' and midwives' experiences and existential considerations after involvement in traumatic childbirth. Acta Obstet Gynecol Scand. 2016b;95(7):735–45.
87. Shaeri S, Delavar MA, Bakouei F, Azizi A, Karbalaeizadeh M. Impact of midwife-led counseling for women who have experienced traumatic childbirth: a clinical trial. Midwifery. 2025;148:104467.
88. Silva YAP, Araújo FG, Amorim T, FranciscaMartins E, Felisbino-Mendes MS. Obstetric analgesia in labor and its association with neonatal outcomes. Rev Bras Enferm. 2020;73:e20180757.
89. Steele H, Bate J, Steele M, Dube SR, Danskin K, Knafo H, et al. Adverse childhood experiences, poverty, and parenting stress. Can J Behav Sci. 2016;48(1):32.
90. Taylor A, Fisk NM, Glover V. Mode of delivery and subsequent stress response. Lancet. 2000;355(9198):120.
91. Tew M. Safer childbirth? A critical history of maternity care. New York: Springer; 2013.
92. Thomas K. Birth trauma inquiry report. Listen to Mums: ending the postcode lottery on perinatal care. 2024. https://www.theo-clarke.org.uk/sites/www.theo-clarke.org.uk/files/2024-05/Birth%20Trauma%20Inquiry%20Report%20for%20Publication_May13_2024.pdf.
93. Trevathan WR. Human birth: an evolutionary perspective. London: Routledge; 2017.
94. Vega-Sanz M, Berastegui A, Sanchez-Lopez A. Perinatal posttraumatic stress disorder as a predictor of mother-child bonding quality 8 months after childbirth: a longitudinal study. BMC Pregnancy Childbirth. 2024;24(1):1–14.
95. Westergren A, Edin K, Nilsson B, Christianson M. Invisible but palpable–gender norms in childbirth: a focused ethnography on woman-midwife interaction and birth practices in two Swedish hospital labour wards. BMC Pregnancy Childbirth. 2025;25:419.
96. WHO. World Health Organization recommendations: Intrapartum care for a positive childbirth experience. 2018. https://www.who.int/reproductivehealth/intrapartum-care/en/.
97. Yildiz PD, Ayers S, Phillips L. The prevalence of posttraumatic stress disorder in pregnancy and after birth: a systematic review and meta-analysis. J Affect Disord. 2017;208:634–45.

A Brief Introduction to Infant Temperament and Parent-Infant Bonding

2

Early infant behaviour can be viewed as an expression of the baby's physiological and neurobiological wellbeing [9]. It is the baby speaking to its caregivers in a clear, if nonverbal, language. Therefore, if we want to study the potential impacts of childbirth on the baby, it is arguably necessary to examine their earliest behaviours and how their so-called "inborn" temperament continues to develop outside the womb.

2.1 Infant Temperament: What Is It and Why Does It Matter?

The concepts of neonatal states of conscious awareness and individual differences in infant temperament were first proposed by Dr. Peter Wolff [67] following his minutely detailed observations of newborn babies. Wolff was a medical doctor and psychiatrist who pioneered this method of researching the infant psyche by collecting lengthy observational data (up to 12 hours at a time) of the neonate's behaviour in their home environment, gradually introducing the new concept of neuropsychology: the study of how our brain affects our behaviour. During this period, a general interest in the seemingly inborn behavioural differences between babies was emerging among eminent developmental psychologists. For the first time, in contrast to the previously popular philosophy, which involved seeing the infant as a "tabula rasa" or blank slate, children were seen to possess unique differences in their physiological and emotional states from the moment of birth [12].

Traditionally, infant temperament was viewed as a purely genetic and hereditary style of behavioural patterns that begin to emerge sometime after childbirth. More recently, according to the two developmental psychologists responsible for designing the popular and widely used Infant Behavior Questionnaire—Martha Gartstein and Mary Rothbart [22]—infant temperament refers to early behavioural differences that emerge in response to internal and external stimuli, describing the child's emotionality (whether positive or negative), self-regulation, attention and activity. Although many would say that temperament is a relatively stable phenomenon due to its basis in genetics [21, 56], Gartstein and Rothbart [22] admit that *early infant* temperament is *less* stable than it later becomes due to the baby's sensitivity to environmental influences and internal regulatory factors. In other words, what the baby experiences and how they are helped to regulate themselves during and after these experiences matters. This chapter presents the idea that infant temperament is still forming during and after childbirth, particularly if the mother and baby's birth experience did not progress as it should and the baby's hypothalamic-pituitary-adrenal (HPA) axis governing their response to stressors has been disturbed [17].

Neurobiological models of temperament based on the conditioning of the nervous system have been around since the 1920s [19]. More recently, temperament has been defined as "a quality that varies among individuals, is moderately stable over time and situation, is under some genetic influence, and appears early in life – a coherent profile of behavior, affect (emotional state), and physiology (neurochemistry of the brain)" [35, p. 38]. It has also been described as "the behavioral style of the individual, the characteristic pattern of experiencing and reacting to the external and internal environment" [13, p. 26]. In other words, temperament is a biologically based behavioural style that characterises the baby's interactions with the world around them and is influenced by their internal nervous system, as well as their external environment (i.e. it has both genetic and environmental components). Emerging temperament, therefore, involves both biological and psychological influences [42]. The current consensus is to view infant temperament as a behavioural style that regulates the infant's developing social behaviour [13].

The thinking around the foundations of temperament, however, was not always clear. A "Roundtable" discussion during the 1980s debated the proportion of baby behaviour that might be governed by the child's temperament [25]. There was also wide disagreement—the classic "nature-nurture" debate—around whether temperament was inherently genetic or whether it emerged in response to the baby's environment. Thomas and Chess [63], founders of the New York Longitudinal Study, where information from parents was collected at various time points across the child's early years, believed that infant temperament could be bidirectional, adapting to the environmental context while the parents (a significant part of the environment) adapted to their child [25].

2.2 Where It All Began: The Origins of Infant Temperament Research

At the forefront of the newfound interest in young infant temperament during the 1950s was the landmark New York Longitudinal Study (NYLS). This began in 1956, 3 years before Peter Wolff's [67] neonatal observations. Rather than focusing on the newborn (as Wolff did), it assessed behavioural differences between babies from 3 months [64]. The NYLS was designed to demonstrate the crucial role of infant temperament in child development by examining how babies interact with their social and physical environments. Nine temperament items were defined based on Thomas and Chess' [63] observations of babies and children and interviews with their parents:

1. *Activity*—the amount of physical motion in the baby, e.g. during sleeping, feeding and bathing
2. *Rhythmicity*—the baby's regularity in their sleeping, feeding and elimination routines
3. *Approach and withdrawal*—the baby's initial response to new people or stimuli
4. *Adaptability*—the baby's flexibility in adapting to new people or situations
5. *Intensity*—the baby's energy level in their response to stimuli
6. *Mood*—the baby's pleasant or unpleasant overt behaviours
7. *Persistence and attention span*—the amount of time spent on any given activity
8. *Distractibility*—how easily the baby is distracted by external stimuli
9. *Sensory threshold*—the amount of sensory input (e.g. light or noise) required to elicit a response

Infant temperament was not considered fixed, but rather a complex, interactive unfolding process between the baby, the parents and the environment, whereby the infant learned and developed their personality and intellect [63]. The authors pinpointed five specific baby behaviours that predicted future behavioural and psychiatric problems. These included: regular crying or fussing; irregular feeding, sleeping and elimination (wee and poo) routines; withdrawing from external stimuli; low adaptability to new people or situations; and intense moods involving loud laughter and tantrums. Definitions of "difficult" infant temperament also began to emerge around this time. These involved worrying traits such as negative mood, inconsolability when distressed, irregular routines, inadaptability, high activity and intensity and lack of self-regulation [63]. As noted by Mills and Page [47], babies who seem healthy and "cuddly" and easier to calm and settle are also easier to love initially. In contrast, babies who are hypersensitive to stimuli, more irritable and difficult to settle can pose practical and psychological problems for the new parents. Parents will need to show more sensitivity, compassion and creativity in nurturing temperamentally difficult babies, but this may require early intervention and support [47].

Following the findings of Thomas and Chess [63], temperament development came to be perceived as a "goodness of fit" between parents and their babies, and essentially innate rather than merely shaped by the environment. Parents were regarded as participants in a reciprocal relationship instead of being perceived as solely responsible for their baby's behaviour. However, depending on the child's behavioural style, specific difficulties in infant temperament were thought to require different responses from parents, as parents' response could help or hinder the child's development. Thomas and Chess suggested that excessive stress or tension in the parent-infant relationship, stemming from a lack of understanding of the child's natural disposition, might lead to developmental delays and future behavioural problems [63]. Therefore, parents had a vital role to play—the onus was on them to gently modify (rather than quash) their child's behaviour from a point of understanding rather than Victorian-style discipline.

Parental Mental Health, Infant Temperament and Parent-Infant Bonding
Expanding on Thomas and Chess' [63] theory about how the baby's temperament contributes to the parent-child relationship (and vice versa), other social scientists considered that the baby's behavioural style might influence how well-equipped parents felt to care for them. This, in turn, may affect bonding and attachment, as well as the baby's ability to adapt to their environment [24]. More recently, there is evidence that this relationship is bidirectional—mother-infant bonding influences infant temperament—and this relationship between bonding and infant temperament is affected by maternal mental health issues such as depression or anxiety [14].

While there is ample research on the impacts of poor postnatal mental health on bonding, the mother's mental health during pregnancy may also play a significant role [36]. Pregnancy can influence infant temperament through early (pre-birth) bonding issues and foetal programming, where maternal stress results in the foetus receiving high levels of cortisol, affecting their later stress response and psychopathology via epigenetic changes and alterations to the baby's microbiome [20, 23]. These effects of maternal stress on the baby's health and wellbeing will be discussed in more detail in later chapters, but they highlight the complexity of the parent-infant relationship and the need for early interventions that support the mother's mental health alongside bonding, baby behaviour and temperament development, from pregnancy onwards.

2.3 Neonatal Behavioural Assessment Scale

Running parallel to the famed 20-year NYLS, and directly inspired by Wolff's [67] newborn observations, a paediatric doctor named Berry Brazelton conducted his own detailed "Neonatal Observations" [7]. These examined a typical newborn baby's 6-day period of "recovery" following childbirth. Brazelton also investigated the frequent delay in "normal" breastfeeding behaviours following pain relief or other childbirth medications. He believed that the way a baby reacts to their birth could set a "prototype" for their future stress response. Based on his ongoing observations, Brazelton developed the Neonatal Behavioural Assessment Scale (NBAS; [8]), a rigorous method still used for assessing physiological, neurobiological and behavioural differences in newborn babies, particularly those born preterm or with a complex obstetric history. The NBAS was designed to measure babies' recuperation post-birth, and this detailed examination of the newborn included measures of the baby's physiological state and their ability to regulate themselves. Unsurprisingly, it correlated with the 5-min Apgar score, a widely used measure of neonatal physiological wellbeing during the first 5 min after birth [43].

Agreeing with Thomas and Chess [63], Brazelton believed that each baby responds differently to its environment and caregivers due to inborn differences in temperament. Brazelton, however, felt that babies might also be influenced by their birth experience and later added some neonatal behaviours to the original physiological measures, such as "crying and fussing", "irritability", "consolability", "self-quieting", "cuddliness", "smiles", "quality of alertness", "low adaptability" and "high intensity" [9]. As the old paediatrician explained with a beaming smile on his 96-year-old face at a WAIMH conference in Edinburgh in 2014 (flying over from America after his doctor had firmly told him *not* to travel), Brazelton firmly believed in the newborn baby's sociable instincts and ability to communicate and interact with their parents from day 1. Similar to the New York Longitudinal Study, he also believed that the baby's innate, individual character differences would influence their personality development and the parent-infant relationship throughout infancy and early childhood [9]. Working alongside him to incorporate these measures of baby behaviour, psychologists Wolke and James-Roberts [69, 70] designed the "Mother and Baby Scales", which were used in the survey presented later (see Chaps. 7 and 8).

Although there's not enough space here to explore every baby behaviour scale in detail, most behaviour measures that have since been designed originated from these two figureheads—the NYLS and the NBAS—and it is important to note that newer definitions of temperament continue to reflect a combination of genetic influence and early adjustment to life outside the womb (i.e. both *nature* and *nurture*). Temperament is generally quite stable from infancy into childhood [56], though there are some exceptions to general understandings about baby behaviour—most notably, the enduring mystery surrounding the condition known as "colic". Typically characterised by prolonged bouts of inconsolable crying, colic tends to emerge around 6 weeks of age and often resolves spontaneously by the time the baby reaches 3 months. Although colic is relatively common in babies, its underlying causes remain largely unexplained. Some studies suggest that it can be alleviated by dietary changes or feeding practices, such as switching to a non-dairy formula or, if breastfeeding, the mother eliminating common allergens like dairy or gluten from their diet [33]. However, these interventions are not always effective, and in many cases, symptoms appear and disappear abruptly without a clear cause [39]. As a result, colic is not generally considered to be a stable or enduring feature of infant temperament [30]. It is also worth noting that, although I asked parents whether their baby had suffered colic in the survey, it was one of the few seemingly important factors that was *not* linked to any of the multiple perinatal variables that we listed [55].

2.4 Why Is It Important to Protect Infant Temperament Development?

So far in this chapter, we have seen how infant temperament may be largely genetic but is also influenced by environmental factors, such as parents' responses to their child's behaviour [63]. In turn, the baby's behaviour and overall temperament affect many aspects of their social and emotional development [78]. For example, the behavioural traits of "high emotionality" and "high activity" in infants aged

12 months predict the behavioural scores, emotional difficulties, conduct problems and activity and attention levels of 5-year-olds [2].

The notion of early infant temperament as "easy" or "difficult" was based mainly on a somewhat dated Western idea of "normal" infant routines, especially around breastfeeding and sleeping [10, 26], and there is a widely held view that breastfeeding may disrupt a baby's sleeping habits due to breast milk's easy digestibility and thus the extra feeding required to satisfy the baby's hunger. This idea is countered by the fact that breastfed babies tend to have fewer feeding and digestive issues, better overall physical health and improved cognitive and behavioural development [71]. Nonetheless, having a baby with irregular feeding and sleeping routines can be problematic for the parents, especially if this occurs alongside frequent crying, fussing and difficulty in being soothed.

Babies who frequently fuss and cry are less able to regulate their internal and external (behavioural) states, including how these behaviours manifest in feeding, sleeping and elimination routines [31]. However, only *persistent* regulatory problems between infancy and preschool age (3–4 years) seem to predict future problems, such as cognitive and motor impairment, behavioural issues and an increased likelihood of attention deficit hyperactivity disorder [59]. Therefore, although there is a strong connection between multiple regulatory problems at 5 months and preschool age (2-5 years) [68], reassuringly, transient regulatory problems in infancy are not believed to predict hyperactivity at school age [59].

2.5 Parent-Infant Bonding and Its Relationship to Infant Behaviour and Temperament

Parent-infant bonding has been defined as the "emotional, behavioural, cognitive and neurobiological tie of the parent to the child" [48]. A parent's ability to form a bond with their baby helps build a strong, secure relationship between parent and child. Both bonding and attachment may play vital roles in the baby's current and future wellbeing, temperament and development [66]. As with many psychological factors, these relationships can be bidirectional, as infant temperament may also influence the mother's attachment to her baby [1].

Parents' stress levels and mental health can have a significant influence on parent-infant bonding, so parents' psychological distress post-birth is a major factor [50]. Given the impacts of parent-infant bonding on infant development, if a mother's feelings about her baby are conflicted because she feels distressed after the birth, this could make her less emotionally available to her baby, with negative consequences for the baby's emotional, behavioural and cognitive outcomes [40, 41]. The mother's subjective birth experience, if it is negative, can therefore adversely affect parent-infant bonding. In fact, it has been found to have even more impact on bonding outcomes than medical complications or current symptoms of psychopathology [34], and one study found that a negative subjective birth experience predicted poorer parent-infant bonding for up to 14 months after childbirth [60]. Another discovered that this relationship was mediated by postnatal depression: adding to the complexity of these intricate and interwoven relationships between the mother's mental health, the subjective birth experience and the mother-infant bonding, *prenatal* depression predicts a more negative birth experience, which in turn predicts poorer mother-infant bonding [18]. According to Australian midwife Cathy Stoodley [61], midwives are ideally positioned to ensure that mothers receive emotionally supportive care, not only to have the best possible birth experience but also to help them bond with their baby during the early postpartum period, no matter what kind of birth experience they've had.

As well as being affected by the birth experience and their mental and emotional health, the parents' ability to bond with their baby may depend on complex factors that are difficult to change during the perinatal period—such as sleep loss, which can lead to profound fatigue and a reduced ability to cope with the new baby [45]. As parent-infant bonding is an essential component of positive infant development, including social-emotional development and behaviour [48], unhealthy parent-infant bonds may lead to developmental issues, such as poorer social and emotional development, lower executive functioning and mental health problems like anxiety or other mood disorders that can persist into childhood, adolescence and even adulthood [37]. Furthermore, a poor parent-infant bond characterised by low levels of parental care, sensitivity and warmth (especially when coupled with high levels of intrusiveness and control) is associated with severe psychopathological outcomes for the infant later in life [57].

Although research on the father's role during the perinatal period has traditionally been lacking, evidence on the psychological importance of father-infant bonding and attachment is finally growing as fathers are steadily becoming more involved in their children's lives from the beginning [16]. Involving fathers is important in a practical sense too. Partners, whether male or female, can feel neglected and dismissed during childbirth and the early postnatal period. Including them in the picture from the very beginning is crucial as they have reported feeling scared, deskilled, lost and inadequate during this time, especially if they (or the mother) are struggling mentally post-birth [32]. Partners need to feel a part of what is happening, rather than being pushed aside. Feeling empowered by health professionals in their vital role as a supportive partner and burgeoning new parent should place them in a better position to support the mother, and accordingly, for both parents to bond with their baby, especially if they are becoming parents for the first time [65].

Traditional ideas on parenting are beginning to shift, and the concept of egalitarian parenting is demanding increasing attention, with a steadily rising demand for greater gender equality around childcare and household duties [58]. Despite this, even in today's "modern" society, most commonly the mother is still the focal point for her newborn baby, and throughout history, a mother's care has been biologically and psychologically essential to the baby's survival. With the exception of a few Scandinavian countries, mothers are still more likely to take time off work, go part-time or stop work altogether after the birth of a child, and this reinforces unequal gender stereotypes, distribution of housework and childcare responsibilities, often creating stress and disharmony between parents [38].

Unresolved and ongoing conflict between a child's parents, in part due to its impact on the parents' moods, has negative outcomes for parental sensitivity, parent-infant bonding and infant wellbeing and development [79]. Once again, these factors tend to be bidirectional with one another as conflict within the couple's relationship and parenting stress both affect and are affected by the baby's behaviour and temperament [5]. Negative cycles of these bidirectional effects, stemming from poor parental functioning and infant temperament, can have long-term consequences for infant development that may need positive interventions to overcome [51]. For example, a parenting training programme called "Mindful with Your Baby" may improve parental functioning, increasing parents' sensitivity, acceptance and synchrony with their baby. This, in turn, enhances the baby's responsiveness and temperament [76] while increasing parents' self-compassion, decreasing their stress levels and reducing depressive and anxiety symptoms [46, 54]. Similar interventions that help parents tune into their baby could also be beneficial to both the baby and to the parent-infant relationship.

The Impacts of Early Neglect and a Lack of Bonding and Attachment Figures

Although the significance of parent-infant bonding and a warm, loving and responsive parent-infant relationship is widely recognised today, this was not always the case. It took a courageous longitudinal study—begun in 2000 and led by medical doctors, psychiatrists and developmental psychologists Charles Zeanah, Nathan Fox and Charles Nelson [72, 73]—to demonstrate this now well-established fact to the world. The team aimed to show Romanian policymakers that the institutionalised care provided for the many thousands of unwanted and abandoned infants in their orphanages caused deep emotional, psychological and physical harm (including stunted growth and decreased brain matter), along with severe developmental damage. Due to the Romanian government's Stalin-initiated policies to increase the population by outlawing contraception and abortion, estimated figures of these abandoned babies from the mid-1950s until the communist government were overthrown in 1989 range between alarming possible totals of 170,000 and 500,000. The actual figures remain unknown.

When Charles Zeanah and his colleagues [72, 73] initiated the Bucharest Early Intervention Project in 2000, thousands of abandoned and orphaned children were still growing up in institutions across Romania, and the government was under pressure to act [74]. The research demonstrated, not only to Romanian policymakers but also to the entire world, that a child spending their early years with minimal social interactions, lacking warm, responsive care and vital sensory stimulation (such as touch), and experiencing no caregiver-infant bonding or any secure attachment figure, resulted in reduced brain matter and impaired cognitive and social-emotional development during infancy. This situation led to an increased risk of psychiatric issues developing in the preschool child [73, 75].

At another World Association for Infant Mental Health (WAIMH) conference in Dublin, Ireland (2023), where the authors of this longitudinal study spoke eloquently about their research, they openly confessed that European ethical controls would almost certainly not allow this type of experiment, involving such a vulnerable population, to occur today. Nonetheless, while adhering to sound scientific practices and doing their utmost to ethically protect the babies and young children they were studying [74], the researchers managed to conduct a well-designed randomised intervention. Their investigation examined the effects of early sensory, social and emotional deprivation on Romanian orphans by comparing the impacts of adverse early life experiences on institutionalised infants' brain and behavioural development with those of infants placed in foster care, as well as a base control group—those who had never left their families or community [49]. As well as the devastating signs of sensory and social-emotional deprivation following severe neglect in Romanian orphanages, the research team identified periods of heightened sensitivity to adverse effects and genetic differences in children's natural resilience—leading to varying degrees of impact.

The research provided important new insights, and in contrast to previous mistaken ideas about children's ability to "bounce back" after their early experiences in institutionalised care involving extreme deprivation, the Bucharest Early Intervention Project effectively showed for the first time that many children never fully recover from the impacts of such early experiences, even if they are later placed in enriched, caring environments [29, 44]. Although the infants placed in foster care before 24 months fared better in terms of brain activity, mental health and attachment to caregivers than those placed after 24 months, sadly, an earlier or later placement didn't seem to influence the degree of psychiatric symptoms if they'd been institutionalised during their early life [74].

Charles Zeanah and his team demonstrated that infants fared better when placed in sensitive foster care in the community than if they were abandoned in neglectful institutions, where the austere atmosphere and staff shortages meant they only received the most basic physical care. As the doctors also had a control group remaining in the community, experiencing everyday family life, they were able to establish that children fared significantly better if they had never been relocated from their original family and community. Since the Bucharest Early Intervention Project, it is now widely accepted that severe neglect and psychosocial deprivation during infancy lead to diminished brain matter, negative behavioural patterns and increased psychopathology. Being placed in a stable foster home with high-quality care as early as possible may help remediate some (but not all) the damage [29].

The Current State of Early Neglect and Parent-Infant Bonding
Despite widespread knowledge and awareness of the damage inflicted by early deprivation due to a lack of bonding and attachment figures, in addition to Bowlby's [6] and Ainsworth's [3] early work on the importance of an engaged, caring and loving parent-infant relationship and a secure attachment figure for the child, this knowledge can sometimes be forgotten. Millions of street children in parts of Asia and Africa still lack access to social care, and millions of abandoned children across the world are growing up in institutions [11, 74]. However, neglect can also occur within the home. With approximately 75% of child abuse cases linked to neglect, infant neglect is the most common form of abuse and is much more likely to occur

when parents have not bonded with their baby [62]. Additionally, infant neglect can occur accidentally in neonatal intensive care units in parts of the world where "kangaroo care" (keeping the newborn in close skin-to-skin contact with a parent) is not always promoted (see Chap. 3 for more about this).

Infant neglect has several risk factors, including parents' postnatal distress or depression, life stress and parenting stress, all of which could create or exacerbate parent-infant bonding issues. Protective factors diminishing the chance of infant neglect include social support, positive parenting attitudes, parenting competence and, of course, parent-infant bonding. All of these can be enhanced through intervention programmes designed to support new parents. One such programme with the aim of benefitting families living in a poor urban American neighbourhood found that children's physical and psychological safety significantly improved, while their externalising and internalising problem behaviours decreased [15]. Such interventions can therefore be effective in promoting parent-child bonding and child wellbeing, although they are not always accessible to the parents who need them most, such as those living in isolated rural communities with limited professional support available.

According to a survey carried out by the Parent-Infant Foundation [53], NICE guidelines on supporting parent-infant bonding in the UK are not currently being followed, and more than one in ten parents are still struggling alone to bond with their baby in the weeks following childbirth. One obvious way to help prevent negative patterns of poor parent-infant bonding and adverse infant behavioural and developmental outcomes would be by providing more focused bonding support for new parents. Parents themselves have stated that they would definitely use this type of resource if it were available within their community, particularly if living in an isolated rural area [52]. Government policies also need to be updated to support parents and mitigate the impact of common external factors that can affect their relationship with their baby after childbirth, such as financial strain and a lack of accessible childcare [38]. Without helpful interventions, these issues may cause huge amounts of stress and conflict within the partnership, particularly for young or first-time parents, potentially affecting parent-infant bonding and the baby's wellbeing and development.

The Impacts of Inter-relationship Conflict on Parent-Infant Bonding

The mother's stress physiology, characterised by increased cortisol reactivity following inter-relationship conflict with a partner, can have a lasting impact on infant physiology. Indeed, scientists have found a corresponding increase in cortisol reactivity in 6-month-old babies [27]. Writing about therapeutic interventions for persistent crying during infancy, Juliet Hopkins [28] highlights babies' responsiveness to positive changes in parents' relationship dynamics, perhaps because these tend to improve the parents' feelings and behaviour towards their child as well. Supporting parents to communicate more effectively with one another may help reduce stress and promote parent-infant bonding. It could also help parents develop positive coping strategies and learn how to co-parent the child together as a team, rather than as two opposing individuals.

This type of support could benefit both the parents' relationship and their relationship with their offspring, leading to a reduction in the behavioural problems associated with increased infant cortisol reactivity [77]. The neurohormonal states of mother and baby are intricately entwined during childbirth and postnatally [17]. During breastfeeding, the baby remains directly connected to their mother's cortisol levels [4]. Therefore, the mother's neurohormonal balance and physiological well-being must be nurtured *throughout* the perinatal period, as it affects everything—from early infant behaviour and the parents' ability to bond with their baby to the child's cognitive and social-emotional development and future wellbeing.

References

1. Abuhammad S, AlAzzam M, AbuFarha R. Infant temperament as a predictor of maternal attachment: a Jordanian study. Nurs Open. 2021;8(2):636–45.
2. Abulizi X, Pryor L, Michel G, Melchior M, Van Der Waerden J, EDEN Mother–Child Cohort Study Group. Temperament in infancy and behavioral and emotional problems at age 5.5: the EDEN mother-child cohort. PLoS One. 2017;12(2):e0171971.
3. Ainsworth MDS. The Bowlby-Ainsworth attachment theory. Behav Brain Sci. 1978;1(3):436–8.
4. Apanasewicz A, Matyas M, Piosek M, Jamrozik N, Winczowska P, Krzystek-Korpacka M, Ziomkiewicz A. Infant temperament is associated with milk cortisol but not with maternal childhood trauma. Am J Hum Biol. 2024;36(11):e24150.
5. Barreto M, Koltermann JP, Crepaldi MA, Vieira ML. Empirical evidence on the relationship between coparenting and temperament: a systematic review of the literature. Trends Psychol. 2019;27:865–78.
6. Bowlby J. Maternal care and mental health. Geneva: World Health Organization; 1951.
7. Brazelton TB. Observations of the neonate. J Am Acad Child Psychiatry. 1962;1(1):38–58.
8. Brazelton TB. Neonatal behavioral assessment scale, Clinics in developmental medicine no. 50. London: Spastics International Medical Publications; 1973.
9. Brazelton TB, Nugent JK. Neonatal behavioral assessment scale. 3rd ed. New York: Cambridge University Press; 1995.
10. Brown A. Breastfeeding uncovered: who really decides how we feed our babies? London: Pinter & Martin; 2016.
11. Browne K, Hamilton-Giachritsis C, Johnson R, Ostergren M. Overuse of institutional care for children in Europe. BMJ. 2006;332(7539):485–7.
12. Carey WB. Measurement of infant temperament in pediatric practice. In: Thomas A, Chess S, editors. Temperament and development. New York: Brunner/Mazel; 1973. p. 212–21.
13. Carey WB, Devitt SC. Child behavioral assessment and management in primary care. 2nd ed. Scottsdale: Behavioral-Developmental Initiatives; 2016. https://www.preventiveoz.org/wp-content/uploads/2018/06/CBAM2-min.pdf.
14. Davies SM, Silverio SA, Christiansen P, Fallon V. Maternal-infant bonding and perceptions of infant temperament: the mediating role of maternal mental health. J Affect Disord. 2021;282:1323–9.
15. DePanfilis D, Dubowitz H. Family connections: a program for preventing child neglect. Child Maltreat. 2005;10(2):108–23.
16. Dikmen-Yildiz P. Father-to-infant attachment and its associated factors during COVID-19 pandemic: a cross-sectional study. J Reprod Infant Psychol. 2025;43(1):151–66.
17. Douglas PS, Hill PS. A neurobiological model for cry-fuss problems in the first three to four months of life. Med Hypotheses. 2013;81(5):816–22.

18. Eitenmüller P, Köhler S, Hirsch O, Christiansen H. The impact of prepartum depression and birth experience on postpartum mother-infant bonding: a longitudinal path analysis. Front Psych. 2022;13:815822.
19. Fox NA, Henderson HA, Perez-Edgar K, White LK. 51 The biology of temperament: an integrative approach. In: Handbook of developmental cognitive neuroscience, vol. 839. Cambridge, MA: MIT Press; 2008.
20. Galbally M, Watson SJ, Lappas M, de Kloet ER, van Rossum E, Wyrwoll C, et al. Fetal programming pathway from maternal mental health to infant cortisol functioning: the role of placental 11β-HSD2 mRNA expression. Psychoneuroendocrinology. 2021;127:105197.
21. Gartstein MA, Rothbart MK. Studying infant temperament via the revised infant behavior questionnaire. Infant Behav Dev. 2003;26(1):64–86.
22. Gartstein MA, Putnam SP, Aron EN, Rothbart MK. Temperament and personality. In: Maltzman S, editor. The Oxford handbook of treatment processes and outcomes in psychology: a multidisciplinary, biopsychosocial approach. Oxford: Oxford Library of Psychology; 2016. p. 11–41.
23. Glover V, O'Donnell KJ, O'Connor TG, Fisher J. Prenatal maternal stress, fetal programming, and mechanisms underlying later psychopathology—a global perspective. Dev Psychopathol. 2018;30(3):843–54.
24. Goldsmith HH, Campos JJ. Toward a theory of infant temperament. In: The development of attachment and affiliative systems. Boston: Springer; 1982. p. 161–93.
25. Goldsmith HH, Buss AH, Plomin R, Rothbart MK, Thomas A, Chess S, Hinde RA, McCall RB. Roundtable: what is temperament? Four approaches. Child Dev. 1987;58(2):505–29.
26. Gopnik A, Meltzoff AN, Kuhl PK. How babies think: the science of childhood. London: Orion Books Ltd; 1999.
27. Hibel LC, Mercado E. Marital conflict predicts mother-to-infant adrenocortical transmission. Child Dev. 2019;90(1):e80–95.
28. Hopkins J. Therapeutic interventions in infancy: two contrasting cases of persistent crying 1. In: Parent-infant psychodynamics. Milton: Routledge; 2018. p. 118–30.
29. Humphreys KL, Fox NA, Nelson CA, Zeanah CH. Psychopathology following severe deprivation: history, research, and implications of the Bucharest early intervention project. In: Child maltreatment in residential care: history, research, and current practice. Cham: Springer; 2017. p. 129–48.
30. James-Roberts IS, Conroy S. Do pregnancy and childbirth adversities predict infant crying and colic? Findings and recommendations. Neurosci Biobehav Rev. 2005;29(2):313–20.
31. James-Roberts IS, Wolke D. Convergences and discrepancies, among mothers' and professionals' assessments of difficult neonatal behaviour. J Child Psychol Psychiatry. 1988;29(1):21–42.
32. Johansson M, Benderix Y, Svensson I. Mothers' and fathers' lived experiences of postpartum depression and parental stress after childbirth: a qualitative study. Int J Qual Stud Health Well Being. 2020;15(1):1722564.
33. Johnson JD, Cocker K, Chang E. Infantile colic: recognition and treatment. Am Fam Physician. 2015;92(7):577–82.
34. Junge-Hoffmeister J, Bittner A, Garthus-Niegel S, Goeckenjan M, Martini J, Weidner K. Subjective birth experience predicts mother–infant bonding difficulties in women with mental disorders. Front Glob Womens Health. 2022;3:812055.
35. Kagan J. Galen's prophecy: temperament in human nature. New York: Routledge; 2018.
36. Khan ZA, Khail SK, Naz H. Assessing the relationship between prenatal mental health disorders and infant bonding postpartum. Res Med Sci Rev. 2024;2(3):179–86.
37. Kidd KN, Prasad D, Cunningham JE, de Azevedo Cardoso T, Frey BN. The relationship between parental bonding and mood, anxiety and related disorders in adulthood: a systematic review and meta-analysis. J Affect Disord. 2022;307:221–36.
38. Kress V, Steudte-Schmiedgen S, Kopp M, Förster A, Altus C, Schier C, et al. The impact of parental role distributions, work participation, and stress factors on family health-related outcomes: study protocol of the prospective multi-method cohort "Dresden Study on Parenting, Work, and Mental Health" (DREAM). Front Psychol. 2019;10:1273.

39. Lam T, Chan PC, Goh LH. Approach to infantile colic in primary care. Singapore Med J. 2019;60(1):12–6.
40. Le Bas GA, Youssef GJ, Macdonald JA, Mattick R, Teague SJ, Honan I, et al. Maternal bonding, negative affect, and infant social-emotional development: a prospective cohort study. J Affect Disord. 2021;281:926–34.
41. Le Bas G, Youssef G, Macdonald JA, Teague S, Mattick R, Honan I, et al. The role of antenatal and postnatal maternal bonding in infant development. J Am Acad Child Adolesc Psychiatry. 2022;61(6):820–9.
42. Lemery-Chalfant K, Kao K, Swann G, Goldsmith HH. Childhood temperament: passive gene–environment correlation, gene–environment interaction, and the hidden importance of the family environment. Dev Psychopathol. 2013;25(1):51–63.
43. Lester BM, Emory EK, Hoffman SL, Eitzman DV. A multivariate study of the effects of high-risk factors on performance on the Brazelton neonatal assessment scale. Child Dev. 1976;47(2):515–7.
44. Mackes NK, Golm D, Sarkar S, Kumsta R, Rutter M, Fairchild G, Mehta MA, Sonuga-Barke EJ, ERA. Young Adult Follow-up team. Early childhood deprivation is associated with alterations in adult brain structure despite subsequent environmental enrichment. Proceedings of the National Academy of Sciences. 2020;117(1):641–9.
45. Mason GM, Cohen ZL, Obeysekare J, Saletin JM, Sharkey KM. Preliminary report: sleep duration during late pregnancy predicts postpartum emotional responses among parents at risk for postpartum depression. Sleep Adv. 2024;5(1):zpae068.
46. Meppelink R, de Bruin EI, Wanders-Mulder FH, Vennik CJ, Bögels SM. Mindful parenting training in child psychiatric settings: heightened parental mindfulness reduces parents' and children's psychopathology. Mindfulness. 2016;7:680–9.
47. Mills BC, Page LA. The growth of human love and commitment. In: The new midwifery: science and sensitivity in practice. Edinburgh: Churchill Livingstone; 2000. p. 223–44.
48. Nakić Radoš S, Hairston I, Handelzalts JE. The concept analysis of parent-infant bonding during pregnancy and infancy: a systematic review and meta-synthesis. J Reprod Infant Psychol. 2024;42(2):142–65.
49. Nelson CA, Zeanah CH, Fox NA, Romer D, Walker EF. The effects of early deprivation on brain-behavioral development: the Bucharest early intervention project. In: Adolescent psychopathology and the developing brain: Integrating brain and prevention science. Oxford: Oxford University Press; 2007. p. 197–215.
50. O'Dea GA, Youssef GJ, Hagg LJ, Francis LM, Spry EA, Rossen L, et al. Associations between maternal psychological distress and mother-infant bonding: a systematic review and meta-analysis. Arch Womens Ment Health. 2023;26(4):441–52.
51. Ortiz RMR, Barnes J. Temperament, parental personality and parenting stress in relation to socio-emotional development at 51 months. Early Child Dev Care. 2019;189:1978–91.
52. Parent Infant Foundation. Securing healthy lives. 2022. https://parentinfantfoundation.org.uk/securinghealthylives/.
53. Parent Infant Foundation. New survey finds NICE guidance on bonding is not being followed. 2023. https://parentinfantfoundation.org.uk/powerful-mums-survey-results-launched-to-mark-start-of-infant-mental-health-awareness-week-2023/.
54. Potharst ES, Kuijl M, Wind D, Bögels SM. Do improvements in maternal mental health predict improvements in parenting? Mechanisms of the mindful with your baby training. Int J Environ Res Public Health. 2022;19:7571.
55. Power C. The influence of maternal childbirth experience on early infant behavioural style. 2021. Available at: https://cronfa.swan.ac.uk/Record/cronfa57276.
56. Prokasky A, Rudasill K, Molfese VJ, Putnam S, Gartstein M, Rothbart M. Identifying child temperament types using cluster analysis in three samples. J Res Pers. 2017;67:190–201.
57. Raffagnato A, Angelico C, Fasolato R, Sale E, Gatta M, Miscioscia M. Parental bonding and children's psychopathology: a transgenerational view point. Children. 2021;8(11):1012.

58. Schaber R, Patella T, Simm J, Garthus-Niegel S. German parents attaining intrapersonal work-family balance while implementing the 50/50-split-model with their partners. J Fam Econ Iss. 2024;46:1–18.
59. Schmid G, Wolke D. Preschool regulatory problems and attention-deficit/hyperactivity and cognitive deficits at school age in children born at risk: different phenotypes of dysregulation? Early Hum Dev. 2014;90(8):399–405.
60. Seefeld L, Weise V, Kopp M, Knappe S, Garthus-Niegel S. Birth experience mediates the association between fear of childbirth and mother-child-bonding up to 14 months postpartum: findings from the prospective cohort study DREAM. Front Psych. 2022;12:776922.
61. Stoodley C, McKellar L, Ziaian T, Steen M, Fereday J, Gwilt I. The role of midwives in supporting the development of the mother-infant relationship: a scoping review. BMC Psychol. 2023;11(1):71.
62. Strathearn L. Maternal neglect: oxytocin, dopamine and the neurobiology of attachment. J Neuroendocrinol. 2011;23(11):1054–65.
63. Thomas A, Chess S. Temperament and development. New York: Brunner/Mazel; 1977.
64. Thomas A, Chess S, Birch HG, Hertzig ME, Korn S. Behavioral individuality in early childhood. New York: New York University Press; 1963.
65. van Vulpen M, Heideveld-Gerritsen M, van Dillen J, Maatman SO, Ockhuijsen H, van den Hoogen A. First-time fathers' experiences and needs during childbirth: a systematic review. Midwifery. 2021;94:102921.
66. Winston R, Chicot R. The importance of early bonding on the long-term mental health and resilience of children. London J Prim Care. 2016;8(1):12–4.
67. Wolff PH. Observations on newborn infants. Psychosom Med. 1959;21(2):110–8.
68. Wolke D. Crying as a sign, a symptom, and a signal. Clinical, emotional and developmental aspects of infant and toddler crying. Child Adolesc Ment Health. 2002;7(3):147–8.
69. Wolke D, James-Roberts I. Multi-method measurement of the early parent-infant system with easy and difficult newborns. In: Psychobiology and early development, vol. 46. Amsterdam: Elsevier; 1987a. p. 49–70.
70. Wolke D, James-Roberts I. Mother and baby scales (MABS). Appendix 2. In: Brazelton TB, Nugent JK, editors. Neonatal behavioral assessment scale. 3rd ed. London: Mac Keith Press; 1987b. p. 135–7). (1995).
71. Wolke D, Schmid G, Schreier A, Meyer R. Crying and feeding problems in infancy and cognitive outcome in preschool children born at risk: a prospective population study. J Dev Behav Pediatr. 2009;30(3):226–38.
72. Zeanah CH, Nelson CA, Fox NA, Smyke AT, Marshall P, Parker SW, Koga S. Designing research to study the effects of institutionalization on brain and behavioral development: the Bucharest early intervention project. Dev Psychopathol. 2003;15(4):885–907.
73. Zeanah CH, Egger HL, Smyke AT, Nelson CA, Fox NA, Marshall PJ, Guthrie D. Institutional rearing and psychiatric disorders in Romanian preschool children. Am J Psychiatry. 2009;166(7):777–85.
74. Zeanah CH, Fox NA, Nelson CA. The Bucharest early intervention project: case study in the ethics of mental health research. J Nerv Ment Dis. 2012;200(3):243–7.
75. Zeanah CH, Humphreys KL, Fox NA, Nelson CA. Alternatives for abandoned children: insights from the Bucharest early intervention project. Curr Opin Psychol. 2017;15:182–8.
76. Zeegers MA, Potharst ES, Veringa-Skiba IK, Aktar E, Goris M, Bögels SM, Colonnesi C. Evaluating mindful with your baby/toddler: observational changes in maternal sensitivity, acceptance, mind-mindedness, and dyadic synchrony. Front Psychol. 2019;10:753.
77. Zemp M, Bodenmann G, Cummings EM. The significance of interparental conflict for children. Eur Psychol. 2016;21(2):99–108.
78. Zentner M, Bates JE. Child temperament: an integrative review of concepts, research programs, and measures. Int J Dev Sci. 2008;2(1-2):7–37.
79. Zietlow AL, Ditzer J, Garthus-Niegel S. From partners to parents: the influence of couple dynamics on parent-infant bonding and child development. J Reprod Infant Psychol. 2024;42(5):785–8.

3

How Is Childbirth Related to Bonding and Baby Behaviour? *Physical Factors That Might Influence the Course of Childbirth and Infant Outcomes*

As we have established over the past two chapters, early infant behaviour is the baby attempting to communicate with its caregivers, occasionally in a very loud and vocal way. In preterm, small or low birthweight babies who may not have the strength to cry, however, communication may instead occur through a more subtle, silent, non-verbal language relayed via tiny bodily movements and minuscule facial expressions [24, 76]. To study the impacts of childbirth on the baby, it is therefore necessary to study babies' earliest behaviours as well as their ongoing behavioural style known as temperament. And yet, in scientific circles, there is still very little research—or even an active conversation—about the possibility of a link between the baby's experience of being born and their early behavioural patterns. When beginning to explore the topic, it quickly became clear that, if such a connection existed, there were probably multiple mechanisms at work behind the scenes. It was very difficult to find any substantial, evidence-based answers to the simple question of whether the birth experience might influence a baby's behaviour. It was only when more specific questions were asked about *how* the birth might affect the baby's behaviour that possible answers began to emerge. They eventually slotted into place like very small pieces finding their place in a large and complex jigsaw puzzle.

    This chapter presents research linking various common physical elements of childbirth to infant behaviour and temperament, covering a wide array of subtopics that came up during these initial investigations. It has since been updated to capture the latest evidence around each topic and provides a historical overview where this adds something of significance to the picture. Childbirth can and should be a transformative event, and every woman deserves accessible and high-quality healthcare during the perinatal period. The World Health Organization [204] has emphasised a "positive experience" as an important indicator of good outcomes for mother and baby. A recent randomised controlled trial confirms that following this model of care reduces the duration of labour and the use of synthetic oxytocin. In addition, women with this positive intervention experienced less fear of childbirth and more comfort during labour while perceiving the care they received as more

© The Author(s), under exclusive license to Springer Nature Switzerland AG 2025
C. Power, *Birth, Bonding and Baby Behaviour*,
https://doi.org/10.1007/978-3-032-05845-4_3

supportive [128]. Reducing fear of childbirth is vital as this common condition is associated with negative physical and psychological birth outcomes for mother and baby [53]. Mangır Meler and Çankaya's [128] research emphasises the rapidly growing idea that everyone giving birth should feel supported, physically and psychologically safe, respected and in control of their own experience [110]. The way that healthcare providers behave towards, interact with and support women during childbirth is crucial. Only then will mothers feel able to relax and allow themselves to succumb to the natural physiological processes of labour and birth.

This chapter also begins to explore some of the ways in which childbirth can become a difficult, complex or traumatic event and the problems that may arise for mother and baby when it does. It examines the existing research evidence linking different types of childbirth experience with infant behaviour and temperament, with a focus on physical factors such as birth mode, birthplace and pain relief medication used during labour and birth. Although physical and psychological aspects of childbirth experience are intertwined, this chapter focuses mainly on objective physical birth events, while the next chapter (Chap. 4) emphasises the more subjective psychological features and potential impacts of childbirth on mother and baby. As one influences the other, many of the psychological outcomes are initially mentioned here.

3.1 Birth Mode: How the Type of Birth Can Affect Mother and Baby

The way a baby enters the world can affect both the mother and the baby in multiple ways. A spontaneous physiological vaginal birth is the way that most parents like to imagine their baby will be born, for several reasons, including established notions of safety and a feeling of being more "natural" [57]. This includes first-time fathers' birth preferences for their partner and baby [9], although it is not necessarily the case for parents who have previously experienced or witnessed their partner having a traumatic vaginal birth. In this situation, they may instead prefer the idea of a planned caesarean section, viewing it as somehow less stressful and more predictable in terms of potential outcomes [74]. However, childbirth, like all aspects of human life, has and will always have some aspects of unpredictability. For example, we still don't know enough about the possible long-term impacts of caesarean sections (and the subsequent course of antibiotics mothers receive to prevent infection) on the baby's health, wellbeing and life expectancy. Therefore, how we or the person we love gives birth to a baby can become a very complex and highly emotive topic because, in the end, there are no rights or wrongs that apply to absolutely everybody. Thankfully, in the UK and many other countries, birthing parents have the right to choose how they give birth.

Spontaneous Physiological Birth
Typically, a spontaneous physiological birth follows a natural progression without any medical interventions, including epidural analgesia (a form of complete pain

relief that numbs all bodily sensations from the waist down). It is the most likely birth mode to lead to a state of "flow" in the person giving birth [47]. This is where the mother becomes completely immersed in labour and less aware of herself and the outside world. Women tend to experience higher levels of birth satisfaction after physiological births compared to operative births [164]. According to the American College of Obstetricians and Gynecologists, spontaneous physiological birth also tends to result in a shorter duration of labour, fewer complications and quicker recovery than other types of birth [3]. It is an involuntary process that generally arises when the baby is ready to be born. If all is going well, the woman's body stimulated by an increase in birthing hormones—a surge in oxytocin, prolactin and beta-endorphins—will progress naturally through labour and birth. Strong involuntary uterine muscle contractions work to dilate the cervix and move the baby down through the birth canal [30, 31]. Engaging in activities that include emotional support and massage may help to increase the natural production of oxytocin and prolactin, and such practices can be especially calming and therefore beneficial for women with a history of previous trauma [79].

As birth that doesn't disturb the body's natural physiology increases the chance of positive birth outcomes, it therefore also increases the mother's sense of empowerment and psychological wellbeing [154]. The spontaneous progression of labour is optimised when a woman feels safe, listened to and supported. In this situation, she is likely to experience a decrease in pain, stress and fear due to the positive impacts of a calm, supportive environment on her neurohormonal system including oxytocin production [155]. Oxytocin is perhaps the best known of the hormones exchanged by mother and baby during childbirth and the perinatal period. Manufactured in both the body and brain, it has a dual purpose, first as an essential hormone for the reproductive processes of birth and breastfeeding and second as a neurotransmitter affecting a wide range of behaviours that include maternal love and bonding, and when combined with dopamine—a hormone linked to the body's pleasure and reward system—motivates these behaviours [123]. Endogenous oxytocin produced in the woman's body calms her nervous system, reducing pain sensations during labour while stimulating powerful contractions and hormonally preparing the new mother for successful caregiving [30]. Playing a vital role in the transition to motherhood, oxytocin buffers mother and baby against stress reactivity, supports positive maternal mood, and regulates healthy mothering behaviours such as breastfeeding and bonding [201]. Together with dopamine, oxytocin also encourages pro-social baby behaviours, such as cooing and smiling.

Although spontaneous labour may be shorter and more efficient with a reduced likelihood of complications in comparison to induced or augmented labours, augmentation is often chosen as the best solution to a prolonged or obstructed labour, either of which may cause further complications with potentially negative outcomes, especially in lower- or middle-income countries where resources are scarce [208]. However, as the length of physiological labour varies, a longer labour should not automatically be a cause for instant augmentation of labour without looking at the wider picture—for example, how the baby is presenting—as scientists have now established that healthy mothers and babies can experience longer first and second stages without any adverse perinatal outcomes than was previously believed [2]. Therefore, the harms of interfering too soon may sometimes outweigh the intended benefits [204]. For example, providing the foetus is not distressed, the mother is coping with contractions well and labour is not *excessively* prolonged, spontaneous physiological childbirth is thought to reduce the overall risk of postpartum complications such as infections, excessive bleeding or perineal trauma including third- or fourth-degree tears [77]. Although spontaneous births may still result in perineal tears, these risks can be minimised with appropriate support and management during labour [174]. Reducing risk factors during spontaneous physiological labour and birth can lead to a healthier and more fulfilling experience for both mother and baby. At times, however, intervention is needed, but there is not the necessary staff or technology available—a situation which unfortunately still occurs frequently in many low- and middle-income countries [18, 20, 22] as well as increasingly in high-income countries due to staff shortages and generally over-stretched resources.

During physiological childbirth, the undisturbed flow of endogenous oxytocin between mother and baby facilitates a smoother birth and breastfeeding transition, thereby helping to ensure effective maternal caregiving behaviours postpartum and promoting mother-infant bonding and attachment [37, 63, 64, 196]. Skin-to-skin contact and breastfeeding following a spontaneous birth may help regulate the interconnected mother's and baby's oxytocin systems and reduce HPA axis (stress response system) activity. Skin-to-skin care, therefore, improves the newborn's neurobiological state by modulating the mother's and baby's stress reactivity. This has far-reaching consequences for the baby's emotional and cognitive development, encouraging healthy development of their immature nervous system [37]. Similar neurobiological studies on fatherhood have found that fathers' testosterone levels decrease alongside an increase in oxytocin levels when holding their newborn, whether or not this contact is skin-to-skin. These complex interactions of the two prominent hormones contribute to positive postnatal fathering behaviours [71].

Immediate skin-to-skin or "kangaroo care" post-birth can facilitate the physiological management of third stage of labour (delivery of the placenta) by increasing uterine involution (where the uterus contracts and returns to its pre-pregnancy state) and reducing postpartum blood loss [6]. Following a spontaneous, physiological labour and birth without complications, most people should experience a straightforward physical recovery, quickly returning to their normal everyday activities, such as walking or driving. A positive birth experience contributes to better overall mental health and wellbeing postnatally, with lower depression rates reported after physiological birth [87]. This could be largely due to the neurobiological benefits of physiological birthing hormones: endogenous oxytocin, prolactin, dopamine and beta-endorphins [30].

There are some distinct physical benefits of being born vaginally to the baby, who is exposed to all the beneficial bacteria in the birth canal as they descend and make their way to the exit. This journey helps them to establish a healthy gut microbiome, which is crucial for building their immune system [55]. The human microbiome, also known as "microbiota", refers to the microorganisms that live on and within the human body, influencing overall health by affecting pathways between the immune, endocrine and neural networks within the body [213]. These pathways form a bidirectional connection between the brain and the gut and are therefore known as the gut-brain axis. The gut microbiota influence physical and psychological health and ideally should be plentiful and diverse throughout a lifetime [124]. Notably, if a mother is stressed during pregnancy or postpartum, this could affect both her own and the baby's microbiome, thereby increasing the risk of future metabolic, neurobehavioral and immunologic disorders in the baby [171].

A healthy balance of gut microbiota plays a crucial role in digestion, food metabolism, the immune system, cognition and behaviour [46]. Yet, mode of birth, exposure to antibiotics and infant feeding style (breast or formula) may all affect the baby's microbiome [213], with possible impacts on the baby's behaviour. Being born without ever entering the birth canal (i.e. by planned caesarean section) could deprive the newborn of the first step of gut colonisation believed to be so vital for their future health [55, 80], although this can be at least partially compensated for with skin-to-skin care or breastfeeding post-birth. Breast milk not only contains the prebiotics and probiotics essential for good health but also microbes that effectively increase the infant's microbiota [102]. However, receiving antibiotics after a caesarean birth or for a postpartum infection reduces these natural benefits of breast milk.

Another physical element of spontaneous physiological birth for the baby is linked to respiration. Vaginal births encourage compression of the baby's chest, helping to expel amniotic fluid from their lungs and reducing the risk of respiratory issues at birth, although the liquid is not entirely expelled until the baby takes his first breath [120]. Added to this, immediate skin-to-skin care and early initiation of breastfeeding are easier and therefore more likely after a straightforward vaginal birth. The initial health and wellbeing of the newborn baby born spontaneously without medicalisation—in contrast to the increased likelihood of requiring analgesia or anaesthesia during an assisted or surgical birth—is reflected in their tendency to have higher Apgar scores than babies born by other means [180].

Assisted Birth

Assisted or "instrumental" births now account for over a third of all UK births [188]. Assisted births require the use of forceps—a surgical instrument used to encircle the baby's head to assist birth—or vacuum extraction (commonly known as "ventouse"), a cup-shaped suction device that is applied to the baby's head for a similar effect. According to the Royal College of Obstetricians and Gynaecologists [166], both of these methods increase the risk of maternal and neonatal trauma. Nonetheless, an assisted birth may be required after a prolonged or challenging labour or where there are concerns about foetal distress. Prolonged labour can cause significant maternal distress and physical exhaustion, depleting the mother's energy reserves and rendering it more challenging for her to cope with the demands of labour and postpartum recovery, in some instances leading to temporary emotional detachment from the newborn [152]. It also comes with an increased risk of a low Apgar score for the newborn at 5 minutes post-birth [8]. Understandably, therefore, health professionals may become concerned if labour does not appear to be progressing. However, intervening too soon entails a different set of risks for mother and baby, and parents should be fully informed of these risks before making any decisions.

General risks of instrumental birth for the mother include a higher chance of experiencing an episiotomy (surgical cut to the perineum) and vaginal, perineal or uterine trauma [127], potentially leading to bladder or anal incontinence or, at the extreme end, pelvic organ prolapse requiring surgical repair [118]. Notably, approximately 20% of American women will require surgery for pelvic floor disorders at some point in their lives, with the majority of injuries caused by instrumental birth (forceps or ventouse) or by pushing against contracted pelvic floor muscles [52]. According to these authors, avoiding damage to the pelvic floor is key. Suggested preventative measures include educating women about perineal massage during pregnancy; encouraging slow, gradual perineal stretching; and *not* instructing women to push against a contracted pelvic floor during labour. The World Health Organization [204] guidelines "Intrapartum Care for a Positive Childbirth Experience" recommend various techniques for reducing perineal trauma during the second pushing stage of labour, such as perineal massage, warm compresses and manual perineal protection. For example, the Ritgen manoeuvre, where the midwife applies pressure to the baby's head during crowning to control the speed of birth, can effectively reduce severe perineal tears [174]. However, this "Finnish intervention" is a contentious issue as it means women cannot adopt different positions. Furthermore, exerting pressure against the baby's head as it descends through the birth canal could disturb its natural orientation towards the place of least resistance, instead leading the head towards the perineum, increasing risk of OASIS (obstetric anal sphincter injury or severe third- or fourth-degree tear) [148]. Indeed, many midwives would argue that the best way to reduce perineal damage is through alternative positions, such as all fours (providing the woman is happy with this), supporting spontaneous "bearing down" while discouraging pushing during crowning, thereby allowing slow perineal stretching. Having a good rapport with the woman is considered essential to achieving this.

Forceps births in particular increase the risk of urinary or faecal incontinence and pelvic organ prolapse up to 26 years later, with detrimental consequences for women's health and wellbeing [78]. Urinary incontinence is the most prevalent of these disorders, and although it is most common in women who are older or overweight, have diabetes or had an episiotomy, it can be a debilitating issue for many new mothers, with negative impacts on their self-esteem and ability to care for the newborn baby [117]. Unfortunately, routine episiotomies are still common obstetric practice in many parts of the world (e.g. in Ukraine) despite their association with higher rates of wound complications and severe perineal injury. It would be preferable in these countries for each potential episiotomy case to be individually assessed [16]. Although some research regarding the perineum considers spontaneous vaginal birth to be equally risky [38, 111], overall, trauma relating to mode of birth and obstetric interventions such as episiotomy is associated with a higher risk of postpartum haemorrhage [66].

Due to these inherent risks attached to instrumental birth, the recovery time afterwards may be prolonged, and the new mother could find it difficult to go about her usual daily activities (including child-rearing) due to severe perineal pain [212]. Understandably, mothers who experience an instrumental birth are more prone to depression, anxiety and general distress post-birth [51], although the evidence on this varies, with some scientists claiming that postnatal mood disorders are linked only to caesarean sections, while others declare there are no links at all between birth mode and postnatal maternal mood. Despite this, a recent study confirmed that perineal tears can seriously impact mothers' mental health after the birth, potentially causing stress and depression and making women less able to cope with their baby [165]. When weighing up all the mixed evidence, it certainly seems likely that having an instrumental birth could easily interfere with the initial stages of mother-infant bonding and breastfeeding as the mother may be suffering mentally or distracted by postnatal pain.

The baby is also directly at risk during an instrumental birth, and forceps births in particular are associated with higher rates of neonatal injuries [33]. Serious physical complications and neonatal trauma that may occur include facial or cranial injuries [166], such as bruising, lacerations, brachial plexus injury (damage to nerves in the shoulder, arm or hand), cephalohematoma (bleeding under the scalp), intracranial haemorrhages and skull fracture or—at the extreme end—neonatal death [146]. As discussed in Chap. 1, birth injuries are highly likely to cause pain and distress to the newborn. This could lead to increased crying, fussing and irritability post-birth although unsettled neonatal behaviour in an injured baby may also be affected by factors such as low birthweight or preterm birth and how much the baby is held [132]. Even without suffering any major injuries, newborn infants born by instrumental delivery have higher cortisol levels than those born by other means [135], reflecting the mother's raised pain and stress levels as well as the baby's own sensations of pain and distress.

It's recommended that clinicians conducting a complicated assisted delivery such as a rotational forceps avoid excessive compression of the baby's skull [88] as, if the pressure becomes too forceful, the baby's safety can be compromised in the urgency of the moment. Consequently, assisted birth in full-term infants is moderately associated with neonatal intracranial haemorrhage [59, 88] and cranial brain injury [160], with potentially severe consequences. Babies born by forceps or vacuum extraction may also have other difficulties due to the circumstances necessitating the intervention. Importantly, the need for medical assessment and intervention following an assisted birth increases the chance of immediate mother-infant separation, with delays to the skin-to-skin contact, breastfeeding and bonding processes that are so crucial to newborn wellbeing, behaviour and development. When these instinctive early mother and baby behaviours are hindered by separation, the new mother becomes more susceptible to developing postpartum depression, whereas mothers who experience immediate and prolonged skin-to-skin contact with their baby have fewer depressive symptoms [43].

Caesarean Birth

If an instrumental birth proves difficult, or there are signs of foetal distress before the baby has fully descended, meaning the birth needs to be expedited, a caesarean section—the increasingly common though major abdominal surgical procedure to birth the infant—may be the best choice. Caesarean births have been on a rising trajectory since 1990, with current trends set to continue into the 2030s. The rates in lower-income countries vary from just 5% in sub-Saharan Africa to approximately 40% in the Caribbean and Latin America, illustrating the global problem of unmet need alongside overuse (or "too little too late" versus "too much too soon"), with both scenarios leading to unnecessary and avoidable morbidity and mortality in women and babies [18–20, 139]. Caesarean section rates above 10–15% are considered counter-productive and in some cases harmful, leading to strong recommendations from the WHO to bring spiralling global rates back under control to reduce risk as well as decreasing the massive burden on our healthcare systems [157].

Caesarean sections come in two forms—planned ("elective") or unplanned ("emergency")—and these have fundamental differences, including potentially disturbing terminology, that may affect the mother's stress levels, postnatal distress and depression [75]. A planned caesarean section either occurs in response to a mother's request or because there is a pressing medical reason for the baby to be born early. Parents can plan their life around the elective caesarean date and so for obvious reasons are less likely to feel stressed than if it ends up being carried out in an emergency. Lower levels of childbirth stress are reflected in lower umbilical cortisol levels for babies born by elective caesarean [135], which correspond with lower cortisol levels in mothers during and after a planned caesarean [184].

Rising caesarean birth rates could be the result of us living in societies with a more risk-averse birth culture while also dealing with a rising fear of childbirth, exacerbated by the increasingly public visibility of negative birth stories on the media. Fear and pain-reducing interventions—including in some countries the caesarean section—are therefore often recommended for an easier birth experience [157]. However, caesarean sections involve multiple risk factors for mother and baby, including an increased possibility of uterine rupture for the mother and respiratory disease in the newborn [147]. Caesarean sections also come with higher rates of postpartum infection, haemorrhage and a longer recovery time than vaginal birth. Overall, they carry a higher risk of severe and possibly life-threatening maternal morbidity, while other factors such as maternal age and weight play a smaller though significant role [112]. Importantly, pre-labour elective caesarean sections prevent the final surge of catecholamines (including epinephrine, commonly known as adrenaline—responsible for the "fight, freeze or flight" response—and norepinephrine or noradrenaline, a neurotransmitter that plays an essential role in stress reactions), and these hormones are necessary for the baby's respiratory system to fully operate after birth [182].

As discussed in the section on spontaneous physiological birth, another potential issue is that a baby who is born surgically may miss out on vital exposure to the mother's healthy vaginal bacteria and consequently experience a delay or imbalance in their microbiome development. The long-term consequences of this are not yet fully known [84]. We are only just beginning to understand how the human microbiome may affect behaviour right from early infancy. Healthy infant gut microbiota at 2.5 months correlates with infant and toddler temperament traits such as positive emotionality, while greater gut diversity is linked to reduced fear reactivity at 6 months and to increased extroversion (considered a positive social trait) at 18–27 months [1, 45]. Therefore, to avoid the negative outcomes of an underdeveloped microbiome in the young infant following caesarean section birth, early interventions to improve gut flora diversity could be helpful in the prevention of future physical and mental health problems [45, 177]. Because of this link to a less healthy microbiome, the increasing use of caesarean section as a mode of birth is also associated with negative impacts on babies' developing immune systems. This is thought to be contributing to an "epidemic" of atopic inflammatory disorders such as respiratory tract infections, asthma, eczema, obesity, type 1 diabetes and coeliac disease [44, 181].

Postoperative pain or complications may be experienced after a surgical birth, sometimes affecting the mother's ability to initiate breastfeeding within the first hour. This first hour is thought to be the "golden time" or "sensitive period" as, when placed naked and unhindered on the mother's bare abdomen, the full-term healthy unmedicated newborn will follow an instinctive set of movements called the "breast crawl", pulling themselves up to the mother's breast to take their first feed [207]. The early skin-to-skin contact between mother and baby that this behaviour entails helps to stabilise the newborn baby's heart rate, body temperature and stress levels while it also exerts a positive influence on social-emotional and neurodevelopmental outcomes. If the first feed is postponed for whatever reason, breastfeeding may take longer and become more difficult to successfully establish. In this way, having a caesarean section might affect breastfeeding success, even in mothers who were set on breastfeeding their baby beforehand, which could have negative follow-on consequences for infant nutrition and how well the mother feels able to bond with and care for her newborn. These effects could be even more likely if the mother has experienced extreme pain, fear, stress and anxiety, fatigue and a prolonged recovery or if she has been separated from her baby so that one of them can receive urgent medical treatment following the birth [106].

Similar to assisted birth, perhaps the most significant issue for mother and baby after a caesarean section is this risk of separation in the important hours and days post-birth due to the increased risk of physical issues, as discussed above. The baby may need to spend time in a neonatal intensive care unit (NICU), which inevitably decreases the opportunities for early skin-to-skin contact and breastfeeding, potentially affecting parent-infant bonding, at least in the short term. Recent studies have provided strong evidence that mother and baby separation at birth increases infant morbidity and mortality in sick or preterm babies, especially in lower- and middle-income countries where separation may increase infant mortality by up to 33% [17]. While India is now a developing economy, there are still huge wealth disparities and pockets of extreme poverty [195]. A large randomised controlled trial conducted by the WHO [206] across five hospitals in poorer regions of India and Africa had similar findings, with survival rates of preterm newborns increasing so dramatically after immediate sustained skin-to-skin contact that the trial had to be stopped for ethical reasons. Immediate "kangaroo care" was instantly recommended for all babies involved in the trial. Kangaroo care is defined as continuous skin-to-skin contact of the newborn baby with the mother's chest rather than being placed in an incubator. If the mother requires urgent medical care, another parent or caregiver such as the father or partner can be encouraged to have skin-to-skin time with the baby.

Temporary separation may seem unavoidable if a baby is born prematurely. However, when a newborn is taken to NICU, the new mother may subsequently struggle to care for her baby or develop a strong attachment to them. She is therefore more likely to feel alien to the baby [210] and has an increased risk of developing postpartum depression [192]. The WHO [209] now strongly recommends kangaroo care for all preterm and low birthweight newborns, a move that is especially pertinent in low-resource settings for physical health reasons, but equally important in all settings for both the mother's and baby's long-term psychological health. This recommendation can be facilitated by creating "Mother-NICUS", where the mother or other caregiver remains with the baby at all times.

Kangaroo care also reduces mortality and morbidity of preterm or low birthweight infants in high-income countries and, due to the huge benefits of synchronised physiological exchanges between parent and baby (including breathing, heartbeat and hormonal synchrony), it should become a fundamental aspect of newborn care for both term and preterm infants globally [126]. As one of the world's most progressive countries, Sweden, with an acute awareness of the physical and psychological benefits of keeping the neonate in close proximity to its parents, has adopted a *zero-separation* policy for all newborns [91, 104]. Alongside saving lives, kangaroo care promotes breastfeeding, bonding and more settled newborn behaviours as it stabilises the newborn's physiology, reducing pain and distress in the neonate while promoting parent-infant closeness [93] and alleviating pain, stress and depressive symptoms in the mother [103]. Notably, in a study of mothers of very low birthweight newborns after just 7 days of kangaroo care, mother-infant bonding significantly improved across various domains of the Postpartum Bonding Questionnaire including "Anger and rejection" and "Confidence and anxiety" [108].

Because assisted or caesarean births often delay this first contact between mother and baby, some scientists believe they may have a negative impact on early interactions, maternal mood and mother-infant bonding. Although the widely accepted associations between birth mode and parent-infant bonding are inconclusive, probably because they are so individual and complex, the parents' subjective birth experience also matters [54]. Therefore, it is vital to ensure that parents are emotionally well-supported in medicalised or emergency birth situations. The opportunity to bond as soon as possible after childbirth is important for the baby's early social, emotional and cognitive development as well as their future physical and mental wellbeing [92, 168]. In addition, there are benefits for the mother's physical and psychological wellbeing when able to hold her baby immediately after birth, and skin-to-skin contact helps to activate oxytocin by effectively blocking the stress response and reducing the circulation of catecholamines [14]. Although

Maggie Redshaw and her colleagues [168] found the positive effects of baby holding on maternal postnatal mood didn't apply after caesarean births, perhaps due to some associated shock or trauma, mothers who held their baby within 5 minutes of an emergency caesarean section were more likely to be breastfeeding at 3 months than those who held their baby later. Therefore, parents should always be facilitated to hold their baby as soon as possible after a caesarean birth.

Caesarean Birth and Mental Health
When this is not possible, a further complication with potentially detrimental impacts on mother and baby can be the broader impact of having a caesarean section on the mother's mental health. An operative delivery may not be the birth she envisaged for herself or her baby. Emergency caesarean sections in particular are associated with higher rates of postnatal depression and post-traumatic stress disorder in new mothers, emphasising the need for adequate support during and after this type of birth [202]. While experiencing birth as traumatic reduces parents' psychological wellbeing post-birth, another interesting finding is that giving birth by caesarean section may reduce first-time mothers' sense of social identity [60]. A string of associated factors could have detrimental consequences for mother and baby wellbeing. While a new mother following an emergency caesarean section may begin her journey of motherhood blaming herself for "failing" at giving birth, her newborn might be experiencing after-effects of the epidural normally used during caesarean births, and a fractious baby recovering from an emergency birth could lead to a further crisis of confidence for the mother, especially if she has breastfeeding issues [85].

Establishing successful breastfeeding brings many benefits to the mother's and baby's health and wellbeing; therefore, it needs to be publicly and socially accepted, protected and promoted [27]. Mothers who are experiencing pain and discomfort after a surgical birth, or difficulty breastfeeding their baby after separation and the anxiety this brings, sometimes stop before they are ready, sometimes leading to postnatal depression [29]. This situation happens more frequently after an induction or caesarean section where the natural flow of endogenous oxytocin has been disrupted, interfering with the mother's neurobiological system, which is geared towards bonding and breastfeeding [197]. Consequently, mothers who've experienced a caesarean section may need extra support to breastfeed and bond with their babies. This can help to stimulate the oxytocin system and reduce mother and baby's pain and stress post-birth [197, 199].

Summing Up the Evidence on Birth Mode
A major factor in how a mother feels after she has given birth to her baby is whether she felt fully informed about all the possible modes and methods of childbirth, provided with unbiased information about the risks and benefits of medicalised options, and whether she had autonomy in decision-making rather than being unduly influenced by an obstetrician's or midwife's recommendation [131]. As we've seen here, the overuse of medical interventions may result in unnecessary stress and trauma to mother and baby. Unnecessary interventions disturb the progression of spontaneous

physiological labour and birth [199] as well as instinctive neonatal behaviours that make it easier for mother and infant to bond and breastfeed post-birth [207]. Research also shows that obstetric interventions can adversely affect a child's health and wellbeing up to the age of 5 [159]. Although relatively little is known about the possible continuing consequences of a medicalised birth on developing infant temperament, it has been suggested that certain high-impact obstetric interventions such as assisted birth (using forceps or vacuum extraction) could potentially have longer-term effects on infant behaviour and functioning [49, 56]. Therefore, women need to be fully informed about the risks and benefits of any intervention suggested to them during labour and birth.

3.2 Birthplace

One of the major decisions that parents have to make is *where* their baby should be born. If there is something amiss with the pregnancy or an underlying health problem in mother or baby, they will probably be advised to register for a hospital birth. For many years, women always birthed at home, and this is still common in some countries. Childbirth was brought into hospitals on the assumption that it would be safer. However, in 2011, an innovative prospective cohort study known as "The Birthplace Study" was conducted across NHS England over a 2-year period to examine differences in outcomes between nearly 65,000 healthy mothers with low-risk pregnancies depending on their *planned* choice of birthplace [26]. The study looked at women planning to give birth at home (with access to hospital transfer if needed), at a "freestanding" or "alongside" midwife-led unit (including *all* midwife-led units in England) or at one of a randomly selected sample of obstetric units (hospitals). Unplanned homebirths, planned caesarean sections and caesarean sections carried out before labour began were excluded. The 250 different outcomes examined involved perinatal mortality and birth-related neonatal morbidity. This included stillbirth after care had begun in labour or neonatal death post-birth, meconium aspiration syndrome and physical injuries, such as a fractured humerus or clavicle.

In total, 4.3 out of 1000 births were adversely affected. Remarkably, given all the fear-mongering around homebirths, the study found that, overall, there were no significant differences for healthy mothers with low-risk pregnancies between giving birth in an obstetric unit and a non-obstetric setting (i.e. home or midwife-led unit). However, *first*-born babies had slightly better outcomes when born in a hospital or midwife-led unit, and transfers from non-obstetric to obstetric settings were more frequent for first-time mothers. There were no significant differences in adverse baby outcomes based on *planned* place of birth for women having their second or subsequent child. For these mothers, planning to give birth at home, in a midwife-led unit and in hospital were all safe options, providing they had a positive relationship with their team of community midwives and agreed to transfer if needed. Women experienced fewer obstetric interventions in non-obstetric settings, allowing them to have a better and more fulfilling birth experience. The authors concluded that all women with healthy pregnancies should be offered a choice of where they give birth, although first-time mothers must be made aware of the slightly increased risk of adverse perinatal outcomes [26].

Although it is debateable whether the birth of a new human being should ever be calculated in monetary terms, a Norwegian study has calculated the difference in costs between planned homebirths and planned hospital births for healthy women with low-risk pregnancies. Planned homebirth for these mothers is a cost-effective option (approximately €2842 as opposed to €4077 for hospital births including any birth-related complications) when the midwives are part of a team covering multiple mothers (i.e. not just one midwife covering one mother) or when they are based at a hospital that facilitates homebirths [96]. We currently have a severe lack of funds for providing good-quality National Health Service (NHS) healthcare across the board, and this includes our currently inhumane Accident and Emergency queues of up to 24 hours in some parts of the UK, leading to unnecessary mortality. At the moment, our homebirth rate is very low at approximately 1%, while, although Holland's previously high rate of over 35% has dropped in recent years, it still lingers around the 16% mark [69]. Dutch midwives are highly trained to recognise any complications if they arise and to "cooperate smoothly" with their colleagues, including paramedics and obstetricians, working closely together to care for the patient and arrange an efficient and speedy hospital transfer if required [205]. Perhaps given the evidence, the well-known psychosocial benefits to mothers[1] and the cost-effectiveness of providing a *choice* to give birth in non-obstetric settings, it is time to think about making better provisions for expert midwifery teams attached to the NHS to cover more homebirths in the UK. Otherwise, there is a risk that facilitating safe homebirths and other physiological births could become a "dying art".

3.3 Induction of Labour and Its Potential Impacts on Mother and Baby

According to a recent cross-sectional survey of maternity units, induction of labour rates in the UK and elsewhere have been on a continuous rise over the past couple of decades, with figures varying between 19% and 54% in the UK. The survey also found that, in many trusts, induction rates fell outside recommended guidelines [188], while a Tanzanian study found that time scarcity led to more inductions. In this study, augmenting labour also deviated from the guidelines, coinciding more with shift turnovers and ward rounds than with actual labour progression [107]. This overuse of induction and augmentation based on time constraints could increase the risk of perinatal harm as birth attendants may also lack time to monitor the mother's and baby's condition during an artificially induced labour.

A Danish national cohort study contributed to the recent exponential rise of inductions of labour. This research found that, while induction rates had more

---

[1] Natural birth physiology may work best if parents are relaxed and supported in their familiar home environment.

than doubled during a 12-year period, stillbirth rates had fallen by one per thousand newborns [81], leaving the authors to conclude that pregnancies should not be allowed to run much past their due dates. However, there was one important factor they had not taken account of—smoking also increases the risk of stillbirth, and the number of women smoking in pregnancy had halved during the same period. In addition, more *high-risk* women were being induced, meaning that the drop in stillbirth rates could be more attributable to these factors than to the soaring rates of blanket inductions at 41 weeks. Potentially, therefore, the findings from Hedegaard et al. [81] are misleading. Whether they promote or detract from neonatal health and wellbeing, it is clear that for "prolonged pregnancies" from 41 weeks, in aiming to prevent a slightly increased risk for stillbirth, over 400 births must be induced (with all the other risks this entails) for one life to be saved [138].

A counter Danish study, finding the adverse outcomes of induction outweighed the benefits, concluded that booking inductions before 42 weeks for low-risk pregnancies goes against the World Health Organization's [204] recommendations, which are for the expected benefits of a medical intervention to outweigh potential harms [173]. Although risks increase for certain obstetric complications (e.g. a larger baby or shoulder dystocia) if parents decide *not* to rush into an early induction [119], they deserve to be given balanced, unbiased information and sufficient time to decide. In our increasingly risk-averse culture, however, and despite the increased risks of maternal and neonatal birth trauma following induction [33], many women in the UK are now automatically booked in for an induction at 41 weeks.

There are many routes to inducing labour. These include inserting a pessary of prostaglandins to ripen the cervix and initiate labour or performing an amniotomy—breaking the baby's waters (amniotic sack), known as artificial rupture of membranes. Although the question of whether induction rates are driving up emergency caesarean rates remains under debate [67], overall they are associated with an increase in caesarean sections [173] and have been linked to a rise in instrumental births [138]. Routine induction procedures such as early rupture of membranes raise the rate of foetal heart abnormalities, increasing the chance of the baby needing urgent assistance to be born [151]. Preliminary methods of induction are not always successful and may result in needing to place the mother on an intravenous drip of Pitocin or Syntocinon, synthetic forms of the natural birth, bonding and breastfeeding hormone and neurotransmitter oxytocin. This increases the need for careful monitoring to avoid risks such as hyperstimulation leading to foetal distress and paediatric effects, including short- and long-term impacts on behaviour [32]. Continuous electronic foetal monitoring restricts the mother's mobility and potentially increases the risk of perineal tears due to the strength of contractions and the mother's stationary physical position on the bed. It may also result in an instrumental or surgical birth if labour "fails to progress". Despite these concerns, and although a Cochrane review concluded that continuous electronic foetal monitoring does *not* improve overall perinatal mortality or cerebral palsy rates compared to more traditional intermittent auscultation methods [4], its routine use has continued without any real evidence to support it.

For the mother, as mentioned earlier, induction of labour is associated with a higher incidence of severe perineal trauma [153]. Such injuries may lead to urinary or anal incontinence after childbirth—distressing conditions that impact heavily on women's day-to-day life, sense of identity and emotional wellbeing [100]. Providing some counter-evidence to this, a medical review and meta-analysis of induction of labour outcomes across eight randomised trials found no increase in third- or fourth-degree tears after induction and, perhaps surprisingly, *lower* caesarean section rates following the intervention [179]. Meanwhile, a large-scale Swedish study confirmed associations between induction of labour and high vaginal tears, along with findings that vacuum extraction—which is more likely to follow an induction—increases the risk of obstetric anal sphincter injuries [90]. Taken as a whole, the current evidence on induction-related risks seems to be inconsistent, contradictory and occasionally alarming.

Ongoing medical debates aside, induced or augmented labours can mean depleted energy reserves and physical exhaustion for the person giving birth, and this added intensity of the birth experience could extend the mother and baby's recovery time. Higher levels of medical intervention and the increased possibility of complications during induced or augmented labours may also raise the mother's stress and anxiety levels, increasing her chance of developing postnatal depression. For the baby, induced labour could be more stressful due to more forceful contractions and the increased potential for interventions. A large-scale 16-year population-based study including a whopping 474,652 births established several adverse risks of induction for the babies including an increased need for resuscitation at birth, respiratory disorders and, remarkably, increased hospital admissions for nose, ear, throat and respiratory infections up to the age of 16 [50]. The physical impacts of induction on the child, therefore, can be long-term. In addition, foetal and neonatal pain and distress arising from birth complications and interventions may cause changes to the baby's central nervous system and their delicate neuroendocrine and immune systems, potentially affecting the baby's temperament and future susceptibility to pain, stress and illness [158].

Synthetic Oxytocin
Synthetic oxytocin is now widely used during childbirth to initiate or accelerate labour and birth, although communications to parents about its potentially harmful side effects can be quite unclear. These may include psychological symptoms, for example, an increase in maternal anxiety, interfering with natural childbirth physiology [41]. Medical risks include umbilical cord prolapse or hyperstimulation of the uterus, potentially causing foetal bradycardia (a sustained low heart rate), both of which could result in emergency caesarean section [15]. Other major problems that can occur following synthetic oxytocin administration include neonatal acidosis, asphyxia and uterine rupture [95]. Synthetic oxytocin is frequently used to avoid the increased mortality and morbidity risks associated with prolonged labour, but although it tends to shorten labour duration, it generally makes the experience more intense, painful and dangerous for mothers and babies in other ways. For example, there appear to be dose-dependent associations between synthetic oxytocin and

caesarean section rates [101]. In another study comparing routine oxytocin infusion with discontinuation during the active phase of labour, stark differences were found in outcomes. Although early discontinuation prolonged the first stage of labour for nearly an hour, there were significant reductions in foetal distress, hyperstimulation, caesarean section and admission to NICU—meaning newborns were healthier at birth [40]. Other studies comparing low and high doses of synthetic oxytocin concluded that a low dosage was as effective but had far fewer side effects of intrauterine and neonatal complications leading to instrumental or caesarean births, postpartum haemorrhage or neonatal mortality [145, 167]. Therefore, high doses that over-stimulate the uterus and cause pain and distress to mother and baby should become a thing of the past.

In spite of these side effects, synthetic oxytocin is generally considered an effective way to induce labour and reduce the time of a prolonged labour that may have stalled for some reason, for example, if the mother has arrived at the hospital feeling anxious and fearful (although there are plenty of healthier ways to try and re-start labour less abruptly, such as social support or massage). It is also used to prevent and treat postpartum haemorrhage [163]. As we have seen, however, the intensity of contractions can seriously elevate pain and stress levels, which increases the body's release of stress hormones and neurotransmitters such as cortisol and catecholamines. These travel directly to the foetus via the placenta, meaning the baby is likely to be born with higher than normal cortisol levels. Moreover, while the aim can be for endogenous oxytocin to take over once labour is underway, in reality, synthetic oxytocin is thought to block the natural (endogenous) form. This may encourage increased stress reactivity in response to labour rather than the contractions generating the calming and pain-relieving benefits to mother and baby that endogenous oxytocin is renowned for—decreasing stress levels by downregulating the mother's HPA axis [198].

If a mother has become highly stressed during an induced or augmented birth, it is likely this will impact the baby's stress response, which is linked to their temperament and behaviour. Increases in physiological and psychological stress also interfere with the mother's endogenous oxytocin production, affecting breastfeeding and bonding. Although research on the effects of exogenous (synthetic) oxytocin on mother-infant outcomes is fairly sparse and inconsistent, rather counter-intuitively, a Romanian study led by obstetricians suggests it may actually *lower* postnatal depression rates [156]. Furthermore, some small-scale evidence suggests it could actually *improve* mother-infant bonding [58]. This seems unlikely, however, as higher cortisol levels in the newborn after the administration of synthetic oxytocin are associated with increased irritability and negative behaviours such as crying and fussing, and this early stress could affect the infant's ongoing stress responsiveness and ability to self-regulate [211].

Epidural analgesia is often called for during an intense or painful induction as it is essential to limit such intense and unnatural pain for the mother to prevent short- and long-term distress (see Sect. 3.6). The impact of epidural on the neonate's nervous system may be more pronounced when used in conjunction with synthetic oxytocin. A prospective US-Swedish study of 63 low-income American mothers found that normal neonatal behaviours, including the "breast crawl" and suckling, were adversely affected by the combination of synthetic oxytocin and the fentanyl contained in epidural analgesia [25], probably because these combined medications interfere with the mother's endogenous production of oxytocin and prolactin and may therefore inhibit breastfeeding and bonding [61, 68].

We know that the endogenous oxytocin system modulates fear and anxiety in the mother, including memories of fear and trauma, but the impacts of synthetic oxytocin on the baby's central nervous system and long-term mental health are still largely unknown and understudied. A lack of endogenous oxytocin could contribute to diminished sociability and an increased incidence of neurodevelopmental disorders such as autism spectrum disorder (ASD) and attention deficit hyperactivity disorder (ADHD) during early childhood [144, 176]. Meanwhile, the influence of *synthetic* oxytocin on the development of infant and child mental disorders such as ASD has mainly remained uninvestigated for many years [163], despite some early research indicating that it could be implicated in less sociable, "aloof" autistic children [142]. More recent studies have explored these potential links between the use of synthetic oxytocin and neurodevelopmental outcomes with mixed results. An extensive cohort study involving 12,503 participants found no significant associations between the use of synthetic oxytocin and later developmental and behavioural issues such as ADHD and ASD [109]. However, a study on the long-term effects of epidural analgesia and Pitocin (synthetic oxytocin) during labour found a 37% increased risk of ASD after epidural. Notably, in this study, the initial associations between Pitocin and ASD disappeared when epidural analgesia use was taken into account [162]. The main risk of Pitocin here could be that it increased the mother's need for opiate-based pain relief interventions such as epidural analgesia, and it may be the *combination* of these two medical interventions that is most damaging.

According to the World Health Organization [204], this ever-increasing "medicalisation" of childbirth is "undermining" women's natural capacity to give birth without interventions and negatively impacting women's birth experience. Similarly, the Royal College of Obstetricians and Gynaecologists [166] have stated that interventions do *not* necessarily lead to improved outcomes for mother and baby and may cause decreased birth satisfaction or even trauma for the mother-infant pair. Consequently, it is worth considering that the overuse of synthetic oxytocin in cases where it is not needed, compounded by its association with further interventions such as epidural analgesia, assisted birth and possibly caesarean section, could be having detrimental effects on the behaviour, social-emotional development and mental health of the next generation. Given its blockade of endogenous oxytocin, and the positive effects that stimulating this powerful hormone and neuropeptide (e.g. through skin-to-skin contact) has on infant physiology and behaviour, some neurobiological scientists specialising in this field are concerned that overly medicalised or stressful births could be affecting the oxytocinergic system on an epigenetic level. This means that subtle biological changes occurring during childbirth (such as increased DNA methylation) could be passed unknowingly onto the next generation, potentially dysregulating the baby's HPA axis and adversely impacting their long-term physiological health, wellbeing and behaviour [200].

In the meantime, while synthetic oxytocin is an important tool for managing labour when it is necessary to intervene, caution should be exercised around blanket rollouts of such highly impactful and potentially dangerous obstetric interventions. With our soaring induction rates fast approaching 50%, it's possible that we're creating both short- and long-term problems for up to half the future generation. More research is needed to reach a fuller understanding of the relationship between different types of induction and mother-infant outcomes so that labour practices that best support maternal and neonatal health can be optimised.

3.4 Pain Relief and Its Relationship to Obstetric Interventions and Infant Outcomes

Obstetric pain relief has a chequered history. Many early forms of analgesia and anaesthesia, using what was known as "twilight sleep" or chloroform for a "painless childbirth", often left the mother either unconscious or semi-conscious with no real memory of the birth [73, 187]. These initial versions of pain relief for labouring women were later found to be harmful to both the mother and newborn baby [118]. Since then, research has demonstrated the adverse effects of certain types of pharmacological pain relief that are often used in labour. When enduring an intense labour, it can be challenging to balance these physical risks against the potentially damaging impacts of acute labour pains, as extreme pain is considered a public health issue that may lead to adverse outcomes for mother and baby [140]. Reducing pain and distress during labour and childbirth is essential for several reasons, but especially when the person giving birth is experiencing medical interventions. When women feel stressed or in unbearable pain during labour, this increases their fear, further intensifying their perceptions of pain, with negative impacts on their mental health post-birth [190]. Meanwhile, a seminal systematic review in the early 2000s found that women who chose not to use any pain relief during labour experienced greater birth satisfaction [86].

It's not easy to separate out the early research on pain relief and obstetric interventions during childbirth. Some women requiring an induction may manage to use only breathing techniques or Entonox (a mix of oxygen and laughing gas known as "gas and air") to birth their baby, while others might feel the need for pethidine or an epidural to help relieve their pain. However, complications, obstetric interventions and pharmacological pain relief often go hand in hand as the mother's experience of pain and stress in these situations can rise to unmanageable levels, and a sedative may help them to cope. There was a small spate of research in the 1970s and 1980s led by a group of scientists interested in newborn infant outcomes after difficult childbirth experiences involving obstetric interventions and pharmacological pain relief. Lester and his colleagues [113] first began investigating these potential risk factors for altered baby behaviour post-birth five decades ago. With an ongoing focus on the *physical* aspects of labour and birth, they discovered cumulative effects of pharmacological substances used during labour on the newborn baby's central nervous system, especially when this was compounded by a long labour or medical interventions during the birth [114]. Their research focused on the impacts of epidural anaesthesia, using the Neonatal Behavioural Assessment Scale (NBAS) designed by Brazelton [23] to assess the newborn baby's physiological wellbeing, recovery from childbirth and behavioural style. They also compared their results with the widely used medical measure—the Apgar score.

The Apgar score was designed by the obstetrical anaesthesiologist Virginia Apgar in the early 1950s to assess the newborn baby's overall physical condition and wellbeing at 1 and 5 minutes post-birth [11]. Although recently there has been a call for a different system of neonatal assessment, for many decades, Apgar scores have been considered a good indicator of the newborn's physiological and neurobiological state. This post-birth state is likely to affect neonatal behaviour and wellbeing following birth. Newborn babies with healthy Apgar scores (7–10 at 5 minutes post-birth) might be expected first to let out a cry, then to have a period of being quiet and alert and finally to settle. Lester and colleagues [113, 114] found associations between the 5-minute Apgar score and the NBAS measurement of "arousal", demonstrating that the newborn baby's neurobiological state (and therefore their Apgar score) can be affected by pharmacological pain relief, a prolonged labour or a challenging birth experience. Lower Apgar scores may indicate elevated stress hormones and potential complications in the baby. For example, low Apgar scores are associated with neurological and psychiatric disorders such as cerebral palsy or intellectual disability and, more recently, autism [141].

Alongside these negative neonatal outcomes of a long, challenging or medicalised birth, Lester and colleagues [114] suggested that the baby's mother might not be in an optimal position to care for her newborn if she is in pain after obstetric interventions. They also noted that the baby may take a few days to become alert after a medicated birth, and, combined with the mother's difficulties in adjusting, this could make it difficult for the mother-infant pair to synchronise their communications, with negative impacts on bonding and breastfeeding. Later researchers concluded that many of the physical impacts of childbirth on the baby (e.g. mode of birth and pain relief medication) are naturally transient or else quickly overshadowed by other environmental and sociodemographic variables such as poverty, deprivation and diet [36]. Similarly, Figueiredo and colleagues [65] found that previous associations between birth mode, pain relief and mother-infant bonding and attachment were no longer significant after accounting for sociodemographic variables and other influences from the baby's environment outside the womb. Therefore, the postnatal environment is probably *at least* as significant as the birthing environment in its impact on early infant behaviour and development.

Epidural Analgesia
Research on the potential impacts of pharmacological pain relief on the newborn baby has resurfaced as an important issue that requires parents' and health professionals' full consideration before childbirth. The effects of epidural analgesia are particularly well researched. While providing a highly effective form of pain relief

with its numbing effect from the waist down, epidurals may also prolong labour, particularly the second stage, where, under the influence of an epidural, the mother may have no pushing sensations and therefore find it difficult to tune into her body. As mentioned earlier, the rise in "assisted" or "instrumental" births, requiring the use of forceps or ventouse to deliver the baby, has been largely attributed to the increased use of epidurals during labour [94], although some later evidence disputes this connection [10, 134]. Regardless of potential associations, it is reasonable to suppose there might be extra challenges for mother and baby during the post-birth recovery period following an epidural. Anecdotally, for example, the mother may experience an increase in back pain afterwards, making it more challenging to care for her newborn, though research on this particular outcome is very mixed. Nonetheless, epidurals have been linked to an array of postnatal physical issues, including motor blockade, hypotension, fever and urinary retention [94]. Furthermore, newborns have a higher risk of admission to NICU and an Apgar score of less than the ideal 7 at 5 minutes following epidural use [105, 112, 113], which could mean that newborn behaviour is also temporarily affected by epidural analgesia.

Although administration methods and dosage for epidural analgesia have been constantly updated and refined to make them more effective while having less adverse impacts [133], many parents understandably still fear the possibility of negative side effects on themselves and their baby. Worryingly, Mellon [136] found anaesthesia during labour to be "neurotoxic" for the foetus, possibly altering the structure and function of the central nervous system, and there is accumulating evidence that neurotoxicity levels may contribute to neurodevelopmental abnormalities, unless the drug is administered using low-dose strategies [133]. Counter to this, a large-scale population-based study, conducted by a consultant anaesthetist and her research team across all Scottish hospitals between 2007 and 2019, found that the use of epidural analgesia during labour among 22% of the 567,216 women giving birth (either vaginally or by unplanned caesarean section) had some *positive* outcomes. According to this study, the incidence of severe maternal morbidity and admission to critical care was reduced by 35% [99]. Although these effects were especially pronounced for those with preterm labour or a medical indication for epidural analgesia, the researchers concluded that providing all women with access to epidural analgesia during childbirth could, in fact, *improve* overall maternal health and wellbeing.

Although there might be negative consequences to this type of easy-access rollout, and perhaps we need to step back and look at the wider picture, it is essential that women do have access to pain relief when they want it or feel the need for it. However, the perceived need for pharmacological forms of pain relief, such as epidural analgesia, should also be explored. One of the reasons behind the ever-increasing use of strong pain relief during labour could be linked to the way that labour is managed in modern maternity wards. Higher induction rates than ever before, alongside equally high maternal stress levels, may be contributing to complications as stress-induced hormonal changes can lead to dysfunctional labour patterns [30]. This could mean an increase in augmentations of labour, with the associated risks of hyperstimulation and uterine rupture, further exacerbating pain, stress and complications. In these types of situations, epidurals could provide a highly effective form of pain relief and reduce cortisol levels during a long, painful or distressing labour while lowering the risk of "baby blues" afterwards due to the impacts of excessive pain on the mother's mental health [89]. The efficacy of epidurals makes them an important addition to the obstetric toolbox. While reducing the mother's stress response during childbirth may go a considerable way towards reducing the neonate's stress response too, open discussions and better education about the risks and benefits of epidurals and the variety of options available should be improved, and women should always be offered effective alternative strategies for pain relief.

Pethidine
Probably the most widely used form of analgesic for pain relief during labour is pethidine, a powerful opiate that may come with some unpleasant effects such as drowsiness and nausea [94]. Pethidine readily crosses the placenta and acts as a depressant to the newborn's immature respiratory system, negatively impacting the baby's Apgar and neurobehavioural scores while adversely affecting their muscle tone, suckling ability and social responsiveness [169, 183]. Using pethidine during labour can also increase newborn crying and discourage early breastfeeding behaviours [28]. Babies with respiratory depression after exposure to pethidine are more likely to be taken to NICU and consequently separated from their mother immediately post-birth [143]. In addition to disrupting breastfeeding and bonding, as discussed earlier, the separation of mother and baby during this critical period may impede the newborn's early social responsiveness. Pethidine's analgesic properties have been much disputed over the years. Some have described it as merely a relaxant, acting more as an anxiety-reducing sedative than effective pain relief [73]. This means its benefits may only extend as far as a psychological remedy, soothing anxious and fearful mothers [5].

Gas and Air
In contrast to pethidine and epidurals, nitrous oxide or Entonox (commonly known as "gas and air") is generally considered a safe and effective form of pain relief for use in labour [150]. In a "gold standard" double-blind, clinical, randomised controlled trial, although Entonox caused nausea, sickness, drowsiness and dizziness in 25% of cases, it was found to reduce pain severity and subsequently the need for pethidine [12]. Another randomised controlled trial found Entonox to be more effective than pethidine during the early stages of labour, and there were no differences in pain severity 60 minutes after using either form of pain relief [140]. Moreover, women using gas and air to help with labour pains often appreciate the self-administration aspect of it [118]; but despite all these positive attributes, the possibility of Entonox affecting child development has been called into question. Therefore, although I am definitely not advocating for childbirth without pain relief unless that is the mother's explicit wish, more research on the safety of supposedly harmless methods is needed before they continue to be promoted in maternity care without any words caution about their possible impacts on the baby [130].

3.5 Alternatives to Using Medical Pain Relief During Childbirth

Various forms of non-pharmacological pain relief can be used during childbirth with fewer known side effects than epidural, pethidine or Entonox. Some of these, including the frequently used TENS (transcutaneous electrical nerve stimulation) machine, are thought to work via the "Pain Gate Control Theory". This is when another physical sensation, such as water, light massage or—in the case of TENS machines—electrical nerve impulses, distracts from and interferes with the transmission of pain signals to the brain while stimulating the body to release endorphins, its own natural painkillers [34]. Chaillet and colleagues [39] found that, in conjunction with continuous support, techniques based on the Pain Gate Control Theory, which inhibit sensations of pain, may offer multiple benefits by providing alternative, non-noxious sensations (e.g. massage and water immersion). These other, more pleasant sensations travel at a faster speed, blocking pain signals from being transmitted to the central nervous system, including the brain [137]. Incorporating sensory, physiological and psychological theories of pain [34], the benefits of this method include reducing obstetric interventions such as synthetic oxytocin, epidural and instrumental or caesarean birth while shortening the length of labour.

Other natural forms of pain relief that work well for some people include relaxation techniques, breathing exercises, hydrotherapy, hypnotherapy, acupuncture, acupressure, massage, the rebozo technique and, notably, continuous social and emotional support. Music therapy has recently been used and tested in some Irish maternity care settings as a strategy to promote the mother's relaxation, reduce symptoms of anxiety and depression and encourage parent-infant attachment postbirth [42]. Including methods such as these in clinical settings could be part of a wider aim to "humanise" the childbirth experience [115].

Trials of different types of "alternative" or more traditional relaxation and pain relief methods have found no adverse outcomes while these methods can effectively reduce perceptions of pain and stress, increase satisfaction with the birth experience and empower the mother to take an active role in her own pain management [94]. For example, alongside creating a safe, secure and reassuring birth environment, learning self-hypnosis during pregnancy can be an effective tool, especially for women who *fear* childbirth. Attending a certified course and learning and practising hypnobirthing during pregnancy can make women feel more empowered and "in control" of their birth as they manage their pain through a combination of techniques: taking long deep breaths (with a focus on the outbreath, triggering relaxation via the parasympathetic nervous system); light massage strokes from a partner (based on the Pain Gate Control Theory and encouraging the release of oxytocin and endorphins, the body's natural and effective painkillers); and visualisations, which serve as distraction techniques. Using these techniques can help prevent the mother from getting locked into a negative fear-tension-pain cycle. Hypnobirthing practices have finally been validated and a recent randomised controlled trial (which is widely considered the "gold standard" of research evidence) has demonstrated that practising hypnobirthing techniques significantly lessens the fear that many mothers experience during labour and birth while also reducing perceptions of pain, especially in first-time mothers [98]. Although, anecdotally, hypnobirthing can encourage a more efficient labour and birth and a calmer, more content baby, no one technique can ever guarantee positive birth outcomes. Still, if practising hypnobirthing during childbirth helps women to remain calm and in control enough to take part in decision-making (e.g. making an informed choice to have a caesarean section), they can feel empowered and positive about this.

Although acupuncture is also used to effectively reduce maternal pain and stress during childbirth, some non-pharmacological pain alleviation strategies have an evidence base that is rather more mixed and inconclusive, with the exception of one extremely beneficial and potentially low-cost intervention: providing continuous physical and emotional support to mother and baby by a team of known and trusted midwives throughout the perinatal period is known as "continuity of care" [48]. Professor Jane Sandall, a leading figure in continuity of care based at King's College London, has recently released an updated Cochrane review of the evidence, as discussed below.

Continuity of Care

Sandall and colleagues [175] emphasise the role of midwife continuity of care in promoting spontaneous physiological birth and a positive birth experience, alongside lowering rates of caesarean sections, instrumental births and, to some extent, episiotomies. Women generally prefer to know their caregivers [86, 87], and having a known midwife helps to reduce fear and perceptions of pain while increasing information sharing, joint decision-making and perceptions of control [82]. The caregiver-patient relationship and the mother's involvement in decision-making are central to her satisfaction with the birth experience [86]. These benefits may not be easy to achieve without continuity of care, although midwife Claire Feeley [62] argues they should still be possible.

Continuity of care (CoC) is, by its very nature, a more person-centred model as a small group of midwives get to know each mother, including her cultural background, medical history and wishes regarding the birth. CoC is designed to meet women's individual preferences, needs and values. Notably, when pregnant women do not receive continuity of care, instead seeing a different health professional at each antenatal visit, this is associated with lower rates of shared decision-making, less respectful maternity care and an increased risk of instrumental birth [7]. Although it may be difficult to fully implement CoC in our current resource-scarce maternity care settings, despite all the known benefits and the distinct possibility it will lessen the need for an emergency caesarean section or any of the other high-intensity resources used during obstetric interventions, it is still considered possible—and arguably essential—to be person-centred in situations where care is fragmented and CoC isn't available [62]. Enabling an extra support person (e.g. a doula) for the person giving birth helps create a more respectful and person-centred experience, thereby enhancing the quality of care, birth satisfaction and mother-baby outcomes [149].

Continuity of care centres around providing continuous, *respectful* care and support to mother and baby. "Respectful maternity care" is based on international and regional laws while being grounded in human rights during pregnancy, childbirth and the postnatal period. It benefits mother and baby through providing equitable healthcare at the highest attainable level [203]. Reflecting Sandall's [175] findings regarding CoC, respectful maternity care promotes a positive birth experience by ensuring that several vital elements of childbirth are met—physical and psychological safety (i.e. freedom from abuse or mistreatment, known as "obstetric violence"); privacy, autonomy and confidentiality; dignity and respect; equitable treatment and justice; and communication, shared decision-making and informed consent [35]. Providing respectful, one-to-one midwifery care and emotional support during childbirth lowers the mother's perceptions of pain, helps prevent negative birthing experiences and increases overall birth satisfaction [164]. One study found that following a model of respectful maternity care also increases the mother's release of prostaglandins, which soften and dilate the cervix, facilitating physiological labour [170]. Sadly, however, there is often a gap between midwives' and other health professionals' *intention* to provide supportive, woman-centred care and the new mother actually feeling that she has received it [116].

Research in low-income countries also echoes Sandall's [175] findings, in particular within sub-Saharan Africa, where maternal and neonatal mortality rates are consistently high [97]. Two separate studies based on large samples of women living in Ethiopia, where neonatal mortality rates are the highest in the world, standing at an estimated 227.13 per 1000 live births in 2022 [194], found that lower rates of person-centred care were associated with mothers with no formal education, fewer antenatal visits and increased birth complications, reinforcing global inequalities [97, 186]. Based on the rapidly accumulating evidence of its benefits for good physical and psychological birth outcomes, personalised continuity of care models are now recommended by the World Health Organization [204] as highly effective contributors to the safe and positive birth experience that every pregnant mother is entitled to. These methods of maternity care could go a long way towards reducing maternal and neonatal morbidity and mortality; therefore, they must be implemented if we are to achieve global targets for maternal and neonatal health and wellbeing [70]. Having continuous social support during childbirth is particularly important in under-resourced countries or areas with a shortage of health professionals.

A key aspect of continuity of care is the continuous psychological and emotional support it provides. This helps prevent complications from occurring as midwives are tuned into the individual needs of the mother, making her feel listened to and cared for so she can more easily relax into physiological labour. It is imperative to have continuous social and emotional support in place when challenges do arise as, together with improving labour outcomes, this will help reduce maternal stress, perceptions of pain and risk of postnatal depression [125] and birth trauma [185]. Providing continuous emotional support alongside standard physical care during labour and birth is therefore an essential component of the effort to reduce maternal pain and distress and raise overall birth satisfaction. The support may come from several sources, including midwives and other health professionals, doulas, family members and partners, who also have a supportive role to play in reducing maternal anxiety [214]. Bilingual, community-based doulas could be a useful provision for migrant or refugee women, facilitating communication between them and health professionals while enabling them to feel calm and safe during and after childbirth [161].

3.6 Why Is It Essential to Reduce Pain and Distress During Labour?

During the early stages of labour, experiencing fear may temporarily halt spontaneous physiological progression as—depending partly on how well-established labour is—the mother's body may instinctively stall when she senses danger [122]. High stress levels lead to elevated stress hormones in both mother and baby, increasing the risk of complications and impacting neonatal behaviour. Therefore, managing maternal fear, stress and pain through a personalised combination of pharmacological and non-pharmacological methods and tailoring these wherever possible to the mother's pre-birth wishes and current needs in collaboration with her partner is probably the most effective way to reduce stress, diminish pain and ensure the mother's voice is heard.

As we know from the recent Birth Trauma Inquiry [189] and previous research, if mothers are not listened to when they are in pain, or they are refused pain relief in response to their requests, instead made to wait until they are at the standard level of dilation for the official "start" of labour (4 cm dilated), this contributes to a traumatic birth experience. If, instead, mothers' needs are fully honoured and respected during labour and birth, they are spoken to with kindness and warmth and they are met as equal people with the fundamental human rights to make their own informed decisions and give birth as they wish, this should enable them to feel calm, relaxed, heard, understood, and physically and emotionally safe while optimising physical and mental health outcomes for both mother and baby [62]. Access to respectful and emotionally supportive care and pain management is especially critical in countries where pain relief is lacking. In Tanzania, for instance, non-pharmacological methods are sometimes the only option available. Unfortunately, there is also a prevailing cultural belief that enduring pain is an essential part of the process, which can leave women feeling very much alone with their labour pain [191]. Given what we know about optimising physiological and psychological outcomes for mother and baby by reducing stress and pain, this style of practice is unlikely to be conducive to their positive physical and mental health or to infant development post-birth.

3.7 Labour Positions

It is only since modern obstetrics entered the birth room that women began to be placed on their backs in a "supine" position for childbirth. It's hardly surprising that labour often stalls in this position as the labouring mother quite literally has to push her baby uphill to give birth, rather than allowing a combination of involuntary internal uterine muscles and gravity to play their part. What is surprising is that the majority of women (over 77%) are still expected to give birth in this position despite all the evidence stacked against its efficacy. Understandably, women tend to have lower childbirth satisfaction in the supine position, particularly if they have been directed into it by medical staff [178].

Childbirth in recumbent or semi-recumbent positions can be a laborious and painful process as the ability of the sacral and coccygeal bones in the pelvis to move and rotate is restricted, impacting mother and baby's comfort and outcomes [193]. In these positions, compared to more flexible sacrum positions, the pelvic outlet is reduced due to the physical constraints imposed by the pressure of the bed (or other hard surface). Giving birth in the supine or semi-recumbent position—as has become the convenient norm in maternity wards across the world—therefore lessens the beneficial effects of gravity and increased pelvic space. Instead, these positions could make it more difficult for the baby to descend, possibly resulting in perineal tears and prolonged, stalled or obstructed labours that require medical assistance. A major concern is that the weight of the uterus could compress major blood vessels, reducing the flow of blood and oxygen to the foetus and increasing risks of maternal hypotension, foetal distress and neonatal hypoxia while inevitably reducing comfort and exacerbating pain [193].

Although stirrups can be helpful for health professionals as they provide easy visual and physical access to the perineum and birth canal, facilitating the use of continuous electronic monitoring and other interventions, overall, giving birth lying down may be detrimental to mother and baby's health and wellbeing. Conceivably, a supine position where the birth often becomes directed by the health professionals rather than by the woman's intuitive needs and desires could also induce feelings of anxiety and a frightening sense of losing control for the labouring mother. In turn, a heightened state of anxiety increases the risk of dystocia (abnormal labour progression), negatively impacting the birth [83].

"Active birth" positions such as kneeling, squatting, standing or sitting, with gravitational force leading to more efficient contractions, facilitate the baby's journey down the birth canal and out into the world. Active births are aided by the expansion of the pelvic diameter in upright positions, creating more space for the baby to descend while reducing pain and the need for obstetric interventions such as forceps, vacuum extraction or caesarean birth [72]. However, these positions have risks and benefits that need ongoing and individualised assessment. While they appear to significantly reduce rates of instrumental birth in women who have not had an epidural, blood loss over 500 mL is more likely [215]. Risks of episiotomy and use of epidural analgesia or synthetic oxytocin are lower in upright compared to supine positions, and there is no apparent variance in the risk of perineal tears or vaginal and labial trauma [21]. If the person giving birth needs to rest, lying on the left side (to avoid compression of major blood vessels on the right) rather than on the back, and with a pillow between the legs if needed, can also lead to a more controlled and comfortable labour and birth.

Labour positions may affect both the newborn baby and the mother, as the improved oxygenation and blood flow associated with upright positions reduce the risk of foetal distress. A smoother descent through the birth canal should result in a less stressful birth process, meaning less overall stress for both mother and baby. Despite some mixed results regarding neonatal outcomes, research by Bodner-Adler et al. [21] found no effects on Apgar scores or umbilical cord PH balance, suggesting that the differences in ease of birth for the mother do not necessarily make a significant difference to the newborn infant's physiological wellbeing and cortisol levels. Given what we now know about mother-baby hormonal exchanges, however, these results might need updating.

Giving birth is a very personal and individual major life event with the possibility of long-lasting repercussions for mother and baby. Ideally, women should be encouraged to "listen to their bodies" and give birth in a position that feels most comfortable for them. Birth positions chosen by the mother in response to the baby's and her own body's instinctive needs will give her more physical and psychological freedom, leading to a sense of control and confidence in her body, and ultimately enabling a more positive birth experience. Midwives are in a unique position to empower women by facilitating such "active" birth experiences [121].

3.8 Conclusion: Where Does This Leave Us Now?

The evolution of modern obstetrics has made an essential contribution to the safety and wellbeing of mothers and babies. Modern obstetric technology and expertise are absolutely vital in an emergency as they can rescue a distressed baby quickly, or both mother and baby if labour becomes stalled or obstructed. However, when it is so readily available and nobody is willing to balance the risks of intervening "too much too soon" or "too little too late" in a careful and considered way before proceeding (often due to fear of litigation), it can be very difficult to determine exactly when "helpful" medical care ends and "unnecessary interventions" begin and where the delicate balance is unwittingly tipped towards long-term physical and psychological harm to mother and baby [204].

In this chapter, we have explored how unnecessary interventions may lead to unnecessary trauma for mother and baby, particularly if emotional support is lacking. Taylor and colleagues [187] first suggested the possibility that a mother's subjective experience of birth and how this affects her postnatally might mitigate some of the physical impacts of being born on the baby's behaviour. Similarly, a meta-analysis led by Professor Susan Ayers [13], a renowned world expert on the causes and effects of birth trauma, found that the mother's *subjective* experiences had more impact on her perceptions of a traumatic birth than the objective (physical) experiences did. Therefore, investigating the mother's subjective birth experience could be key to uncovering whether, and if so how, childbirth might affect early baby behaviour. This concept became the main focus of my research, leading me to explore the way mothers view their birth experience, the impacts this has on the way they perceive and bond with their babies, and the way their babies behave post-birth. As the subjective birth experience is linked to the mother's mental health, and we know this affects mother-baby bonding as well as the baby's behaviour and development [129], it became important to include psychological aspects of childbirth and maternal mental health in my investigations around how the birth experience might relate to bonding and baby behaviour post-birth. These concepts are further explored in Chap. 4.

References

1. Aatsinki AK, Lahti L, Uusitupa HM, Munukka E, Keskitalo A, Nolvi S, O'Mahony S, Pietilä S, Elo LL, Eerola E, Karlsson H, Karlsson L. Gut microbiota composition is associated with temperament traits in infants. Brain Behav Immun. 2019;80:849–58.
2. Abalos E, Oladapo OT, Chamillard M, Díaz V, Pasquale J, Bonet M, et al. Duration of spontaneous labour in 'low-risk' women with 'normal' perinatal outcomes: a systematic review. Eur J Obstet Gynecol Reprod Biol. 2018;223:123–32.
3. ACOG, Caughey AB, Cahill AG, Guise JM, Rouse DJ. Safe prevention of the primary cesarean delivery. Am J Obstet Gynecol. 2014;210:179–93.
4. Alfirevic Z, Gyte GM, Cuthbert A, Devane D. Continuous cardiotocography (CTG) as a form of electronic fetal monitoring (EFM) for fetal assessment during labour. Cochrane Database Syst Rev. 2017;2017:CD006066.
5. Allameh Z, Tehrani HG, Ghasemi M. Comparing the impact of acupuncture and pethidine on reducing labor pain. Adv Biomed Res. 2015;4:46.
6. Almutairi WM, Raidi DK. The effect of immediate kangaroo mother care during third stage of labor on postpartum blood loss and uterine involution: a quasi-experimental comparative study. Healthcare. 2024;12:2548. MDPI.
7. Alruwaili TA, Crawford K, Fooladi E. Shared decision-making in maternity care in Saudi Arabia: a cross-sectional study. Midwifery. 2024;138:104147.
8. Altman M, Sandström A, Petersson G, Frisell T, Cnattingius S, Stephansson O. Prolonged second stage of labor is associated with low Apgar score. Eur J Epidemiol. 2015;30:1209–15.
9. Altunay Davran GB, Serçekuş Ak P. Fathers' emotions, thoughts on childbirth, and coping with childbirth stress: a qualitative study. J Educ Res Nurs. 2024;21:1–7.
10. Apfelbaum JL, Hawkins JL, Agarkar M, Bucklin BA, Connis RT, Gambling D, Mhyre J, Nickinovich DG, Sherman H, Tsen LC, Yaghmour ET. Practice guidelines for obstetric anesthesia: an updated report by the American Society of Anesthesiologists Task Force on obstetric anesthesia and the Society for Obstetric Anesthesia and Perinatology. Anesthesiology. 2016;124:270–300.
11. Apgar V. A proposal for a new method of evaluation of the newborn infant. Anesth Analg. 1953;32:260–7.
12. Attar AS, Feizabadi AS, Jarahi L, Feizabadi LS, Sheybani S. Effect of entonox on reducing the need for pethidine and the relevant fetal and maternal complications for painless labor. Electron Physician. 2016;8:3325.
13. Ayers S, Bond R, Bertullies S, Wijma K. The aetiology of post-traumatic stress following childbirth: a meta-analysis and theoretical framework. Psychol Med. 2016;46:1121–34.
14. Badr HA, Zauszniewski JA. Kangaroo care and postpartum depression: the role of oxytocin. Int J Nurs Sci. 2017;4:179–83.
15. Baker PN, Kenny LC, editors. Obstetrics by 10 teachers. 19th ed. London: Hodder Arnold; 2011.
16. Beniuk, V., Lastovetska, L., Shcherba, O., Kovaliuk, T., Venzovka, Y., & Thadayoose, M. (2024). Episiotomy as vaginal surgery during childbirth.
17. Bergman NJ. New policies on skin-to-skin contact warrant an oxytocin-based perspective on perinatal health care. Front Psychol. 2024;15:1385320.

18. Betrán AP, Ye J, Moller AB, Zhang J, Gülmezoglu AM, Torloni MR. The increasing trend in caesarean section rates: global, regional and national estimates: 1990–2014. PLoS One. 2016;11:e0148343.
19. Betrán AP, Temmerman M, Kingdon C, Mohiddin A, Opiyo N, Torloni MR, Regina M, Zhang J, Musana O, Wanyonyi SZ, Gülmezoglu AM, Downe S. Interventions to reduce unnecessary caesarean sections in healthy women and babies. Lancet. 2018;392:1358–68.
20. Betran AP, Ye J, Moller AB, Souza JP, Zhang J. Trends and projections of caesarean section rates: global and regional estimates. BMJ Glob Health. 2021;6:e005671.
21. Bodner-Adler B, Bodner K, Kimberger O, Lozanov P, Husslein P, Mayerhofer K. Women's position during labour: influence on maternal and neonatal outcome. Wien Klin Wochenschr. 2003;115:720–3.
22. Bohren MA, Vogel JP, Hunter EC, Lutsiv O, Makh SK, Souza JP, et al. The mistreatment of women during childbirth in health facilities globally: a mixed-methods systematic review. PLoS Med. 2015;12:e1001847.
23. Brazelton TB. Neonatal behavioral assessment scale. Clinics in developmental medicine no. 50. London: Spastics International Medical Publications; 1973.
24. Brazelton TB, Nugent JK. Neonatal behavioral assessment scale. 3rd ed. New York: Cambridge University Press; 1995.
25. Brimdyr K, Cadwell K, Widström AM, Svensson K, Phillips R. The effect of labor medications on normal newborn behavior in the first hour after birth: a prospective cohort study. Early Hum Dev. 2019;132:30–6.
26. Brocklehurst P, Hardy P, Hollowell J, Linsell L, Macfarlane A, McCourt C, et al. Perinatal and maternal outcomes by planned place of birth for healthy women with low risk pregnancies: the birthplace in England national prospective cohort study. BMJ. 2011;343:d7400.
27. Brown A. Breastfeeding as a public health responsibility: a review of the evidence. J Hum Nutr Diet. 2017;30:759–70.
28. Brown A, Jordan S. Impact of birth complications on breastfeeding duration: an internet survey. J Adv Nurs. 2013;69:828–39.
29. Brown A, Rance J, Bennett P. Understanding the relationship between breastfeeding and postnatal depression: the role of pain and physical difficulties. J Adv Nurs. 2016;72:273–82.
30. Buckley SJ. Executive summary of hormonal physiology of childbearing: evidence and implications for women, babies, and maternity care. J Perinat Educ. 2015;24:145–53.
31. Buckley S, Uvnäs-Moberg K. Nature and consequences of oxytocin and other neurohormones in the perinatal period. In: Downe S, Byrom S, editors. Squaring the circle: normal birth research, theory and practice in a technological age. London: Pinter and Martin; 2019. p. 19–31.
32. Burguet A, Rousseau A. Oxytocin administration during spontaneous labor: guidelines for clinical practice. Chapter 6: Fetal, neonatal and pediatric risks and adverse effects of using oxytocin augmentation during spontaneous labor. J Gynecol Obstet Human Rep. 2017;46:523–30.
33. Cabrera Vega P, Castellano Caballero G, Reyes Suárez D, Urquía Martí L, Siguero Onrubia M, Borges Luján M, et al. Birth trauma: incidence and associated risk factors: a case–control study. Future. 2024;2:126–34.
34. Campbell TS, Johnson JA, Zernicke KA. Gate control theory of pain. In: Gellman MD, editor. Encyclopedia of behavioral medicine. Cham: Springer; 2020. p. 914–6.
35. Cantor AG, Jungbauer RM, Skelly AC, Hart EL, Jorda K, Davis-O'Reilly C, et al. Respectful maternity care: dissemination and implementation of perinatal safety culture to improve equitable maternal healthcare delivery and outcomes. Bethesda, MD: NIH National Library of Medicine; 2024. https://www.ncbi.nlm.nih.gov/books/NBK599318/.
36. Carey WB, Devitt SC. Child behavioral assessment and management in primary care. 2nd ed. Scottsdale: Behavioral-Developmental Initiatives; 2016. https://www.preventiveoz.org/wp-content/uploads/2018/06/CBAM2-min.pdf
37. Carter CS. Oxytocin pathways and the evolution of human behavior. Annu Rev Psychol. 2014;65:17–39.

38. Cattani L, Decoene J, Page AS, Weeg N, Deprest J, Dietz HP. Pregnancy, labour and delivery as risk factors for pelvic organ prolapse: a systematic review. Int Urogynecol J. 2021;32:1623–31.
39. Chaillet N, Belaid L, Crochetière C, Roy L, Gagné GP, Moutquin JM, et al. Nonpharmacologic approaches for pain management during labor compared with usual care: a meta-analysis. Birth. 2014;41:122–37.
40. Chakraborty B, Basu M, Debangshi M, Mondal PK. Routine oxytocin infusion versus discontinuation during active phase of labour: does it make a difference in outcome—a prospective longitudinal study. J Indian Med Assoc. 2024;122:46–9.
41. Chapman V, Charles C, editors. The midwife's labour and birth handbook. 2nd ed. Oxford: John Wiley & Sons; 2009.
42. Cheung PS, McCaffrey T, Tighe SM, Mohamad MM. Healthcare practitioners' experiences and perspectives of music in perinatal care in Ireland: an exploratory survey. Midwifery. 2024;132:103987.
43. Cho H, Jeong IS. The relationship between mother-infant contact time and changes in postpartum depression and mother-infant attachment among mothers staying at postpartum care centers: an observational study. Nurs Health Sci. 2021;23:547–55.
44. Cho CE, Norman M. Cesarean section and development of the immune system in the offspring. Am J Obstet Gynecol. 2013;208:249–54.
45. Christian LM, Galley JD, Hade EM, Schoppe-Sullivan S, Kamp Dush C, Bailey MT. Gut microbiome composition is associated with temperament during early childhood. Brain Behav Immun. 2015;45:118–27.
46. Clarke G, O'Mahony SM, Dinan TG, Cryan JF. Priming for health: gut microbiota acquired in early life regulates physiology, brain and behaviour. Acta Paediatr. 2014;103:812–9.
47. Dahan O, Zibenberg A, Goldberg A. Birthing consciousness and the flow experience during physiological childbirth. Midwifery. 2024;138:104151.
48. Dahlberg U, Aune I. The woman's birth experience—the effect of interpersonal relationships and continuity of care. Midwifery. 2013;29:407–15.
49. Dahlen HG, Kennedy HP, Anderson CM, Bell AF, Clark A, Foureur M, Ohm JE, Shearman AM, Taylor JY, Wright ML, Downe S. The EPIIC hypothesis: intrapartum effects on the neonatal epigenome and consequent health outcomes. Med Hypotheses. 2013;80:656–62.
50. Dahlen HG, Thornton C, Downe S, De Jonge A, Seijmonsbergen-Schermers A, Tracy S, et al. Intrapartum interventions and outcomes for women and children following induction of labour at term in uncomplicated pregnancies: a 16-year population-based linked data study. BMJ Open. 2021;11:e047040.
51. Dekel S, Ein-Dor T, Berman Z, Barsoumian IS, Agarwal S, Pitman RK. Delivery mode is associated with maternal mental health following childbirth. Arch Womens Ment Health. 2019;22:817–24.
52. DeLancey JO, Masteling M, Pipitone F, LaCross J, Mastrovito S, Ashton-Miller JA. Pelvic floor injury during vaginal birth is life-altering and preventable: what can we do about it? Am J Obstet Gynecol. 2024;230:279–94.
53. Dencker A, Nilsson C, Begley C, Jangsten E, Mollberg M, Patel H, et al. Causes and outcomes in studies of fear of childbirth: a systematic review. Women Birth. 2019;32:99–111.
54. Döblin S, Seefeld L, Weise V, Kopp M, Knappe S, Asselmann E, et al. The impact of mode of delivery on parent-infant-bonding and the mediating role of birth experience: a comparison of mothers and fathers within the longitudinal cohort study DREAM. BMC Pregnancy Childbirth. 2023;23:285.
55. Dominguez-Bello MG, Costello EK, Contreras M, Magris M, Hidalgo G, Fierer N, Knight R. Delivery mode shapes the acquisition and structure of the initial microbiota across multiple body habitats in newborns. Proc Natl Acad Sci. 2010;107:11971–5.
56. Douglas PS, Hill PS. A neurobiological model for cry-fuss problems in the first three to four months of life. Med Hypotheses. 2013;81:816–22.
57. Downe S, Finlayson K, Oladapo O, Bonet M, Gülmezoglu AM. What matters to women during childbirth: a systematic qualitative review. PLoS One. 2018;13:e0194906.

58. Edwards H, Buisman-Pijlman FT, Esterman A, Phillips C, Orgeig S, Gordon A. Exogenous oxytocin administered to induce or augment labour is positively associated with quality of observed mother-infant bonding. Compr Psychoneuroendocrinol. 2024;20:100262.
59. Ekéus C, Högberg U, Norman M. Vacuum assisted birth and risk for cerebral complications in term newborn infants: a population-based cohort study. BMC Pregnancy Childbirth. 2014;14:1–10.
60. El-Salahi S, Knowles Bevis R, Hogg L. The relationship between traumatic childbirth and first-time mothers' social identity and wellbeing: a cross-sectional observational study. BMC Pregnancy Childbirth. 2024;24:437.
61. Erickson EN, Emeis CL. Breastfeeding outcomes after oxytocin use during childbirth: an integrative review. J Midwifery Womens Health. 2017;62:397–417.
62. Feeley C. Skilled heartfelt midwifery practice: safe. Springer Nature: Relational Care for Alternative Physiological Births; 2023.
63. Feldman R, Weller A, Zagoory-Sharon O, Levine A. Evidence for a neuroendocrinological foundation of human affiliation: plasma oxytocin levels across pregnancy and the postpartum period predict mother-infant bonding. Psychol Sci. 2007;18:965–70.
64. Feldman R, Zagoory-Sharon O, Weisman O, Schneiderman I, Gordon I, Maoz R, Shalev I, Ebstein RP. Sensitive parenting is associated with plasma oxytocin and polymorphisms in the OXTR and CD38 genes. Biol Psychiatry. 2012;72:175–81.
65. Figueiredo B, Costa R, Pacheco A, Pais Á. Mother-to-infant emotional involvement at birth. Matern Child Health J. 2008;13:539–49.
66. Fitzgerald I, Corcoran P, McKernan J, Connell RO, Greene RA. Trends, causes and factors associated with primary postpartum haemorrhage (PPH) in Ireland: a review of one million hospital childbirths. Eur J Obstet Gynecol Reprod Biol. 2024;301:258–63.
67. Fonseca MJ, Santos F, Afreixo V, Silva IS, do Céu Almeida, M. Does induction of labor at term increase the risk of cesarean section in advanced maternal age? A systematic review and meta-analysis. Eur J Obstet Gynecol Reprod Biol. 2020;253:213–9.
68. French CA, Cong X, Chung KS. Labor epidural analgesia and breastfeeding: a systematic review. J Hum Lact. 2016;32:507–20.
69. Galková G, Böhm P, Hon Z, Heřman T, Doubrava R, Navrátil L. Comparison of frequency of home births in the member states of the EU between 2015 and 2019. Global Pediatric Health. 2022;9:2333794X211070916.
70. Getahun SA, Muluneh AA, Seneshaw WW, Workie SG, Kassa ZY. Person-centered care during childbirth and associated factors among mothers who gave birth at health facilities in Hawassa city administration Sidama region, Southern Ethiopia. BMC Pregnancy and Childbirth. 2022;22:584.
71. Gettler LT, Kuo PX, Sarma MS, Trumble BC, Burke Lefever JE, Braungart-Rieker JM. Fathers' oxytocin responses to first holding their newborns: interactions with testosterone reactivity to predict later parenting behavior and father-infant bonds. Dev Psychobiol. 2021;63:1384–98.
72. Gizzo S, Di Gangi S, Noventa M, Bacile V, Zambon A, Nardelli GB. Women's choice of positions during labour: return to the past or a modern way to give birth? A cohort study in Italy. Biomed Res Int. 2014;2014:638093.
73. Goodson C, Martis R. Pethidine: to prescribe or not to prescribe? A discussion surrounding pethidine's place in midwifery practice and New Zealand prescribing legislation. NZ Coll Midwives J. 2014;49:21–8.
74. Greer J, Lazenbatt A, Dunne L. Fear of childbirth' and ways of coping for pregnant women and their partners during the birthing process: a salutogenic analysis. Evidence Based Midwifery. 2014;12:1–12.
75. Grisbrook MA, Dewey D, Cuthbert C, McDonald S, Ntanda H, Giesbrecht GF, Letourneau N. Associations among caesarean section birth, post-traumatic stress, and postpartum depression symptoms. Int J Environ Res Public Health. 2022;19:4900.
76. Grunau RV, Craig KD. Pain expression in neonates: facial action and cry. Pain. 1987;28:395–410.

77. Gurol-Urganci I, Cromwell DA, Edozien LC, Mahmood TA, Adams EJ, Richmond DH, et al. Third-and fourth-degree perineal tears among primiparous women in England between 2000 and 2012: time trends and risk factors. BJOG Int J Obstet Gynaecol. 2013;120:1516–25.
78. Hagen S, Sellers C, Elders A, Glazener C, MacArthur C, Toozs-Hobson P, et al. Urinary incontinence, faecal incontinence and pelvic organ prolapse symptoms 20–26 years after childbirth: a longitudinal cohort study. BJOG Int J Obstet Gynaecol. 2024;131:1815–23.
79. Haim-Dahan R, Bachner-Melman R, Lev-Ran H. Women friendly: the effectiveness of a woman-centered childbirth intervention in Israel. Midwifery. 2024;140:104212.
80. Harman T, Wakeford A. The microbiome effect: how your baby's birth affects their future health. London: Pinter & Martin; 2016.
81. Hedegaard M, Lidegaard Ø, Skovlund CW, Mørch LS, Hedegaard M. Reduction in stillbirths at term after new birth induction paradigm: results of a national intervention. BMJ Open. 2014;4:e005785.
82. Hildingsson I, Rubertsson C, Karlström A, Haines H. A known midwife can make a difference for women with fear of childbirth-birth outcome and women's experiences of intrapartum care. Sex Reprod Healthc. 2019;21:33–8.
83. Hishikawa K, Kusaka T, Fukuda T, Kohata Y, Inoue H. Anxiety or nervousness disturbs the progress of birth based on human behavioral evolutionary biology. J Perinat Educ. 2019;28:218–23.
84. Hoang DM, Levy EI, Vandenplas Y. The impact of caesarean section on the infant gut microbiome. Acta Paediatr. 2021;110:60–7.
85. Hobbs AJ, Mannion CA, McDonald SW, Brockway M, Tough SC. The impact of caesarean section on breastfeeding initiation, duration and difficulties in the first four months postpartum. BMC Pregnancy Childbirth. 2016;16:1–9.
86. Hodnett ED. Pain and women's satisfaction with the experience of childbirth: a systematic review. Am J Obstet Gynecol. 2002;186:S160–72.
87. Hodnett ED, Gates S, Hofmeyr GJ, Sakala C. Continuous support for women during childbirth. Cochrane Database Syst Rev. 2013;7:CD003766.
88. Horan MA, Murphy DJ. Operative vaginal delivery. Obstet Gynaecol Reprod Med. 2016;26:358–63. https://www.england.nhs.uk/mat-transformation/implementing-better-births/mat-review/
89. Ioscovich AM, Riazanova OV, Alexandrovich YS. The relationship between labor pain management, cortisol level and risk of postpartum depression development: a prospective non-randomized observational monocentric trial. Rom J Anaesth Intensive Care. 2018;25:123–30.
90. Jansson MH, Franzén K, Hiyoshi A, Tegerstedt G, Dahlgren H, Nilsson K. Risk factors for perineal and vaginal tears in primiparous women–the prospective POPRACT-cohort study. BMC Pregnancy Childbirth. 2020;20:1–14.
91. Johansson MW, Lilliesköld S, Jonas W, Thernström Blomqvist Y, Skiöld B, Linnér A. Early skin-to-skin contact and the risk of intraventricular haemorrhage and sepsis in preterm infants. Acta Paediatr. 2024;113:1796–802.
92. Johnson K. Maternal-infant bonding: a review of literature. Int J Childbirth Educ. 2013;28:17–23.
93. Johnston C, Campbell-Yeo M, Disher T, Benoit B, Fernandes A, Streiner D, et al. Skin-to-skin care for procedural pain in neonates. Cochrane Database Syst Rev. 2017;2017:CD008435.
94. Jones L, Othman M, Dowswell T, Alfirevic Z, Gates S, Newburn M, et al. Pain management for women in labour: an overview of systematic reviews. Cochrane Database Syst Rev. 2012;2012:CD009234.
95. Jonsson M, Nordën-Lindeberg S, Östlund I, Hanson U. Acidemia at birth, related to obstetric characteristics and to oxytocin use, during the last two hours of labor. Acta Obstet Gynecol Scand. 2008;87:745–50.
96. Joranger P, Huitfeldt AS, Bernitz S, Blix E. Cost minimisation analyses of birth care in low-risk women in Norway: a comparison between planned home birth and birth in a standard obstetric unit. BMC Health Serv Res. 2024;24:1150.

97. Kabale WD, Bekele GG, Gonfa DN, Yami AT. Person-centered maternity care during childbirth and associated factors at public hospitals in Central Ethiopia. SAGE Open Med. 2024;12:20503121241257790.
98. Kamalimanesh B, Moradi M, Fathi M, Afiat M, Rezazadeh MB, Shakeri MT. Effect of self-hypnosis on fear and pain of natural childbirth: a randomized controlled trial. J Complement Integr Med. 2025;22(2):353–62. https://doi.org/10.1515/jcim-2024-0353.
99. Kearns RJ, Kyzayeva A, Halliday LOE, Lawlor DA, Shaw M, Nelson SM. Epidural analgesia during labour and severe maternal morbidity: population-based study. Obstet Anesth Dig. 2025;45:3–4.
100. Keighley MRB, Perston Y, Bradshaw E, Hayes J, Keighley DM, Webb S. The social, psychological, emotional morbidity and adjustment techniques for women with anal incontinence following obstetric anal sphincter injury: use of a word picture to identify a hidden syndrome. BMC Pregnancy Childbirth. 2016;16:1–12.
101. Khezerdoost S, Mahdavi R, Hantoushzadeh S, Ghaemi M, Borna H, Arman M, Ghalandarpoor-Attar SM. Determinants of higher oxytocin dose need during labor induction. Fertility Gynecol Androl. 2024;4:e148579.
102. Kim H, Sitarik AR, Woodcroft K, Johnson CC, Zoratti E. Birth mode, breastfeeding, pet exposure, and antibiotic use: associations with the gut microbiome and sensitization in children. Curr Allergy Asthma Rep. 2019;19:1–9.
103. Kirca N, Adibelli D. Effects of mother-infant skin-to-skin contact on postpartum depression: a systematic review. Perspect Psychiatr Care. 2021;57:2014–23.
104. Klemming S, Lilliesköld S, Westrup B. Mother-newborn couplet care from theory to practice to ensure zero separation for all newborns. Acta Paediatr. 2021;110:2951–7.
105. Kraft F, Wohlrab P, Meyer EL, Helmer H, Leitner H, Kiss H, et al. Epidural analgesia and neonatal short-term outcomes during routine childbirth: a 10-year retrospective analysis from the national birth registry of Austria. Minerva Anestesiol. 2024;90:491–9.
106. Kuguoglu S, Yildiz H, Tanir MK, Demirbag BC. Breastfeeding after a cesarean delivery, vol. 121. Rijeka: InTech; 2012.
107. Kujabi ML, Maembe L, Nkungu D, Maaløe N, D'mello BS, van Roosmalen J, et al. Temporalities of oxytocin for labour augmentation: a mixed-methods study of time factors shaping labour practices in a busy maternity unit in Tanzania. BMC Pregnancy Childbirth. 2024;24:1–12.
108. Kulkarni A, Manerkar S, Paul N, Gupta A, Mondkar J. Impact of kangaroo mother care on mother-infant bonding in very low birth weight infants. J Neonatal Nurs. 2025;31:206–9.
109. Kurth L, O'Shea TM, Burd I, Dunlop AL, Croen L, Wilkening G, et al. Intrapartum exposure to synthetic oxytocin, maternal BMI, and neurodevelopmental outcomes in children within the ECHO consortium. J Neurodev Disord. 2024;16:26.
110. Leinweber J, Fontein-Kuipers Y, Karlsdottir SI, Ekström-Bergström A, Nilsson C, Stramrood C, Thomson G. Developing a woman-centered, inclusive definition of positive childbirth experiences: a discussion paper. Birth. 2023;50:362–83.
111. Leng B, Zhou Y, Du S, Liu F, Zhao L, Sun G, Zhao Y. Association between delivery mode and pelvic organ prolapse: a metaanalysisof observational studies. Eur J Obstet Gynecol Reprod Biol. 2019;235:19–25.
112. Leonard SA, Main EK, Carmichael SL. The contribution of maternal characteristics and cesarean delivery to an increasing trend of severe maternal morbidity. BMC Pregnancy Childbirth. 2019;19:1–9.
113. Lester BM, Emory EK, Hoffman SL, Eitzman DV. A multivariate study of the effects of high-risk factors on performance on the Brazelton neonatal assessment scale. Child Dev. 1976;47:515–7.
114. Lester BM, Als H, Brazelton TB. Regional obstetric anesthesia and newborn behavior: a reanalysis toward synergistic effects. Child Dev. 1982;53:687–92.
115. Levett KM, Salomons E, Shenoy P, Kaur I, Fernandez E. Humanising childbirth–maternity acupressure training for healthcare providers at the Fernandez foundation hospitals,

Hyderabad, India. Evaluation of program delivery in one region of India. Women Birth. 2024a;37:101819.
116. Levett KM, Sutcliffe KL, Vanderlaan J, Kjerulff KH. The first baby study: what women would like to have known about first childbirth. A mixed-methods study. Birth. 2024b;51:795–805.
117. Liang Y, Chen Y, Yu X, Li X. Quality of life among women with postpartum urinary incontinence: a cross-sectional study. Gynecol Obstet Clin Med. 2021;1:164–8.
118. Lim G, Facco FL, Nathan N, Waters JH, Wong CA, Eltzschig HK. A review of the impact of obstetric anesthesia on maternal and neonatal outcomes. Anesthesiology. 2018;129:192–215.
119. Lindquist AC, Hastie RM, Hiscock RJ, Pritchard NL, Walker SP, Tong S. Risk of major labour-related complications for pregnancies progressing to 42 weeks or beyond. BMC Med. 2021;19:1–8.
120. LoMauro A, Aliverti A. Physiology masterclass: extremes of age: newborn and infancy. Breathe. 2016;12:65–8.
121. Lopes MI, Vieira M, Cardoso A. Women's empowerment for active labor: a qualitative study with nurse-midwives in antenatal education for childbirth. European Journal of Midwifery. 2024;8:10–18332.
122. Lothian JA. Do not disturb: the importance of privacy in labor. J Perinat Educ. 2004;13:4.
123. Love TM. Oxytocin, motivation and the role of dopamine. Pharmacol Biochem Behav. 2014;119:49–60.
124. Lozupone CA, Stombaugh JI, Gordon JI, Jansson JK, Knight R. Diversity, stability and resilience of the human gut microbiota. Nature. 2012;489:220–30.
125. Lunda P, Minnie CS, Benadé P. Women's experiences of continuous support during childbirth: a meta-synthesis. BMC Pregnancy Childbirth. 2018;18:1–11.
126. Maguire L, Male F, Clarke H, Ndlovu B, Harris J, Chintende JM, Claudine BU. Skin-to-skin contact. Are we doing enough? J Neonatal Nurs. 2025;31:125–8.
127. Man R, Morton VH, Morris RK. Childbirth-related perineal trauma and its complications: prevalence, risk factors and management. Obstet Gynaecol Reprod Med. 2024;34:252–9.
128. Mangır Meler K, Çankaya S. The effect of intrapartum care model given in line with world health organization (WHO) recommendations on labor pain, fear of labor, comfort of labor, duration of labor, administration of oxytocin and perception of midwifery care: a randomized controlled study. Postgrad Med. 2025;37:379–95. https://doi.org/10.1080/00325481.2025.2501943.
129. Mäntymaa M, Puura K, Luoma I, Salmelin RK, Tamminen T. Early mother–infant interaction, parental mental health and symptoms of behavioral and emotional problems in toddlers. Infant Behav Dev. 2004;27:134–49.
130. Markley JC, Rollins MD. Non-neuraxial labor analgesia: options. Clin Obstet Gynecol. 2017;60:350–64.
131. Mascarenhas Silva CH, Laranjeira CLS, Pinheiro WF, de Melo CSB, Campos e Silva VDO, Brandão AHF, et al. Pregnant women autonomy when choosing their method of childbirth: scoping review. PLoS One. 2024;19:e0304955.
132. Maunu J, Kirjavainen J, Korja R, Parkkola R, Rikalainen H, Lapinleimu H, et al. Relation of prematurity and brain injury to crying behavior in infancy. Pediatrics. 2006;118:e57–65.
133. McCann ME, Matthes K, Greco C, editors. Essentials of anesthesia for infants and neonates. Cambridge: Cambridge University Press; 2018.
134. McKenzie CP, Cobb B, Riley ET, Carvalho B. Programmed intermittent epidural boluses for maintenance of labor analgesia: an impact study. Int J Obstet Anesth. 2016;26:32–8.
135. Mears K, McAuliffe F, Grimes H, Morrison JJ. Fetal cortisol in relation to labour, intrapartum events and mode of delivery. J Obstet Gynaecol. 2004;24:129–32.
136. Mellon RD, Simone AF, Rappaport BA. Use of anesthetic agents in neonates and young children. Anesth Analg. 2007;104:509–20.
137. Melzack R. Gate control theory: on the evolution of pain concepts. Pain Forum. 1996;5:128–38. Churchill Livingstone
138. Middleton P, Shepherd E, Crowther CA. Induction of labour for improving birth outcomes for women at or beyond term. Cochrane Database Syst Rev. 2018;5:CD004945.

139. Miller S, Abalos E, Chamillard M, Ciapponi A, Colaci D, Comandé D, et al. Beyond too little, too late and too much, too soon: a pathway towards evidence-based, respectful maternity care worldwide. Lancet. 2016;388:2176–92.
140. Mobaraki N, Yousefian M, Seifi S, Sakaki M. A randomized controlled trial comparing use of Entonox with pethidine for pain relief in primigravid women during the active phase of labor. Anesthesiol Pain Med. 2016;6:e37420.
141. Modabbernia A, Sandin S, Gross R, Leonard H, Gissler M, Parner ET, et al. Apgar score and risk of autism. Eur J Epidemiol. 2019;34:105–14.
142. Modahl C, Green LA, Fein D, Morris M, Waterhouse L, Feinstein C, Levin H. Plasma oxytocin levels in autistic children. Biol Psychiatry. 1998;43:270–7.
143. Moe-Byrne T, Brown JVE, McGuire W. Naloxone for opioid-exposed newborn infants. Cochrane Database Syst Rev. 2018;10:CD003483.
144. Moerkerke M, Peeters M, de Vries L, Daniels N, Steyaert J, Alaerts K, Boets B. Endogenous oxytocin levels in autism—a meta-analysis. Brain Sci. 2021;11:1545.
145. de Moraes FCA, Kelly FA, Leite MGHSJ, Dal Moro L, Morbach V, Burbano RMR. High-dose versus low-dose oxytocin for labor augmentation: a meta-analysis of randomized controlled trials. J Pers Med. 2024;14:724.
146. Muraca GM, Boutin A, Razaz N, Lisonkova S, John S, Ting JY, Scott H, Kramer MS, Joseph KS. Maternal and neonatal trauma following operative vaginal delivery. Cmaj. 2022;194(1):E1–2.
147. Mylonas I, Friese K. Indications for and risks of elective cesarean section. Dtsch Arztebl Int. 2015;112:489.
148. Myrfield K, Brook C, Creedy D. Reducing perineal trauma: implications of flexion and extension of the fetal head during birth. Midwifery. 1997;13:197–201.
149. Nakphong MK, Afulani PA, Beltrán-Sánchez H, Opot J, Sudhinaraset M. Integrating support persons into maternity care and associations with quality of care: a postpartum survey of mothers and support persons in Kenya. BMC Pregnancy Childbirth. 2024;24:425.
150. NHS. Pain relief and medication during labour. 2024. https://www.nhs.uk/start-for-life/pregnancy/preparing-for-labour-and-birth/pain-relief-and-medication-during-labour/#gas-and-air.
151. NHS England. Better births (National Maternity Review): improving outcomes of maternity services in England. London: NHS England; 2016.
152. Nystedt A, Högberg U, Lundman B. Women's experiences of becoming a mother after prolonged labour. J Adv Nurs. 2008;63:250–8.
153. Okeahialam NA, Sultan AH, Thakar R. The prevention of perineal trauma during vaginal birth. Am J Obstet Gynecol. 2023;230:S991–S1004.
154. Olza I, Leahy-Warren P, Benyamini Y, Kazmierczak M, Karlsdottir SI, Spyridou A, et al. Women's psychological experiences of physiological childbirth: a meta-synthesis. BMJ Open. 2018;8:e020347.
155. Olza I, Uvnas-Moberg K, Ekström-Bergström A, Leahy-Warren P, Karlsdottir SI, Nieuwenhuijze M, et al. Birth as a neuro-psycho-social event: an integrative model of maternal experiences and their relation to neurohormonal events during childbirth. PLoS One. 2020;15:e0230992.
156. Onuc S, Rus M, Badiu D, Delcea C, Tica V. Intrapartum synthetic oxytocin as a potential mediator for postpartum depression. Psychiatry Int. 2025;6:26.
157. Opiyo N, Kingdon C, Oladapo OT, Souza JP, Vogel JP, Bonet M, et al. Non-clinical interventions to reduce unnecessary caesarean sections: WHO recommendations. Bull World Health Organ. 2020;98:66.
158. Page GG. Are there long-term consequences of pain in newborn or very young infants? J Perinat Educ. 2004;13:10.
159. Peters LL, Thornton C, de Jonge A, Khashan A, Tracy M, Downe S, Feijen-de Jong EI, Dahlen HG. The effect of medical and operative birth interventions on child health outcomes in the first 28 days and up to 5 years of age: a linked data population-based cohort study. Birth. 2018;45:347–57.

160. Pollina J, Dias MS, Li V, Kachurek D, Arbesman M. Cranial birth injuries in term newborn infants. Pediatr Neurosurg. 2001;35:113–9.
161. Purandare R, Ådahl K, Stillerman M, Schytt E, Tsekhmestruk N, Lindgren H. Migrant women's experiences of community-based doula support during labor and childbirth in Sweden. A mixed methods study. Sex Reprod Healthc. 2024;41:101000.
162. Qiu C, Carter SA, Lin JC, Shi JM, Chow T, Desai VN, et al. Association of labor epidural analgesia, oxytocin exposure, and risk of autism spectrum disorders in children. JAMA Netw Open. 2023;6:e2324630.
163. Rashidi M, Maier E, Dekel S, Sütterlin M, Wolf RC, Ditzen B, et al. Peripartum effects of synthetic oxytocin: the good, the bad, and the unknown. Neurosci Biobehav Rev. 2022;141:104859.
164. Ratislavová K, Janoušková K, Hendrych Lorenzová E, Martin CR. The process of childbirth as a factor influencing women's satisfaction. Central Eur J Nurs Midwifery. 2024;15:1100–6.
165. Rattaz V, Cairo Notari S, Avignon V, Achtari C, Horsch A. Parenting stress after perineal tear during childbirth: the role of physical health and depressive symptoms. Front Psychol. 2025;16:1477316.
166. RCOG. Operative vaginal delivery. Green-top guideline no. 26. 2020. https://www.rcog.org.uk/en/guidelines-research-services/guidelines/gtg26/.
167. Reddy UM, Sandoval GJ, Tita AT, Silver RM, Mallett G, Hill K, et al. Oxytocin regimen used for induction of labor and pregnancy outcomes. Am J Obstet Gynecol MFM. 2024;6:101508.
168. Redshaw M, Hennegan J, Kruske S. Holding the baby: early mother–infant contact after childbirth and outcomes. Midwifery. 2014;30:e177–87.
169. Reynolds F. Labour analgesia and the baby: good news is no news. Int J Obstet Anesth. 2011;20:38–50.
170. Rusnawati MS, Chalid MT, Saleh A, Mappaware NA, Saidah Syamsuddin JJ, Nur A, Halisah AT. Effectiveness of the application of respectful midwifery care on prostaglandin (Pge2) levels and maternal pain perception level in normal childbirth. Pak J Life Soc Sci. 2024;22:348–54.
171. Ryan N, O'Mahony S, Leahy-Warren P, Philpott L, Mulcahy H. The impact of perinatal maternal stress on the maternal and infant gut and human milk microbiomes: a scoping review. PLoS One. 2025;20:e0318237.
172. Please delete ref 170 and renumber accordingly, thank you
173. Rydahl E, Eriksen L, Juhl M. Effects of induction of labor prior to post-term in low-risk pregnancies: a systematic review. JBI Evid Synth. 2019;17:170–208.
174. Salusest S, Salvi S, Aprile FT, Rubini A, Stollagli F, Buongiorno S, et al. Ritgen's maneuver in childbirth care: a case-control study in a central Italian setting. Eur J Midwifery. 2024;8:10–18332.
175. Sandall J, Turienzo CF, Devane D, Soltani H, Gillespie P, Gates S, et al. Midwife continuity of care models versus other models of care for childbearing women. Cochrane Database Syst Rev. 2024;2024:CD004667.
176. Sasaki T, Hashimoto K, Oda Y, Ishima T, Kurata T, Takahashi J, et al. Decreased levels of serum oxytocin in pediatric patients with attention deficit/hyperactivity disorder. Psychiatry Res. 2015;228:746–51.
177. Schmidt C. Mental health: thinking from the gut. Sci Am. 2015;312:S12–5.
178. Scholten N, Strizek B, Okumu MR, Demirer I, Kössendrup J, Haid-Schmallenberg L, et al. Birthing positions and mothers satisfaction with childbirth: a cross-sectional study on the relevance of self determination. Arch Gynecol Obstet. 2025;311:591–8.
179. Sigdel M, Burd J, Walker KF, Wennerholm UB, Berghella V. Severe perineal lacerations in induction of labor versus expectant management: a systematic review and meta-analysis of randomized controlled trials. Am J Obstet Gynecol MFM. 2024;6:101407.
180. Simon LV, Shah M, Bragg BN. APGAR score. NIH National Library of Medicine, National Centre for Biotechnology Information; 2019. https://www.ncbi.nlm.nih.gov/books/NBK470569/#:~:text=The%20score%20is%20recorded%20at,to%2010%20are%20considered%20reassuring

References

181. Słabuszewska-Jóźwiak A, Szymański JK, Ciebiera M, Sarecka-Hujar B, Jakiel G. Pediatrics consequences of caesarean section—a systematic review and meta-analysis. Int J Environ Res Public Health. 2020;17:8031.
182. Sotiriadis A, Makrydimas G, Papatheodorou S, Ioannidis JP, McGoldrick E. Corticosteroids for preventing neonatal respiratory morbidity after elective caesarean section at term. Cochrane Database Syst Rev. 2018;8:CD006614.
183. Sprung J, Flick RP, Wilder RT, Katusic SK, Pike TL, Dingli M, Gleich SJ, Schroeder DR, Barbaresi WJ, Hanson AC, Warner DO. Anesthesia for cesarean delivery and learning disabilities in a population-based birth cohort. Anesthesiology. 2009;111(2):302.
184. Stjernholm YV, Nyberg A, Cardell M, Höybye C. Circulating maternal cortisol levels during vaginal delivery and elective cesarean section. Arch Gynecol Obstet. 2016;294:267–71.
185. Suarez A, Yakupova V. Past traumatic life events, postpartum PTSD, and the role of labor support. Int J Environ Res Public Health. 2023;20:6048.
186. Tarekegne AA, Giru BW, Mekonnen B. Person-centered maternity care during childbirth and associated factors at selected public hospitals in Addis Ababa, Ethiopia, 2021: a cross-sectional study. Reprod Health. 2022;19:199.
187. Taylor A, Fisk NM, Glover V. Mode of delivery and subsequent stress response. Lancet. 2000;355:120.
188. Taylor B, Cross-Sudworth F, Rimmer M, Quinn L, Morris RK, Johnston T, et al. Induction of labour care in the UK: a cross-sectional survey of maternity units. PLoS One. 2024;19:e0297857.
189. Thomas K. Listen to mums: ending the postcode lottery on perinatal care. A report by The All-Party Parliamentary Group on Birth Trauma. 2024. https://www.theo-clarke.org.uk/sites/www.theo-clarke.org.uk/files/2024-05/Birth%20Trauma%20Inquiry%20Report%20for%20Publication_May13_2024.pdf.
190. Thomson G, Feeley C, Moran VH, Downe S, Oladapo OT. Women's experiences of pharmacological and non-pharmacological pain relief methods for labour and childbirth: a qualitative systematic review. Reprod Health. 2019;16:1–20.
191. Thorgaard-Rasmussen K, Alvesson HM, Pembe AB, Mselle LT, Unkels R, Metta E, Alwy Al-beity FM. Women's and maternity care providers' perceptions of pain management during childbirth in hospitals in southern Tanzania. BMC Pregnancy Childbirth. 2024;24:417.
192. Topal S, Çaka SY. The mediating role of postpartum depression between mother-infant contact barriers and maternal attachment: a cross-sectional study from Turkey. Rev Assoc Med Bras. 2025;71:e20241413.
193. Topalidou A, Haworth L, Kaur I, Ahmed M, Chohan A. Assessment of the pelvic and body interface pressure during different recumbent and semi-recumbent birthing positions. Clin Biomech. 2024;119:106328.
194. UNICEF, & World Health Organization. Levels and trends child mortality-report 2023: estimates developed by the United Nations Inter-agency Group for child mortality estimation. 2024. https://data.unicef.org/resources/levels-and-trends-in-child-mortality-2024/.
195. United Nations Development Programme (UNDP). National multidimensional poverty index: a progress review 2023. 2023. https://www.undp.org/india/publications/national-multidimensional-poverty-index-progress-review-2023#:~:text=The%20country%20registered%20a%20significant,from%2032.59%25%20to%2019.28%25.
196. Uvnäs-Moberg K. Oxytocin: the biological guide to motherhood. Praeclarus Press; 2014.
197. Uvnäs-Moberg K. Why oxytocin matters, vol. 16. London: Pinter & Martin Ltd.; 2019.
198. Uvnäs-Moberg K. The physiology and pharmacology of oxytocin in labor and in the peripartum period. Am J Obstet Gynecol. 2024;230:S740–58.
199. Uvnäs-Moberg K, Ekström-Bergström A, Berg M, Buckley S, Pajalic Z, Hadjigeorgiou E, Kotłowska A, Lengler L, Kielbratowska B, Leon-Larios F, Magistretti CM, Downe S, Lindström B, Dencker A. Maternal plasma levels of oxytocin during physiological childbirth–a systematic review with implications for uterine contractions and central actions of oxytocin. BMC Pregnancy Childbirth. 2019;19:285.

200. Uvnäs-Moberg K, Gross MM, Agius A, Downe S, Calleja-Agius J. Are there epigenetic oxytocin-mediated effects on the mother and infant during physiological childbirth? Int J Mol Sci. 2020;21:9503.
201. Walter MH, Abele H, Plappert CF. The role of oxytocin and the effect of stress during childbirth: neurobiological basics and implications for mother and child. Front Endocrinol. 2021;12:742236.
202. Wang T, Pavelko R. Increasing social support for women via humanizing postpartum depression. Health Commun. 2024;40:668–78.
203. White Ribbon Alliance. Respectful maternity care: the universal rights of women and newborns. 2024. https://whiteribbonalliance.org/wp-content/uploads/2022/05/WRA_RMC_Charter_FINAL.pdf.
204. WHO. World Health Organization recommendations: intrapartum care for a positive childbirth experience. 2018. https://www.who.int/reproductivehealth/intrapartum-care/en/.
205. WHO. Europe news item. 2020. https://www.who.int/europe/news/item/31-01-2020-renate-de-bie-a-dutch-midwife-shares-her-experiences-of-safe-and-peaceful-home-births.
206. WHO Immediate KMC Study Group. Immediate "kangaroo mother care" and survival of infants with low birth weight. N Engl J Med. 2021;384:2028–38.
207. Widström AM, Brimdyr K, Svensson K, Cadwell K, Nissen E. Skin-to-skin contact the first hour after birth, underlying implications and clinical practice. Acta Paediatr. 2019;108:1192–204.
208. Wilson S, Ambikapur S. The impact of labor augmentation methods on delivery outcomes: a study of oral misoprostol versus intravenous oxytocin in term pregnancies. Int J Life Sci Biotechnol Pharma Res. 2024;13:508–14.
209. World Health Organization. WHO recommendations for care of the preterm or low birth weight infant. 2022. https://www.who.int/publications/i/item/9789240058262.
210. Worrall S, Silverio SA, Fallon VM. The relationship between prematurity and maternal mental health during the first postpartum year. J Neonatal Nurs. 2023;29:511–8.
211. Wu Q, Feng X. Infant emotion regulation and cortisol response during the first 2 years of life: association with maternal parenting profiles. Dev Psychobiol. 2020;62:1076–91.
212. Yamada A, Takahashi Y, Usami Y, Tamakoshi K. Impact of perineal pain and delivery related factors on interference with activities of daily living until 1 month postpartum: a longitudinal prospective study. BMC Pregnancy Childbirth. 2024;24:446.
213. Yang I, Corwin EJ, Brennan PA, Jordan S, Murphy JR, Dunlop A. The infant microbiome: implications for infant health and neurocognitive development. Nurs Res. 2016;65:76–88.
214. Yulita Ichwan E, Dwi Fitriani C, Nirmala Sari G. Effectiveness of audiovisual media on childbirth support and pregnancy anxiety: a quasi-experimental study. J Holistic Nurs Midwifery. 2024;34:237–44.
215. Zang Y, Lu H, Zhang H, Huang J, Ren L, Li C. Effects of upright positions during the second stage of labour for women without epidural analgesia: a meta-analysis. J Adv Nurs. 2020;76:3293–306.

Psychological Impacts of Childbirth on Mother and Baby

4

> We need to stop just pulling people out of the river.
> We need to go upstream and find out why they're falling in.
> Desmond Tutu

4.1 Introduction to the Psychology of Childbirth

Pregnancy, childbirth and the first year after birth are often presumed to be a happy, transformative time for new parents. However, the perinatal period can also be extremely complex and challenging. Having a negative experience at such a crucial time can have a profoundly adverse impact on the mother and baby and their relationship with each other. These effects may just be fleeting, but need to be considered seriously as they could be temporarily debilitating or even life-changing.

Due to dramatic hormonal and lifestyle changes, the perinatal period is one of the most vulnerable times for psychiatric illness, including perinatal depression, anxiety and post-traumatic stress [112]. Postpartum mood disorders are on the rise. For example, approximately one in eight American women who give birth now suffers from postnatal depression, and these figures increased sevenfold between 2000 and 2015 [69]. As we saw in the previous chapter, multiple factors can influence how parents feel before, during and after childbirth. While we have already touched upon some of the potential psychological outcomes of physical birth events, this chapter explores them in more depth. It also examines what happens to the baby when the parents are not experiencing mental and emotional wellness by exploring the research evidence on perinatal mental health and the possible infant outcomes of poor mental health in either parent.

Postnatal mood disorders may have repercussive effects on mother-baby bonding and infant temperament, as we will explore in this chapter. Parents' mental health issues during the perinatal period may also present problems for the baby's wellbeing and development. Anxiety and depression have attracted the most research to

© The Author(s), under exclusive license to Springer Nature
Switzerland AG 2025
C. Power, *Birth, Bonding and Baby Behaviour*,
https://doi.org/10.1007/978-3-032-05845-4_4

date, perhaps due to the high prevalence of these postnatal mood disorders. Other postpartum psychiatric disorders that might affect the baby's temperament, physiology, development and general wellbeing include childbirth-related post-traumatic stress disorder (CB-PTSD), postpartum psychosis, eating disorders and obsessive-compulsive disorder, to name but a few. Until recently, however, the influence of CB-PTSD on infant behavioural and developmental outcomes has been much less studied, and investigations about its possible implications are still in their "infancy" [41]. This chapter will focus first on the perinatal mood disorders of depression and anxiety, which seem to have the most research linked to adverse outcomes for the baby's behaviour and development, before turning our attention to CB-PTSD as another potential trigger for negative outcomes.

Although research on partners and fathers is gradually expanding, most existing research about childbirth focuses on the mother, and that is reflected here. However, it is increasingly clear that partners of any gender have an essential role to play, and their mental state may also affect the child; therefore, many studies now try to include them. For example, when working in collaboration with Professor Susan Garthus-Niegel and her team of scientists, using their large dataset, we found that both mothers' and fathers' heightened stress levels during the pandemic were associated with poorer mental health in addition to affecting parent-infant bonding [137]. The study, therefore, highlighted the importance of protecting the mental health of *all* parents. Similarly, the Croatian scientist Sandra Nakić Radoš and her colleagues [115] verified that postpartum depression or childbirth-related PTSD in *either* parent may have negative consequences for parent-infant bonding, and a recent systematic review and meta-analysis of the research literature has confirmed this link [144]. However, although paternal depression has been acknowledged as a serious issue for some time, research is only just beginning to explore treatments for childbirth-related PTSD in non-birthing parents [135]. Measurement scales to assess fathers' perceptions of traumatic childbirth are also now being developed [177], and an adapted scale to measure *partners*' birth satisfaction has been published [108].

The two main periods where parents' mental health is already considered crucial to infant outcomes are during pregnancy and the postnatal period. Research specifically on what might be occurring between mother and baby, both physiologically and psychologically, *during* childbirth is still lagging far behind. Nevertheless, there is accumulating evidence that a negative or traumatic birth experience and symptoms of PTSD afterwards may lead to a poorer quality mother-infant relationship [59]. In the qualitative arm of this study, mothers described the main factors contributing to their postnatal symptoms of distress as a lack of effective shared communication by health professionals, intrusive interventions—which may be as simple as an unwarranted, unexplained or unconsented vaginal examination [18], lack of support during childbirth and lack of care postnatally, highlighting the necessity of a caring and openly communicative caregiver-patient relationship for positive perinatal mental health and wellbeing.

In places where health professionals are in short supply, doulas could be an alternative solution for ensuring good communication and emotional care are provided during childbirth and the postnatal period. A prospective cohort study of 445 birthing mothers found that being accompanied by a doula during labour was associated with a better birth experience, increased wellbeing and less distress post-birth [98]. One reason for this could be that doulas provide a communication channel and effective buffer between the labouring woman and health professionals. Harris and Ayers [71] discovered that one of the main "hotspots" for intrapartum distress (overriding medical complications and interventions) was adverse interpersonal experiences with midwives, nurses and obstetricians. Therefore, doulas need to be aware that these professional working relationships are essential to positive outcomes and should therefore always be protected. Indeed, women with PTSD have stated their preference for professional midwife confidants and support over any other form of treatment. The same is true for women with postpartum depression although, for both groups, the support given by personal confidants (e.g. family, friends or doulas) is also vital [79].

Ideally, therefore, a doula should *supplement* rather than replace the emotional aspect of maternity care provided by health professionals. Overall, mothers who have a doula report coping better during labour, experiencing less anxiety or depression and having greater self-esteem post-birth. As postnatal doula support facilitates stronger relationships between parents and their babies, they also report less infant crying and easier, more successful bonding and breastfeeding [172]. All the evidence points towards mothers and babies benefiting enormously from continuous, compassionate, practical and emotional care and support during and after childbirth. This should be the norm rather than the sole privilege of those who can afford it.

The three perinatal periods—pregnancy, birth and postnatal—will now be explored individually. Note there tends to be a general overlap (known as "comorbidity") between the different mental health disorders across the entire perinatal period [12]. Therefore, some of the same outcomes will be mentioned across different sections.

4.2 The Psychology of Pregnancy

Mental health issues in the mother during pregnancy can trigger an inflammatory response in the body, affecting maternal and foetal health and wellbeing. Chronic stress, anxiety or depression during pregnancy leads to elevated cortisol levels that cross the placenta, causing higher cortisol levels in the amniotic fluid. This induces stress-related biological alterations in the pregnant mother and may also affect the foetus [136]. Chronic stress during pregnancy can have negative impacts on infant temperament [25]—an effect known as "foetal programming". For example, an interesting review looking at the impacts of pandemic-related maternal stress on the foetus during pregnancy found direct associations with infant temperament and social-emotional development. The authors thought this could be due to foetal programming, involving epigenetic changes such as permanent alterations in the structure and function of the baby's brain [118]. More specifically, prenatal maternal anxiety is associated with increased infant fearfulness, withdrawal and negative reactivity [150]. However, this connection between maternal anxiety and infant outcomes is mediated by postnatal bonding, highlighting the particular importance of promoting bonding, particularly between anxious mothers and their babies.

Maternal depression during pregnancy is associated with a higher risk of preterm and low-weight infants [66] who are more likely to be admitted to NICU, with all the additional separation issues this entails. Depressed pregnant women tend to have higher levels of inflammatory cytokines than their non-depressed counterparts, and—as with anxiety—this could affect the structure and function of the foetal brain, influencing the baby's immune development, stress response and certain aspects of their social-emotional development such as emotional regulation and processing [105]. Babies born to mothers with high levels of prenatal stress and depression therefore have an increased risk of behavioural issues post-birth, including increased fussiness, crying, irritability and difficulties in stress regulation [117]. Alongside having more challenging temperaments, these babies tend to be less adaptable to new situations, adding to the coping issues for parents who are already struggling with their mental health. Parents in this situation desperately need extra help, support and positive, evidence-based interventions. For example, a recent study found that treating depression with cognitive behavioural therapy may help the mother while encouraging more adaptive emotional regulation in the baby [95].

It's possible that fathers' prenatal mental health could also affect infant outcomes through its potential for indirect impacts on the mother's anxiety and stress levels. In Sweden, a country with very high egalitarian principles and good overall economic support for both parents, a recent study showed that fathers may also suffer mental health issues (such as fear of childbirth) during pregnancy. However, due to social stigma, fathers don't always feel they can reach out and access professional mental health support [121], meaning the figures for fathers' perinatal mental health issues could be much higher than we think [37]. Prenatally and postnatally, fathers are reported to be around half as likely as mothers to suffer from depression, anxiety or PTSD [74]. However, they may find it easier than mothers to escape momentarily for moments of sanity, for example, by maintaining their hobbies or taking outdoor exercise [40]—perhaps because they're not as intimately connected to the physical aspects of pregnancy, birth and breastfeeding that come with having a baby. It might be for this reason that fathers' needs are often overlooked despite their emotional vulnerability and involvement in the birth process [4].

4.3 The Psychology of Childbirth

Alongside medical vigilance regarding *physical* safety during childbirth, improving emotional and psychological safety is vital, and this can only be ensured by providing a high level of psychosocial care and support. In the context of maternity care, emotional and psychological safety can be defined as experiencing supportive and respectful care, feeling heard, feeling well taken care of, feeling secure and being cared for in a calm environment. This involves the parents who enter maternity care having their physical and emotional needs met while also having personal agency to make informed decisions within trusting relationships. Emotional safety positively influences the birth experience, making mothers feel empowered and improving outcomes [124]. When midwives and other health professionals protect a woman's emotional safety, adverse outcomes are reduced for mother and baby, while interestingly, mental health is protected in both the birthing *and* non-birthing parent. A recent study from the Czech Republic showed that mothers who are able to bond with their baby while still in the birth room are the *most* satisfied with their birth experience [17]. Therefore, facilitating skin-to-skin care, breastfeeding and bonding as soon after childbirth as possible would help protect mothers' emotional wellbeing, thereby contributing to positive mental health in both parents.

As recommended by the World Health Organization [175], having an adequate number of available midwives to ensure that a midwifery model of respectful, person-centred care based on human rights is firmly in place (i.e. avoiding unnecessary interventions while providing highly skilled clinical maternity care) helps protect the parents' emotional safety. This includes recognising and referring problems as soon as they arise, so they are dealt with promptly [80]. Respectful, supportive, person-centred midwifery care within a positive birth environment also facilitates trust, dignity and respect, privacy and confidentiality, good communication and autonomy, which again increases women's overall satisfaction with the birth [90] while helping to protect the baby from adverse outcomes.

Esteemed midwifery Professor Soo Downe et al. [48] advised the World Health Organization's [175] intrapartum guidelines for a positive birth experience on the basis of their findings around "what matters to women during childbirth". They established that women *equally* valued physical safety and psychosocial (emotional) wellbeing. Most women wanted to have a physiological birth if possible and give birth to a live baby in a clinically and psychologically safe environment. Their needs included having practical and emotional support from birth companions of their choice as well as kind, competent and reassuring clinical staff. They acknowledged that childbirth might be frightening and unpredictable, and therefore they may need to "go with the flow" to obtain the best outcomes for themselves and, importantly, their baby. Where interventions such as epidural, acceleration of labour or caesarean section were needed, women wanted to retain their sense of achievement and remain "in control" by playing an active role in the decision-making.

The Role of Oxytocin in Childbirth and Mother and Baby Behaviour

As discussed in Chap. 3, the hormone and neuropeptide oxytocin, released in the mother's body and brain during and after childbirth, plays an essential role in childbirth by promoting uterine contractions, breastfeeding and maternal bonding behaviours [26]. It is sometimes referred to as "the love hormone" due to its association with romantic love and other close relationships, even those we have with our pets [162]. Oxytocin lowers anxiety by modulating the body's stress response system and strengthening coping mechanisms [142]. However, the release of natural (endogenous) oxytocin in the birthing person's body can be inhibited by stress. Therefore, women with high anxiety levels are prone to lower oxytocin levels during labour, which could prolong their labour, creating a window of opportunity for complications or interventions to occur [167]. At the same time, a stressed labouring mother is likely to release an abundance of catecholamines (the stress hormones epinephrine and norepinephrine, also known as adrenaline and noradrenaline). Although a certain amount of adrenaline is required to prepare the baby for being born, *excessive* amounts of stress hormones may interfere with the natural progression of labour, as they block the body's endogenous production of calming, anxiety-reducing and pain-relieving oxytocin. This has the effect of reducing blood flow in the uterus and slowing contractions [26].

We know that high maternal cortisol levels during pregnancy negatively impact the foetus' brain and, subsequently, the baby's temperament [25, 136]. Because of this foetal programming effect, a baby born to a mother who is highly stressed or anxious during labour may exhibit higher cortisol levels, distress signals and increased crying. Conceivably, they could also have higher stress reactivity and be more challenging to settle, although research on the potential impacts of childbirth on infant temperament remains relatively sparse.

Obstetric Violence

A significant factor contributing to a negative or traumatic birth experience is obstetric violence, defined as abuse, disrespect and mistreatment during childbirth [140]. Definitions of obstetric violence incorporate over-medicalisation (converting "natural processes" into "pathological" ones), coercion, loss of autonomy, unconsented interventions and dehumanising or inhumane treatment [38]. However, mistreatment during childbirth has a broad compass, which also includes general factors such as a lack of rapport between health professionals and the person they are caring for, stigma or discrimination, and failure to meet professional standards of health and maternity care [29]. It is considered a gender-based and sex-specific form of discrimination against women that has finally been recognised as a violation of human rights and a public health scandal [64]. According to Kahalon and Klein [88], it is the dehumanisation of women in healthcare settings that makes obstetric violence possible and permitted. These authors cite several factors as responsible for the dehumanising perceptions and attitudes leading to obstetric violence: the perception of childbirth as a medical process with an emphasis on women's reproductive functions, ongoing stereotyping of mothers as self-sacrificing, and the current belief that a physically healthy baby is the only important outcome. Given these attitudes, it is perhaps not surprising that obstetric violence is still a widespread phenomenon.

Receiving this type of disrespectful care during childbirth increases mortality and morbidity rates in both mother and baby while dismissing fundamental human rights and displaying a worrying lack of empathy towards the mother's emotional state during labour and birth [106]. Obstetric violence adversely impacts parents' mental health and self-esteem, often leading to symptoms of post-traumatic stress [94]. A Nepalese study also found that women's risk of postnatal depression increased by over 50% following mistreatment during labour and birth, and this figure rose to 70% for adolescent mothers [68], which is especially concerning given the social disadvantages already faced by young parents.

In a Brazilian cross-sectional study, a woman experiencing two or more incidents of mistreatment in the forms of disrespect or abuse was associated with increased susceptibility to postnatal depression, and in countries like Brazil where obstetric violence is very common, the figures for this are alarmingly high [35, 130]. However, it's not just Brazil, Latin America or other developing countries where these problems can occur. Unfortunately, obstetric violence is an ongoing issue across the world. In high-income countries, the prevalence of mistreatment during childbirth it thought to be as high as 45% with the major problems being a lack of information and/or consent, lack of access to analgesia, ignored requests for help, scolding or shouting and the use of fundal pressure known as the "Kristeller manoeuvre" during the second stage of labour [61]. Other research reporting on a global level has found that a third of women in higher-income countries and approximately two-thirds of women in lower- and middle-income countries say they felt disrespected, unsupported or abused during childbirth [86].

Meanwhile, a nationwide French study found that a high percentage of emergency interventions lacked informed consent [81]. An Australian study highlighted the existence of a twofold trauma during and after obstetric violence—to both the woman giving birth and their midwife witnesses [34]. Seeing this kind of traumatic childbirth experience is common for student midwives during clinical training, yet it affects their mental and emotional health as well as plans regarding their career, pregnancies and childbirth [3]. On the whole, the intentions of health professionals are positive and geared towards saving lives during childbirth. However, they may not have taken into account any emotional or psychological factors. Those who try to intervene can find it challenging to navigate their role within the restrictions of obstetric medical care models and may feel that, by intervening, they're putting their own wellbeing and potentially their career on the line [153].

Practical interventions for preventing obstetric violence include increasing the availability of birth companions [70], such as doulas. Providing doulas could therefore be an appropriate response, especially in areas with midwifery shortages. Doulas might enable women's open communication and autonomy, help them to access pain relief when they need it and encourage freedom to choose their birth position while providing the supportive care necessary for a positive childbirth experience [91]. Furthermore, having a birth companion during labour benefits birth outcomes, reducing the duration of labour, alleviating labour fear, increasing birth satisfaction, decreasing pain and lessening the need for painkillers [49, 168]. Despite these benefits, the global rate of implementating birth companionship remains at only 40% [23]. It would also be beneficial to train health professionals to enhance their communication skills, introduce themselves when entering the room, facilitate open discussions and recognise the woman's right to be fully informed while respecting her privacy and confidentiality [176]. However, providing dignified and respectful, patient-centred, more personalised and generally better-quality maternity care in countries where healthcare systems are understaffed and under-resourced (such as the UK) is very challenging [86].

As we've seen in this chapter so far, foetal programming occurs during pregnancy in response to maternal stress and elevated cortisol levels, raising an important question about what might happen during childbirth itself in terms of epigenetic changes to the baby if the mother experiences excessive stress or distress [47]. Therefore, we must all work together to prevent obstetric violence from becoming mainstream and acceptable in maternity care settings if we want to see happy, healthy babies after childbirth. If more midwives cannot be trained or recruited, doulas should be made available on the NHS to support mothers practically and emotionally during the birth and in the immediate postnatal period.

4.4 Postnatal Mental Health

The mother's state of mental health post-birth is all-important to the baby as he tries to make sense of his new surroundings. In the worst-case scenario, poor postnatal mental health may lead to suicide—the leading cause of maternal death during the first year after childbirth across Western countries [156]. The recent MBRRACE-UK (Mothers and Babies: Reducing Risk through Audits and Confidential Enquiries across the UK) report shows that mental health issues continue to rise and are responsible for 34% of maternal deaths, remaining the leading cause of a baby's mother dying between 6 weeks and a year postpartum [109]. Sadly, the well-known UK health disparities around race and deprivation continue to affect vulnerable women disproportionately. Even after all the very public post-pandemic campaigns for more equitable maternity care, Black mothers are still nearly three times more likely to die, and Asian mothers are nearly twice as likely to die as their white British counterparts. This situation would undoubtedly be helped by continuity of carer, where mothers become better acquainted with their midwives, who in turn would be able to provide more personalised treatment and support throughout the perinatal journey if they knew more about the women in their care. It goes without saying that distressed mothers would be more inclined to share their thoughts and feelings with a known and trusted midwife or health visitor.

Even when not resulting in such a tragic outcome as suicide, postpartum mood disorders can have far-reaching and potentially devastating effects on the mother and baby, primarily by impairing the mother's ability to care for herself and her newborn. Negative postnatal mood may also interfere with bonding, which is particularly concerning in cases where the mother and baby lack adequate support [63]. Poor maternal mental health also affects a child's social and emotional development, although the quality of mother-infant bonding mediates these effects [28]. Overall, symptoms of depression may lead to weaker bonding, which in turn is linked to increased psychosocial difficulties in children up to 12 years old [152]. To help reduce these risks, early interventions aimed at supporting parents' postnatal mental health and promoting healthy bonding with their babies are essential, and simple, low-cost interventions can be highly effective. For example, a randomised controlled trial taking place with 54 women in a Turkish hospital found that those attending a course in newborn massage during pregnancy had enhanced mother-infant attachment 6–10 weeks post-birth and a reduced risk of postpartum depression [161].

Postnatal depression and anxiety are probably the most common, and indeed the most studied, mood disorders that can arise during the first year after birth. Between them, they affect 10–20% of new mothers [169, 170]. These two conditions have multiple shared risk factors, including a personal history of depression or anxiety, a family history of psychiatric illness, isolation, lack of social support (including partner support) and stressful life events [141]. The prevalence of postnatal depression is slightly higher in developing countries (15%) compared to developed countries (12%) [102]. It is substantially higher for parents of preterm babies [134], increasing the risk of impaired infant cognitive, social and emotional development [181]. A large-scale meta-analysis involving tens of thousands of participants shows that interventions that focus on increasing parents' self-efficacy can effectively reduce rates of stress, anxiety and depression in the parents of preterm babies [44]. Such programmes should therefore be included in routine care, especially for preterm births, as they would benefit not only the parents but also the baby's future developmental trajectory. They could also reduce parent-infant bonding issues by helping parents to establish positive relationships with their baby [139].

Other key contributors to both depression and anxiety during the postnatal period include pre-birth fear, low confidence, mode of birth, loss of control, suboptimal treatment from staff and negative perceptions of the birth experience [53]. Postnatal depression is explicitly associated with negative physical and psychological birth experiences and poor family support, and mothers suffering from depression during the postnatal period may feel lonely, trapped, frustrated and overburdened by the overwhelming responsibility of looking after a new baby. Both disorders significantly influence baby behaviour and infant temperament development [120] via their negative impacts on breastfeeding, mother-baby interactions, bonding and health [54, 102]. Mothers may also have a poor body image after childbirth, which sometimes leads to self-isolation. Breastfeeding problems can compound this issue, and mothers may be racked with guilt about not being able to breastfeed or care for their newborn baby in the way they would like to or feel they should [84].

Nervous and negative thoughts involving self-doubt and anxiety about breastfeeding or the baby's health and wellbeing are often pervasive in new mothers, but especially during maternity hospitalisation [133], or if the baby has to spend time in NICU [19]. This is a shame as breastfeeding is considered beneficial in preventing or alleviating depression and anxiety as it helps to regulate the circadian rhythm of the hypothalamic-pituitary-adrenal (HPA) axis—the body's stress response system. Combined with the effects of oxytocin and prolactin, breastfeeding promotes emotional closeness, reduces stress and depressive symptoms and helps regulate sleep patterns in the mother and baby [43]. However, only mothers who manage to *successfully* establish breastfeeding experience these mental health advantages [151]. Some mothers may find it very difficult and can struggle with the pressures associated with breastfeeding, such as the hugely emotive and divisive concept of "Breast is Best". Therefore, providing appropriate support is crucial. Increased breastfeeding support, particularly from fathers, may enhance the mother's self-esteem and enable her to establish successful feeding patterns [89, 179, 180].

While postnatal anxiety, with its restlessness, excessive worry and intrusive thoughts, can be crippling for a new mother to deal with, especially if the anxious thoughts concern her baby [141], depression may also feel debilitating as it often includes persistent sadness, lack of interest, sleep and appetite disturbances, low self-esteem, anxiety, irritability and hostility (occasionally directed at the infant), self-blame and—perhaps most worryingly—feelings of hopelessness and despair [28]. Mothers who are depressed are more likely to feel anxious about their baby's health and wellbeing [119]. Various interventions may be helpful; for example, providing psychoeducation about the baby and the postnatal period empowers parents by increasing their knowledge [67].

Excessive stress, anxiety and depression are all linked to a disruption of the mother's microbiome and gut flora during the postnatal period [85]. Consequently, scientific trials are beginning to look at new interventions and treatments for postnatal mental health that involve rebalancing the microbiome—for example, with supplements of *Bifidobacteriales*, *Bifidobacteriaceae* and *Bifidobacterium*, although relationships between these healthy bacteria and a reduction in symptoms are complex [62]. Meanwhile, lack of sleep is the single factor most strongly associated with postnatal depression, so increasing sleep may help to alleviate symptoms [171]—if this were ever possible with a new baby.

Maternal anxiety and depression, especially if severe, may affect the mother's sensitivity, warmth and responsiveness towards her baby, with negative impacts on infant emotional regulation and development [24]. Research on the broader effects of CB-PTSD on infant behaviour and development has yet to catch up [163]. Nonetheless, as anxiety, depression and CB-PTSD are known to be comorbid [12], the impacts of these postpartum mood disorders on infant outcomes are also likely to be shared or at least have some significant similarities with one another. In support of this concept, a recent study found that CB-PTSD in the mother is associated with negative infant mood and lower levels of mother-baby synchrony [113].

The two *postnatal* mood disorders that have been most connected to infant outcomes are postnatal depression and PTSD. Therefore, these disorders will now be further explored, specifically concerning their relationship to bonding and baby behaviour, with suggestions on how to mitigate the potential risks they pose to positive outcomes.

Postnatal Depression

Postnatal depression is characterised by a deterioration in a parent's mental health involving profound sadness and depressive symptoms, often alongside anxiety, lower self-esteem including feelings of worthlessness or excessive guilt, heightened irritability, less ability to control anger, insomnia, fatigue and a general loss of energy, diminished concentration and disinterest in the infant [112]. These symptoms are associated with a decline in quality of life and may disrupt parent-infant bonding, caregiving behaviours and the parent-baby relationship [179, 180].

Untreated perinatal depression can seriously impact a baby's behaviour, although it may lose this effect when adjusted for bonding [60]. However, babies whose mothers manage to engage and bond with them despite their diagnosis can still develop well socially and emotionally, highlighting how important it is to support parent-infant bonding, especially between depressed mothers and their babies. Although mild or fluctuating symptoms of parental depression do not adversely impact the baby, if the condition becomes chronic, it can lead to disruptions in infant stress reactivity and social-emotional development; and, if it persists, there is an increased risk of emotional and behavioural problems in the 2-year-old child [138], possibly because of reduced mother-baby interactions and maternal sensitivity towards the baby's needs [56, 131].

Babies of mothers with postnatal depression have more hospital admissions. They are more likely to cry excessively and have disturbed sleep and temperament problems, which could lead to more difficult mother-baby interactions and interfere with breastfeeding. Infant temperament, physical growth, cognitive development, nutrition and sleep may all be affected [55, 128]. One study found adverse impacts of maternal postnatal depression symptoms on the baby's gut microbiota and neurodevelopment at 6 months [182]. However, supportive interventions may lessen the effects of postnatal mood disorders on the baby's behaviour and physical wellbeing [119]. A simple though effective technique for reducing distress in the baby and depression and sleep deprivation in the mother is kangaroo care, where the depressed parent places their baby in skin-to-skin contact as often as possible [96].

As we saw in Chap. 3, regular and prolonged kangaroo care has numerous positive physiological benefits for the baby, as it facilitates healthier physical, social-emotional and cognitive development while improving the chances of breastfeeding success [32, 160]. Neonates with mothers who are depressed (or have a history of depression) may exhibit fewer socially interactive behaviours during the early days after birth, emphasising the need to protect mothers from exacerbating factors such as traumatic birth or separation from their baby, identify maternal depression as early as possible and intervene to support skin-to-skin care and parent-infant bonding [21]. Providing this type of support benefits mother-infant wellbeing, the mother-baby relationship and infant development by reducing the mother's physiological and psychological stress alongside any depressive symptoms she might be experiencing after a challenging birth [93].

New research shows that depressed mothers and their babies have lower oxytocin levels, while, conversely, parents who practise "mind-mindedness" during parent-infant interactions have higher oxytocin levels [14]. Mind-mindedness is based on the principles of sensitive or "mindful" communication between parents and babies—the ability to understand and acknowledge them as separate beings with their own thoughts and feelings. It involves adapting to meet the baby's evolving needs and facilitating their emotional regulation, as well as the strong mother-infant attachment necessary for healthy social, emotional and cognitive infant development [110, 111]. Additionally, parents' emotional availability encourages the baby's communication skills and language development [126]. Therefore, there are some obvious ways to support mothers and babies postnatally, especially if they have shown signs of stress or depression since birth. Caring for mothers and building their resilience while helping them to become emotionally available and provide calm, sensitive care for their babies might make up for some of the impacts of a negative birth experience.

Studies have consistently shown the power of family support in reducing postnatal depression, and higher perceived social support is associated with lower depression scores [83]. Indeed, research shows that women who have strong social support from their family and partner, as well as a positive birth experience followed by skin-to-skin contact and successful bonding with their baby, have a lower risk of postnatal depression [45]. This research highlights the importance of creating the best possible birth experience and facilitating skin-to-skin contact and parent-infant bonding immediately post-birth. However, birth and postnatal events, mood and behaviour are not always as simplistic or straightforward to prevent, diagnose or treat as they might at first appear. A seminal article that is still frequently discussed in scientific circles and aptly titled "Ghosts in the Nursery" first drew public attention to how we are all influenced for better or worse by our background, upbringing and experiences, all of which may intentionally or unintentionally affect our feelings and behaviour towards our baby [57, 58]. The strength of our attachment relationships during our own infancy and early childhood can affect how we bond with our babies. While this might be difficult to change, it can be helped through supportive interventions and health professionals' greater awareness and support [114]. Midwives are best placed to provide this type of care alongside supportive interventions that facilitate parent-infant bonding after childbirth [157]. However, to achieve this, they need to work within a system that allows them to spend time with mothers and babies. Unfortunately, this is often not the case in the UK and elsewhere, where a shortage of midwives and disruptive hospital routines regularly interfere with—rather than support—parent-infant bonding.

A study of first-time mothers found that higher depression scores in mothers corresponded with lower maternal attachment to their babies. Educated mothers who breastfed their babies and received adequate support from their partners after childbirth had fewer depressive symptoms [129]. Aligning with this, a small-scale Nepalese study found that educating partners about gender-equitable attitudes and norms, helping with household chores and caretaking and providing emotional support could help boost mothers' recovery [20]. However, fathers may also get depressed after the birth of their child. Fathers are more likely to get depressed if their partner is depressed or they have low relationship satisfaction [169, 170]. Fathers' emotional states (including anger and hostility) therefore benefit from higher relationship satisfaction and perceptions of social support [97]. Therefore, health professionals need to include and involve partners and other family members during the perinatal period. This is especially pertinent if they or the mother has any pre-existing mental health issues; otherwise, fathers can easily come to feel marginalised and neglected [123]. Overall, postnatal depression appears to be approximately half as common in fathers as mothers, although this could be partly due to less recognition and therefore lower rates of diagnosis. Notably, postnatal depression in either parent is associated with more behaviour problems and mental health issues in the children, an effect that is even more potent in poorer families [33]. Bolstering financial support for young families, as progressive governments do across the Nordic countries, would effectively reduce some of the inevitable strain parents face during the perinatal period. This would reduce wealth and health inequalities from the outset, benefitting babies and the health, welfare and education systems further down the line. In the UK, however, regardless of which government is in power and despite all the evidence of later cost savings, we seem to have a blind spot when it comes to helping those born into less privileged backgrounds [75].

Postnatal depression is often associated with low socioeconomic status, adverse birth experiences and life stress. This means that poor postnatal mental health tends to be exacerbated for parents and infants living in lower- or middle-income countries where maternal and neonatal morbidity and mortality rates are higher and there are fewer midwives available to improve these adverse outcomes [122]. Over the past decade or so, Professor Prabha Chandra from India has also shed light on the heavy impact of social risk factors such as intimate partner violence, isolation and poor social support on perinatal mood disorders, often leading to poor neonatal outcomes [30]. According to Professor Prabha Chandra, the issues she talks about are more pronounced in areas of social and economic deprivation, which may have inadequate housing, food insecurity and malnutrition, natural disasters, war and conflict. They also occur in rural areas, where there are still poor transport links and limited access to healthcare, combined with traditional cultural norms that dictate the woman must stay home alone to care for the children, which increases social isolation [31].

As we have seen, there are established connections between persistent postnatal depression and adverse impacts on the baby in terms of language, behavioural and social-emotional development [92, 155]. The frequent links between postnatal depression and cognitive or physical development [104] are sometimes thought to be less consistent [8]. However, a recent cross-sectional study of nearly 700 mothers and babies established definite links. In this study, babies of depressed mothers were over 20% more likely to experience developmental delays in fine motor development as well as social-emotional and language development [2].

Meanwhile, a review on breastfeeding in lower- and middle-income countries indicated significant public health benefits to incorporating breastfeeding programmes and policies. These were found to help prevent and alleviate depressive symptoms [103]. However, it's essential to note that a mother can only reap these benefits if she has chosen to breastfeed and received strong support to do so [43]. Pressurising mothers to breastfeed could be counter-productive and have negative impacts on their mental health. On the other hand, Wheeler et al. [174] demonstrated that supporting mothers in their transition to parenthood without judgement or guilt, regardless of *their feeding choices* ,isgenerallyexperiencedasempowering, which is likely to boost the mother's postnatal mental health.

Post-traumatic Stress Disorder After Childbirth

Experiencing a difficult birth, particularly if the person giving birth has a history of mental health issues, means an increased risk of developing anxiety, depression or post-traumatic stress disorder [1, 12, 125]. A European collective of experts led by Professor Susan Ayers has defined a traumatic childbirth experience as *a woman's experience of interactions and/or events directly related to childbirth that caused overwhelming distressing emotions and reactions, leading to short and/or long-term negative impacts on a woman's health and wellbeing*. These symptoms may occur after a birth experience where the mother perceives a threat (whether real or imagined) to her own or her baby's life or to her physical or psychological wellbeing and integrity [101].

PTSD following childbirth fought for a place in the American Psychological Association's *Diagnostic and Statistical Manual of Mental Disorders* (DSM) for a long time before it was eventually accepted that giving birth (or witnessing it) could be a traumatic event. The traumatic symptoms of PTSD following childbirth were finally included in the fifth edition of the manual, known as DSM-5 [5]. Experiencing PTSD after childbirth may have detrimental effects on the mother's mental wellbeing and family relationships [42], although understanding the pathways between a traumatic birth experience and maternal mood is complex. Traumatic birth is most likely to occur after complications, high levels of negative emotions, suboptimal care or mistreatment [12, 13, 22]. Recently, it has also been suggested that the rise in birth trauma rates is associated with increased levels of medical interventions, such as induction of labour. This association occurs particularly if women feel they were not adequately informed or consulted beforehand [127].

Between 20% and 40% of women appraise their birth as traumatic, meeting the DSM-5 criteria for their birth as a traumatic stressor, although only a proportion of these (approximately 12–17%) experience the full range of postnatal traumatic stress symptoms [178]. These include negative cognitions and mood, reliving the birth and re-experiencing symptoms (flashbacks), avoidance of the birth scene or reminders of the birth (e.g. avoiding postnatal visits to the birthplace or the baby's first birthday) and hyperarousal (defined as very anxious, constantly aware of threats and easily startled). Approximately 3–5% of people who give birth are diagnosed with PTSD after these heightened stress response symptoms have remained or worsened for over a month, leading to extreme distress and impaired functioning [178]. Five years after this initial review of studies on PTSD after childbirth, another systematic review and meta-analysis that included *both* parents estimated the figures to be 4.7% in mothers and 1.2% in fathers. At the same time, the rates for experiencing post-traumatic stress *symptoms* without reaching full diagnostic criteria were 12.3% in mothers and 1.3% in fathers [74]. A recent Icelandic study assessing diagnosable levels of PTSD symptoms in around 600 women found an even higher rate of 5.7% for all new mothers [159]. As soon-to-be published research by Susan Ayers' team is showing similar figures in the UK, it appears that traumatic birth experiences are on the rise [173].

According to Professor Susan Ayers, one of the world's leading experts on birth trauma, childbirth as a traumatic stressor is more complex to treat than generic

PTSD because it is likely to affect at least two people—mother and baby (Society for Reproductive and Infant Psychology early career researchers' workshop, June 2024). Cheryl Beck [16], another well-known specialist in postpartum mood disorders, refers to the "ripple effect of birth trauma" outwards from mother to baby and the wider family. In addition to affecting the mother-infant relationship in terms of bonding [131, 164, 165], PTSD symptoms place a strain on the couple's relationship, decreasing the parents' quality of life [42, 72].

In her ground-breaking and comprehensive meta-analysis, Ayers [12] defined how the *type* of birth and birth events (e.g. instrumental or caesarean birth) and the way a mother perceives and evaluates this can dramatically impact her postnatal psychological wellbeing. She also established that the *subjective birth experience*, or how a mother *perceives* the birth, is *at least* as important as the objective experience, which encompasses *events* that occur around the time of and during childbirth. However, there is an overlap: obstetric complications and interventions play an influential role in the mother's subjective experience and evaluation of childbirth and how she responds psychologically post-birth [6, 12]. The meta-analysis also showed that, although birth trauma is not universal, but different for everyone who experiences it, childbirth-related PTSD has four main risk factors: a negative subjective birth experience, operative birth, poor support and dissociation—where the woman experiences a sense of detachment from mind and body during labour and birth as a way of coping with intense pain or stress [12].

The European collective of birth trauma experts is helping to shake the myth that traumatic birth experiences involve a mismatch between expectations and reality [13]. Although, of course, expectations of childbirth have a role to play in outcomes (negative expectations and fear tend to *increase* negative birth experiences), *actual* childbirth experiences are more significant than pre-birth expectations in the development of PTSD symptoms [10, 13, 27]. There are a few obvious high-risk groups for childbirth-related PTSD, such as those who experience pre-eclampsia, preterm birth or stillbirth. Prevalence rates are also higher in women who experience fear of childbirth, poor physical or mental health and complications during pregnancy or postnatally [78].

A longitudinal study has exposed *birth satisfaction* as an important factor, moderating the relationship between the mother's personal characteristics (specifically neuroticism and lack of resilience) and higher levels of PTSD. Previous trauma or abuse also plays a part, leading the authors to recommend screening for vulnerable women during pregnancy and providing trauma-informed maternity care, especially for those with high levels of neuroticism or previous traumatic experiences [116]. The Icelandic study mentioned above [159] found that support during labour, effective communication between mothers and health professionals, shared decision-making and a sense of control boosted mothers' birth satisfaction while simultaneously reducing symptoms of PTSD. Consistent with this, a European survey of over 500 women found that adverse childbirth experiences and lower satisfaction in health professional support during childbirth meant higher levels of PTSD in women with a history of psychological problems, highlighting competent, kind and caring professional support during labour and birth as a powerful preventative measure, especially for vulnerable women [15].

Traumatic births happen at a huge cost to society in the form of postnatal treatments and litigation [13] as well as the very real possibility of increased healthcare and educational costs for the children of traumatic births who develop special educational needs and disabilities related to their birth experience (such as cerebral palsy, autistic spectrum disorder or attention deficit hyperactivity disorder, to name just a few possibilities). In addition to the issue of adverse impacts on mothers and babies, maternity care providers witnessing traumatic birth may suffer emotional burnout. This means they are more likely to leave the profession early, adding to the shortage of one-to-one care for women during childbirth and, therefore, potentially exacerbating the existing problems, including the seemingly ever-rising rates of traumatic childbirth and the extra costs involved in training and recruiting new midwives. Hospitals, therefore, need to implement supportive strategies that build health professionals' resilience and specialist knowledge [146], for example, how to provide trauma-informed care to prevent traumatic birth experiences from happening in the first place. Equally important is the ongoing issue of midwifery shortages in the UK and elsewhere. Given this situation and all the compelling scientific evidence presented here, it is difficult to comprehend why the bursary for trainee midwives was ever abolished.

As well as providing continuous, personalised one-to-one professional midwifery care during childbirth, other protective factors for PTSD include the use of epidural analgesia during painful interventions such as inductions and "humanised" birth practices such as kindness, respecting the mother's birth plans and promoting skin-to-skin contact with the baby immediately post-birth [73]. Women who receive respectful care, are allowed autonomy and encouraged to make their own decisions during childbirth tend to feel more trusting of their care providers and describe their experience as more positive, regardless of their mode of birth [166]. In addition, resilience and the ability to "bounce back" after adversity are helpful qualities for recovery [145]. This can be encouraged by providing appropriate support throughout pregnancy, childbirth and the postpartum period. Professional and social support nurture the woman's resilience and therefore protect against the development of PTSD. Conversely, experiencing a *lack* of support is a major risk factor [10, 77]. Thus during any birth, but particularly when things go wrong, emotional support is an effective buffer against a traumatic response [12, 46]. As outlined in a European-funded project called "DEVOTION: *Optimizing the birth environment*", midwives and obstetricians are best placed to ensure that relationships built on trust are established during childbirth. When this occurs, it enables more positive birth experiences where women's psychological and emotional needs are met by their care providers through empathic, nurturing and trauma-informed, person-centred interactions [100].

Aligning with these quantitative findings, qualitative research exploring birth trauma has established that, among other things, it can involve being treated inhumanely, experiencing a rollercoaster of emotions, feeling invisible or out of control and being trapped in a recurring nightmare about childbirth [51]. A mixed-method study involving over 700 women found that the actions and interactions of health professionals with the women in their care impacted perceptions of mistreatment and birth trauma, highlighting the need to train and support midwives and obstetricians to minimise interpersonal trauma [143]. This further underscores the importance of compassionate care and support, empathetic communication from health professionals, a trusting relationship and shared decision-making during labour and birth [50]. When it comes to PTSD, the attitudes and behaviours of caregivers during childbirth are even more critical than the joint influences of pain and pain relief [76].

Trauma-informed support programmes can effectively reduce stress and post-traumatic stress symptoms in women who have experienced complications during childbirth [7]; therefore, providing such programmes more widely could contribute to improved care for mothers who have suffered trauma. To do this, however, we need to increase public and health professional awareness and education about PTSD after childbirth so that it can be quickly recognised and treated [87]. Due to current stigmas around childbirth-related PTSD and a general fear of treatment, common barriers would need to be tackled through financial subsidies or outreach services to improve access and encourage parents who are suffering from distressing symptoms to seek help [82].

Other qualitative research highlights how traumatic birth experiences may also trigger previous mental health problems, exacerbating the mother's response to trauma, with repercussions for the couple's relationship [42]. The debilitating impacts of birth trauma include a deterioration in physical wellbeing, feeling invaded and violated by what has happened, severe depression or suicidal thoughts, being afraid of future pregnancies (fear of childbirth), sexual dysfunction and experiencing a loss of trust in others [11]. The mothers in this insightful qualitative study felt their experience of a traumatic response to childbirth may have affected their perceptions of and bonding with their baby, and this seemed to develop into anxious or avoidant mother-infant attachments, which we know impact heavily on infant behaviour and development. Despite a lack of statistical evidence to date, therefore, it seems reasonable to suggest the possibility of disrupted baby behavioural outcomes following a traumatic birth. According to a review by Cook et al. [36], however, evidence on the outcomes of parent-infant interactions, parent-infant relationships and infant development is contradictory, although PTSD symptoms *do* appear to affect breastfeeding. This might occur because high cortisol levels are the antithesis of endogenous oxytocin, the powerful neurohormone responsible for birth, bonding and breastfeeding (as detailed earlier).

As was the case for postnatal depression, PTSD in the mother is likely to affect the baby too, due to their intertwined physiology and neurohormonal systems during and after childbirth. The mother's psychological stress, as measured by cortisol, interacts with prolactin, the hormone largely responsible for producing breast milk, and the hormones are transported to the baby through breastfeeding. Therefore, managing the mother's stress response during and after childbirth is vital for successful breastfeeding and bonding. Notably, both hormones are involved in the postnatal programming of early infant behaviour and development: while prolactin bolsters the baby's immune system and metabolism, high cortisol levels may counteract this positive effect [107]. Consequently, high salivary cortisol levels in infants have been linked to adverse clinical outcomes, including adjustment problems involving excessive reactions to stress, negative thoughts, strong emotions and behavioural issues [154]. This effect could involve the baby's HPA axis, microbiome and/or epigenome and therefore might be responsible for the increased "cry fuss" behaviours observed after a challenging birth experience [47]. However, as findings regarding the relationships between postnatal mood disorders and HPA axis dysregulation remain inconclusive [112], more research is needed on the potential baby behaviour outcomes of traumatic birth [163].

Despite the limited evidence on more generic outcomes of PTSD involving the baby's physiological well-being and behaviour, some studies have shown that it can impact their emotional reactivity, regulation and social-emotional and cognitive development [52, 65, 132]. Furthermore, a systematic review [163] found associations between PTSD symptoms, baby behaviour and mother-infant attachment [36]. Meanwhile, research by Professor Antje Horsch's team at Lausanne University Hospital's "Femme-Mère-Enfant" department in Switzerland has found significant links between childbirth-related PTSD and parent-infant bonding [158], which in turn influences the baby's wellbeing, behaviour and development [99]. These associations are likely to be moderated by environmental factors such as parenting style and social risk, including the parents' own adverse childhood experiences. As we saw for postnatal depression, a deterioration in the mother's mental health after childbirth may reduce the mother's sensitivity and responsiveness towards her baby, affecting her ability to provide the intensive, dedicated care required for the baby to thrive. This could have negative consequences for the mother's and baby's interrelated wellbeing. If left untreated, postnatal mood disorders such as depression or PTSD may worsen, with worrying implications for mother-and-baby bonding and attachment, baby behaviour and infant development [28, 163].

The Parents' Relationship Matters to the Baby Too
Given the importance of the parents' relationship dynamics to infant outcomes, and the disruption to a couple's emotional, physical and sexual connection often caused by childbirth and the transition to parenthood [39], parents need to be better informed and supported around how to regain their intimacy after the birth of their child. Receiving appropriate information may help parents to manage unrealistic relationship expectations before childbirth, as more realistic expectations are associated with greater sexual and relationship wellbeing during the postnatal period [149]. Inevitably, emotional, physical and sexual intimacy all influence the new parents' relationship satisfaction, although the findings around this topic are complex, nuanced and heterogeneous due to individual differences. Together with relationship satisfaction, parents' sexual intimacy also influences (and is influenced by) postnatal mood disorders such as depression. Interestingly, and despite the seemingly obvious links between postnatal maternal pain and sexual desire and functioning, Natalie Rosen and her colleagues [147, 148] found that when biomedical physical risk factors (such as induction, episiotomy, epidural, mode of birth or

perineal tear) were considered alongside psychological factors (such as stress, parental fatigue due to poor infant sleep, postnatal depression, discrepancies in desire, mental catastrophising about pain or relationship issues), the physical factors paled into insignificance beside the psychological ones. Therefore, targeting interventions and support towards improving parents' mental health could also help couple and family relationships.

Further research has confirmed the importance of psychological factors in resuming sexual functioning and advocates for better information giving during pregnancy and facilitating partner support postnatally, particularly after perineal injuries affecting the woman's self-image and desire [9]. These findings reinforce the importance of caring for both partners and providing adequate information and support for their emotional, psychological, sexual and physical wellbeing throughout the perinatal period. If parents are well-supported and manage to regain their intimacy and connection, they will be better placed to form a strong bond with their baby.

As we have seen in this chapter, parents' mental health may be affected by the mother's birth and early postnatal experiences, emphasising the need for early screening, intervention and compassionate care for parents with postnatal mood disorders in the postpartum period. Protecting the expectant or labouring person's physiological and psychological state and providing adequate emotional support for both parents is crucial, as this is likely to affect their experience of childbirth and how well they cope with and feel able to care for their baby postnatally. In turn, the parents feeling mentally and emotionally well after the birth is vital for the baby's early behaviour and development.

In the following two chapters (Chaps. 5 and 6), we will explore the two qualitative studies I conducted on perceptions of childbirth experience and baby behaviour. Forty mothers, health professionals and other maternity care providers (such as doulas) were interviewed. I will begin by presenting the profound wisdom and insights shared by maternity care providers, who nurture mothers and babies to the very best of their ability within the constraints of busy and overstretched maternity and neonatal care systems.

References

1. Alcorn KL, O'Donovan A, Patrick JC, Creedy D, Devilly GJ. A prospective longitudinal study of the prevalence of post-traumatic stress disorder resulting from childbirth events. Psychol Med. 2010;40:1849–59.
2. Alfayumi-Zeadna S, Masarwe S, Findling Y, Ereli A, O'Rourke N. The impact of postpartum depression on infant development in the first year of life. J Affect Disord. 2025;388:119558.
3. Altaweli R, Alotaibi SZ, Aldokhi GD, Alotaibi SM, Megari RM, Alobthani NM, Alanazi DH. The prevalence and effect of traumatic childbirth witnessed by midwifery students: a quantitative study. Sex Reprod Healthc. 2025;44:101099. https://doi.org/10.1016/j.srhc.2025.101099.
4. Altunay Davran GB, Serçekuş Ak P. Fathers' emotions, thoughts on childbirth, and coping with childbirth stress: a qualitative study. J Educ Res Nurs. 2024;21:1–7.

5. American Psychological Association. Diagnostic and statistical manual of mental disorders. Am Psychiatric Assoc. 2013;21:591–643. https://seragpsych.com/wordpress/wp-content/uploads/2019/02/DSM5Update_October2018.pdf.
6. Andersen LB, Melvaer LB, Videbech P, Lamont RF, Joergensen JS. Risk factors for developing post-traumatic stress disorder following childbirth: a systematic review. Acta Obstet Gynecol Scand. 2012;91:1261–72.
7. Andersson H, Nieminen K, Malmquist A, Grundström H. Trauma-informed support after a complicated childbirth–an early intervention to reduce symptoms of post-traumatic stress, fear of childbirth and mental illness. Sex Reprod Healthc. 2024;41:101002.
8. Aoyagi SS, Tsuchiya KJ. Does maternal postpartum depression affect children's developmental outcomes? J Obstet Gynaecol Res. 2019;45:1809–20.
9. Artieta-Pinedo I, Paz-Pascual C, Garcia-Alvarez A, Bully P, Espinosa M. Resumption of sexual activity after childbirth and its related factors in Spanish women, a cross-sectional study. Midwifery. 2024;141:104259.
10. Ayers S. Birth trauma and post-traumatic stress disorder: the importance of risk and resilience. J Reprod Infant Psychol. 2017;35:427–30.
11. Ayers S, Eagle A, Waring H. The effects of childbirth-related post-traumatic stress disorder on women and their relationships: a qualitative study. Psychol Health Med. 2006;11:389–98.
12. Ayers S, Bond R, Bertullies S, Wijma K. The aetiology of post-traumatic stress following childbirth: a meta-analysis and theoretical framework. Psychol Med. 2016;46:1121–34.
13. Ayers S, Horsch A, Garthus-Niegel S, Nieuwenhuijze M, Bogaerts A, Hartmann K, et al. Traumatic birth and childbirth-related post-traumatic stress disorder: international expert consensus recommendations for practice, policy, and research. Women Birth. 2024;37:362–7.
14. Baron-Cohen KL, Fearon P, Meins E, Feldman R, Hardiman P, Rosan C, Fonagy P. Maternal mind-mindedness and infant oxytocin are interrelated and negatively associated with postnatal depression. Dev Psychopathol. 2025;37:2026–37. https://doi.org/10.1017/S0954579424001585.
15. Beato A, Alves S, Akik BK, Albuquerque S. Protecting mothers against posttraumatic stress symptoms related to childbirth: what's the role of formal and informal support? Midwifery. 2025;141:104236.
16. Beck CT. Perinatal mood and anxiety disorders: research and implications for nursing care. Nurs Womens Health. 2021;25:e8–e53.
17. Belešová R, Machová A, Mágrová M, Filausová D. Care for women and newborns in south bohemian obstetrics wards. Kontakt. 2025;27:15–22. https://doi.org/10.32725/kont.2025.007.
18. Bergstrom L, Roberts J, Skillman L, Seidel J. "You'll feel me touching you, sweetie": vaginal examinations during the second stage of labor. Birth. 1992;19:10–8.
19. Bernardo J, Rent S, Arias-Shah A, Hoge MK, Shaw RJ. Parental stress and mental health symptoms in the NICU: recognition and interventions. NeoReviews. 2021;22:e496–505.
20. Bhardwaj A, Maharjan SM, Magar AJ, Shrestha R, Dongol A, Hagaman A, et al. Engaging husbands in a digital mental health intervention to provide tailored counseling for women experiencing postpartum depression: a mixed methods study in Nepal. SSM-Mental Health. 2024;6:100340.
21. Bind RH, Biaggi A, Bairead A, Du Preez A, Hazelgrove K, Waites F, et al. Mother–infant interaction in women with depression in pregnancy and in women with a history of depression: the Psychiatry Research and Motherhood–Depression (PRAM-D) study. BJPsych open. 2021;7:e100.
22. Bohren MA, Vogel JP, Hunter EC, Lutsiv O, Makh SK, Souza JP, et al. The mistreatment of women during childbirth in health facilities globally: a mixed-methods systematic review. PLoS Med. 2015;12:e1001847.
23. Bohren MA, Hazfiarini A, Vazquez Corona M, Colomar M, De Mucio B, Tunçalp Ö, Portela A. From global recommendations to (in) action: a scoping review of the coverage of companion of choice for women during labour and birth. PLoS Global Public Health. 2023;3:e0001476.

References

24. Bozicevic L, De Pascalis L, Montirosso R, Ferrari PF, Giusti L, Cooper PJ, Murray L. Sculpting culture: early maternal responsiveness and child emotion regulation–a UK-Italy comparison. J Cross-Cult Psychol. 2021;52:22–42.
25. Bruinhof N, Vacaru SV, van den Heuvel MI, de Weerth C, Beijers R. Prenatal hair cortisol concentrations during the COVID-19 outbreak: associations with maternal psychological stress and infant temperament. Psychoneuroendocrinology. 2022;144:105863.
26. Buckley SJ. Executive summary of hormonal physiology of childbearing: evidence and implications for women, babies, and maternity care. J Perinat Educ. 2015;24(3):145–53.
27. Buyukcan-Tetik A, Seefeld L, Bergunde L, Ergun TD, Dikmen-Yildiz P, Horsch A, et al. Birth expectations, birth experiences and childbirth-related post-traumatic stress symptoms in mothers and birth companions: dyadic investigation using response surface analysis. Br J Health Psychol. 2024;29:925–42.
28. Carlson K, Mughal S, Azhar Y, Siddiqui W. Postpartum depression. In: StatPearls [Internet]. StatPearls Publishing; 2024. https://www.ncbi.nlm.nih.gov/books/NBK519070/.
29. Cayama MR, Vamos CA, Harris NL, Logan RG, Howard A, Daley EM. Respectful maternity care in the United States: a scoping review of the research and birthing people's experiences. J Midwifery Womens Health. 2025;70:212–22. https://doi.org/10.1111/jmwh.13729.
30. Chandra P, Gupta N. The relevance of social factors and "social prescribing" for perinatal mental health. Indian J Soc Psychiatry. 2023;39:195–7.
31. Chandra PS, Ross D, Agarwal PP. Mental health of rural women. In: Mental health and illness in the rural world. Singapore: Springer Nature; 2020. p. 119–49.
32. Chen WY, Wu YY, Xu MY, Tung TH. Effect of kangaroo mother care on the psychological stress response and sleep quality of mothers with premature infants in the neonatal intensive care unit. Front Pediatr. 2022;10:879956.
33. Clément M, Orri M, Ahun MN, Domond P, Moullec G, Côté SM. Parental postpartum depression and children's socioemotional development: the role of socioeconomic inequality. JAACAP Open. 2024;3:663–77. https://doi.org/10.1016/j.jaacop.2024.06.008.
34. Collins EC, Burns ES, Dahlen HG. 'It was horrible to watch, horrible to be a part of': midwives' perspectives of obstetric violence. Women Birth. 2024;37:101631.
35. Conceição HND, Madeiro AP. Association between disrespect and abuse during labor and the risk of postpartum depression: a cross-sectional study. Cad Saude Publica. 2024;40:e00008024.
36. Cook N, Ayers S, Horsch A. Maternal posttraumatic stress disorder during the perinatal period and child outcomes: a systematic review. J Affect Disord. 2018;225:18–31.
37. Darwin Z, Galdas P, Hinchliff S, Littlewood E, McMillan D, McGowan L, et al. Fathers' views and experiences of their own mental health during pregnancy and the first postnatal year: a qualitative interview study of men participating in the UK Born and Bred in Yorkshire (BaBY) cohort. BMC Pregnancy Childbirth. 2017;17:1–15.
38. Davis DA, Casper MJ, Hammonds E, Post W. The continued significance of obstetric violence: a response to Chervenak, McLeod-Sordjan, Pollet et al. Health Equity. 2024;8:513–8.
39. Dawson SJ, Vaillancourt-Morel MP, Pierce M, Rosen NO. Biopsychosocial predictors of trajectories of postpartum sexual function in first-time mothers. Health Psychol. 2020;39:700.
40. Deforges C, Centamori A, Garthus-Niegel S, Horsch A. One birth, two experiences: why is the prevalence of childbirth-related posttraumatic stress disorder four times lower in fathers than in mothers? J Reprod Infant Psychol. 2025;43:227–9.
41. Dekel S, Chan SJ, Jagodnik KM. Childbirth-related post-traumatic stress disorder. In: The Routledge international handbook of perinatal mental health disorders. London: Routledge; 2024. p. 330–57.
42. Delicate A, Ayers S, Easter A, McMullen S. The impact of childbirth-related post-traumatic stress on a couple's relationship: a systematic review and meta-synthesis. J Reprod Infant Psychol. 2018;36:102–15.

43. Dessì A, Pianese G, Mureddu P, Fanos V, Bosco A. From breastfeeding to support in mothers' feeding choices: a key role in the prevention of postpartum depression? Nutrients. 2024;16:2285.
44. Dewi DTK, Nguyen CTT, Chen SR, Lee GT, Tsai SY, Huda MH, Kuo SY. Effectiveness of parenting interventions on self-efficacy, anxiety, stress, and depression among parents of preterm infants: a systematic review and meta-analysis of randomized control trials. Int J Nurs Stud. 2025;169:105128.
45. Diaz-Ogallar MA, Hernandez-Martinez A, Linares-Abad M, Martinez-Galiano JM. Mother-child bond and its relationship with maternal postpartum depression. J Reprod Infant Psychol. 2024:1–24. https://doi.org/10.1080/02646838.2024.2397126.
46. Döblin S, Seefeld L, Weise V, Kopp M, Knappe S, Asselmann E, et al. The impact of mode of delivery on parent-infant-bonding and the mediating role of birth experience: a comparison of mothers and fathers within the longitudinal cohort study DREAM. BMC Pregnancy Childbirth. 2023;23:285.
47. Douglas PS, Hill PS. A neurobiological model for cry-fuss problems in the first three to four months of life. Med Hypotheses. 2013;81:816–22.
48. Downe S, Finlayson K, Oladapo O, Bonet M, Gülmezoglu AM. What matters to women during childbirth: a systematic qualitative review. PLoS One. 2018;13:e0194906.
49. Dubey K, Sharma N, Chawla D, Khatuja R, Jain S, Khaduja R. Impact of birth companionship on maternal and fetal outcomes in primigravida women in a government tertiary care center. Cureus. 2023;15:e38497.
50. Egenberg S, Skogheim G, Tangerud M, Sluijs AM, Slootweg YM, Elvemo H, et al. Clinical decision-making during childbirth in health facilities from the perspectives of labouring women, relatives, and health care providers: a scoping review. Midwifery. 2025;140:104192.
51. Elmir R, Schmied V, Wilkes L, Jackson D. Women's perceptions and experiences of a traumatic birth: a meta-ethnography. J Adv Nurs. 2010;66:2142–53.
52. Enlow MB, Kitts RL, Blood E, Bizarro A, Hofmeister M, Wright RJ. Maternal posttraumatic stress symptoms and infant emotional reactivity and emotion regulation. Infant Behav Dev. 2011;34:487–503.
53. Field T. Postpartum anxiety prevalence, predictors and effects on child development: a review. J Psychiat Psychiatric Disorders. 2017;1:86–102.
54. Field T. Postnatal anxiety prevalence, predictors and effects on development: a narrative review. Infant Behav Dev. 2018;51:24–32.
55. Field T. Paternal prenatal, perinatal and postpartum depression: a narrative review. J Anxiety Depression. 2018;1:1–16.
56. Figueiredo B, Costa R, Pacheco A, Pais Á. Mother-to-infant emotional involvement at birth. Matern Child Health J. 2008;13:539–49.
57. Fraiberg S, Adelson E, Shapiro V. Ghosts in the nursery: a psychoanalytic approach to the problems of impaired infant-mother relationships. J Am Acad Child Psychiat. 1975;14:387–421.
58. Fraiberg S, Adelson E, Shapiro V. Ghosts in the nursery: a psychoanalytic approach to the problems of impaired infant–mother relationships 1. In: Parent-infant psychodynamics. London: Routledge; 2018. p. 87–117.
59. Frankham LJ, Thorsteinsson EB, Bartik W. Factors associated with birth-related post-traumatic stress disorder symptoms and the subsequent impact of traumatic birth on mother–infant relationship quality. Behav Sci. 2024;14:808.
60. Fransson E, Sörensen F, Kallak TK, Ramklint M, Eckerdal P, Heimgärtner M, et al. Maternal perinatal depressive symptoms trajectories and impact on toddler behavior–the importance of symptom duration and maternal bonding. J Affect Disord. 2020;273:542–51.
61. Fraser LK, Cano-Ibáñez N, Amezcua-Prieto C, Khan KS, Lamont RF, Jørgensen JS. Prevalence of obstetric violence in high-income countries: a systematic review of mixed studies and meta-analysis of quantitative studies. Acta Obstet Gynecol Scand. 2025;104:13–28.
62. Gao Z, Zhou R, Chen Z, Qian H, Xu C, Gao M, Huang X. Dissecting causal relationships between gut microbiota, blood metabolites, and postpartum depression: a mendelian randomization study. J Stroke. 2024;25:350–60. https://assets-eu.researchsquare.com/files/rs-4911853/v1/f3dc8e47-7205-41a9-96f4-d8daa301d642.pdf?c=1725973186

63. Garapati J, Jajoo S, Aradhya D, Reddy LS, Dahiphale SM, Patel DJ. Postpartum mood disorders: insights into diagnosis, prevention, and treatment. Cureus. 2023;15:e42107.
64. Garcia LM, Jones J, Scandlyn J, Thumm EB, Shabot SC. The meaning of obstetric violence experiences: a qualitative content analysis of the break the silence campaign. Int J Nurs Stud. 2024;160:104911.
65. Garthus-Niegel S, Ayers S, Martini J, von Soest T, Eberhard-Gran M. The impact of postpartum post-traumatic stress disorder symptoms on child development: a population-based, 2-year follow-up study. Psychol Med. 2017;47:161–70.
66. Ghimire U, Papabathini SS, Kawuki J, Obore N, Musa TH. Depression during pregnancy and the risk of low birth weight, preterm birth and intrauterine growth restriction-an updated meta-analysis. Early Hum Dev. 2021;152:105243.
67. Grubb MD, Wilson CA, Zhang L, Liu G, Lee S, Monk C, Werner EA. Practical Resources for Effective Postpartum Parenting (PREPP): a randomized controlled trial of a novel parent-infant dyadic intervention to reduce symptoms of postpartum depression: RCT of the PREPP intervention for postpartum depression. Am J Obstet Gynecol MFM. 2024;6:101526.
68. Gurung R, Bask M. Does mistreatment during institutional childbirth increase the likelihood of experiencing postpartum depressive symptoms? A prospective cohort study in Nepal. Glob Health Action. 2024;17:2381312.
69. Haight SC, Byatt N, Simas TAM, Robbins CL, Ko JY. Recorded diagnoses of depression during delivery hospitalizations in the United States, 2000–2015. Obstet Gynecol. 2019;133:1216–23.
70. Hameed W, Khan B, Avan BI. The role of birth companionship in women's experiences of mistreatment during childbirth and postpartum depression. medRxiv. 2024;2024:11.
71. Harris R, Ayers S. What makes labour and birth traumatic? A survey of intrapartum 'hotspots'. Psychol Health. 2012;27:1166–77.
72. Hernández-Martínez A, Rodríguez-Almagro J, Molina-Alarcón M, Infante-Torres N, Manzanares MD, Martínez-Galiano JM. Postpartum post-traumatic stress disorder: associated perinatal factors and quality of life. J Affect Disord. 2019;249:143–50.
73. Hernández-Martínez A, Rodríguez-Almagro J, Molina-Alarcón M, Infante-Torres N, Rubio-Álvarez A, Martínez-Galiano JM. Perinatal factors related to post-traumatic stress disorder symptoms 1–5 years following birth. Women Birth. 2020;33:e129–35.
74. Heyne CS, Kazmierczak M, Souday R, Horesh D, Lambregtse-van den Berg M, Weigl T, et al. Prevalence and risk factors of birth-related posttraumatic stress among parents: a comparative systematic review and meta-analysis. Clin Psychol Rev. 2022;94:102157.
75. Hills J. Good times, bad times: the welfare myth of them and us. Bristol: Policy Press; 2017.
76. Hodnett ED. Pain and women's satisfaction with the experience of childbirth: a systematic review. Am J Obstet Gynecol. 2002;186:S160–72.
77. Horn SR, Charney DS, Feder A. Understanding resilience: new approaches for preventing and treating PTSD. Exp Neurol. 2016;284:119–32.
78. Horsch A, Garthus-Niegel S, Ayers S, Chandra P, Hartmann K, Vaisbuch E, Lalor J. Childbirth-related posttraumatic stress disorder: definition, risk factors, pathophysiology, diagnosis, prevention, and treatment. Am J Obstet Gynecol. 2024;230:S1116–27.
79. Horstmann RH, Seefeld L, Schellong J, Garthus-Niegel S. Treatment and counselling preferences of postpartum women with and without symptoms of (childbirth-related) PTSD: findings of the cross-sectional study INVITE. BMC Pregnancy Childbirth. 2024;24:885.
80. International Confederation of Midwives. Philosophy and model of midwifery care. 2014. https://www.internationalmidwives.org/assets/files/definitions-files/2018/06/eng-philosophy-and-model-of-midwifery-care.pdf.
81. Jacques M, Chantry AA, Evrard A, Lelong N, Le Ray C, ENP2021 Study Group, et al. Consent for interventions during childbirth: a national population-based study. Int J Gynecol Obstet. 2025;168:333–42.
82. Jehn V, Seefeld L, Schellong J, Garthus-Niegel S. Access and barriers to treatment and Counseling for postpartum women with and without symptoms of (CB-) PTSD within the cross-sectional study INVITE. 2024. https://assets-eu.researchsquare.com/files/rs-4743317/v1/dac42fda-d20a-4d30-94dd-7de4959aa831.pdf?c=1723100214.

83. Jemini Gashi L, Fetahu D, Sutaj B, Sahatqija M, Selimi X. Prevalence and predictors of postpartum depression in women in Kosovo. Women Health. 2025;21:1–10.
84. Jiaming W, Xin G, Jiajia D, Junjie P, Xue H, Yunchuan L, Yuanfang W. Psychological experience of patients with postpartum depression: a qualitative meta-synthesis. PLoS One. 2024;19:e0312996.
85. Jin W, Li B, Wang L, Zhu L, Chai S, Hou R. The causal association between gut microbiota and postpartum depression: a two-sample mendelian randomization study. Front Microbiol. 2024;15:1415237.
86. Kabale WD, Bekele GG, Gonfa DN, Yami AT. Person-centered maternity care during childbirth and associated factors at public hospitals in Central Ethiopia. SAGE Open Med. 2024;12:20503121241257790.
87. Kahalon R, Handelzalts JE. Investigating the under-recognition of childbirth-related post-traumatic stress disorder among the public and mental health professionals. J Anxiety Disord. 2024;106:102897.
88. Kahalon R, Klein V. Unmasking the role of dehumanization in obstetric violence. Psychol Violence. 2025;15:21–31.
89. Kalli A, Iliadou M, Palaska E, Louverdi S, Dagla C, Orovou E, Dagla M. Mothers' body appreciation and postpartum self-esteem in relation to body changes and breastfeeding difficulties: a cross-sectional survey in Cyprus. Nurs Rep. 2025;15:76.
90. Kamat ML, Kharde S. The satisfaction levels of post-natal mothers with the respectful maternity care (RMC) at a tertiary care hospital, Belagavi. Afr J Biomed Res. 2024;27:622–5.
91. Kaur R, Singh T, Kalaivani M, Yadav K, Gupta SK, Kant S. Respectful maternity care during childbirth among women in a rural area of northern India. Indian J Community Med. 2024;50:93–8.
92. Kc A, Chandna J, Acharya A, Gurung R, Andrew C, Skalkidou A. A longitudinal multicentric cohort study assessing infant neurodevelopment delay among women with persistent postpartum depression in Nepal. BMC Med. 2024;22:284.
93. Kirca N, Adibelli D. Effects of mother–infant skin-to-skin contact on postpartum depression: a systematic review. Perspect Psychiatr Care. 2021;57:2014–23.
94. Kohan S, Mena-Tudela D, Youseflu S. The impact of obstetric violence on postpartum quality of life through psychological pathways. Sci Rep. 2025;15:4799.
95. Krzeczkowski JE, Kousha KY, Savoy C, Schmidt LA, Van Lieshout RJ. Adaptive changes in infant emotion regulation persist three months following birthing parent receipt of cognitive behavioral therapy for postpartum depression. J Affect Disord. 2025;381:467–74.
96. Küçükkaya B, Cihangir Öztürk T, Erginler G, Temiz M, Erçel Ö. The effect of early-initiated half-swaddling and kangaroo care practices on maternal sleep quality and postpartum depression in term infants: a randomized controlled trial. Nurs Health Sci. 2025;27:e70066.
97. Kümpfel J, Weise V, Mack JT, Garthus-Niegel S. Parental relationship satisfaction, symptoms of depression and anger/hostility, and the moderating role of perceived social support—a prospective cohort study in the light of the COVID-19 pandemic. Front Psychol. 2025;16:1470241.
98. Lai X, Chen J, Lu D, Wang L, Lu X, Chen I, et al. The association between doula care and childbirth-related post-traumatic stress disorder symptoms: the mediating role of childbirth experience. Birth. 2024;52:243–51.
99. Le Bas G, Youssef G, Macdonald JA, Teague S, Mattick R, Honan I, et al. The role of antenatal and postnatal maternal bonding in infant development. J Am Acad Child Adolesc Psychiatry. 2022;61:820–9.
100. Leinweber J, Stramrood C. Improving birth experiences and provider interactions: expert opinion on critical links in maternity care. Eur J Midwifery. 2024;8:10-18332.
101. Leinweber J, Fonstein-Kuipers Y, Thomson G, Karlsdottis S, Nilsson C, Ekström-Bergström A, et al. Developing a woman-centred, inclusive definition of traumatic childbirth experiences. In: 21st international normal labour and birth research conference Denmark–Aarhus 2022. September 12th to 14th, 2022, p. 1.

102. Liu X, Wang S, Wang G. Prevalence and risk factors of postpartum depression in women: a systematic review and meta-analysis. J Clin Nurs. 2022;31:2665–77.
103. Lubis PN, Saputra M, Rabbani MW. A systematic review of the benefits of breastfeeding against postpartum depression in low-middle-income countries. J Ment Health. 2024;35:305–17.
104. Lubotzky-Gete S, Ornoy A, Grotto I, Calderon-Margalit R. Postpartum depression and infant development up to 24 months: a nationwide population-based study. J Affect Disord. 2021;285:136–43.
105. Madigan S, Oatley H, Racine N, Fearon RP, Schumacher L, Akbari E, et al. A meta-analysis of maternal prenatal depression and anxiety on child socioemotional development. J Am Acad Child Adolesc Psychiatry. 2018;57:645–57.
106. Martínez-Velasco IG, Jiménez-López R, Gallego-Mora MF, Basilio-Reyes A, Cisneros-Martínez E, Guillén-González MA, Angulo-Arrieta AP. Obstetric violence: women perception during labor in two hospitals in Nahua-Mixteca zone. Perinatol Reprod Hum. 2024;38:1–6.
107. Matyas M, Apanasewicz A, Krzystek-Korpacka M, Jamrozik N, Cierniak A, Babiszewska-Aksamit M, Ziomkiewicz A. The association between maternal stress and human milk concentrations of cortisol and prolactin. Sci Rep. 2024;14:28115.
108. Mazúchová L, Lochmannová A, Hollins Martin CJ, Martin CR. Translation and psychometric validation of the Slovak Partner version of the Birth Satisfaction Scale-Revised (BSS-R). J Reprod Infant Psychol. 2025:1–14. https://doi.org/10.1080/02646838.2025.2508482.
109. MBRRACE-UK. Saving lives, improving mothers' care 2024 – lessons learned to inform maternity care from the UK and Ireland Confidential Enquiries into Maternal Deaths and Morbidity 2020–22. 2024. https://www.npeu.ox.ac.uk/mbrrace-uk/reports/maternal-reports/maternal-report-2020-2022.
110. Meins E, Fernyhough C, Fradley E, Tuckey M. Rethinking maternal sensitivity: mothers' comments on infants' mental processes predict security of attachment at 12 months. J Child Psychol Psychiatry Allied Discip. 2001;42:637–48.
111. Meins E, Fernyhough C, de Rosnay M, Arnott B, Leekam SR, Turner M. Mind-mindedness as a multidimensional construct: appropriate and nonattuned mind-related comments independently predict infant–mother attachment in a socially diverse sample. Infancy. 2012;17:393–415.
112. Meltzer-Brody S, Howard LM, Bergink V, Vigod S, Jones I, Munk-Olsen T, et al. Postpartum psychiatric disorders. Nat Rev Dis Prim. 2018;4:1–18.
113. Messerli-Bürgy N, Sandoz V, Deforge C, Lacroix A, Sekarski N, Horsch A. Stress responses of infants and mothers to a still-face paradigm after traumatic childbirth. Psychoneuroendocrinology. 2024;171:107222.
114. Mills BC, Page LA. The growth of human love and commitment. In: The new midwifery: science and sensitivity in practice. Edinburgh: Churchill Livingstone; 2000. p. 223–44.
115. Nakić Radoš S, Matijaš M, Anđelinović M, Čartolovni A, Ayers S. The role of posttraumatic stress and depression symptoms in mother-infant bonding. J Affect Disord. 2020;268:134–40.
116. Nakić Radoš S, Brekalo M, Žutić M, Matijaš M, Habek D, Marton I, et al. Prospective study of individual characteristics and posttraumatic stress disorder (PTSD) symptoms following childbirth: birth satisfaction as a moderator. Psychol Trauma Theory Res Pract Policy. 2024. https://psycnet.apa.org/record/2025-43882-001.
117. Nazzari S, Fearon P, Rice F, Dottori N, Ciceri F, Molteni M, Frigerio A. Beyond the HPA-axis: exploring maternal prenatal influences on birth outcomes and stress reactivity. Psychoneuroendocrinology. 2019;101:253–62.
118. Nazzari S, Pili MP, Günay Y, Provenzi L. Pandemic babies: a systematic review of the association between maternal pandemic-related stress during pregnancy and infant development. Neurosci Biobehav Rev. 2024;162:105723.
119. Nguyen HTM, Luu DP, Quyet TN, Hoang H, Tran MNP, Le MTP. Postpartum depression in mothers of infants under 12 months at Hai Duong Pediatric hospital and its association on infant health. MedPharmRes. 2024;8:265–73.

120. Nieto L, Lara MA, Navarrete L, Manzo G. Infant temperament and perinatal depressive and anxiety symptoms in Mexican women. Sex Reprod Healthc. 2019;21:39–45.
121. Nordin-Remberger C, Johansson M, Lindelöf KS, Wells MB. Support needs, barriers, and facilitators for fathers with fear of childbirth in Sweden: a mixed-method study. Am J Mens Health. 2024;18:15579883241272057.
122. Nove A, Boyce M, Neal S, Homer CS, Lavender T, Matthews Z, Downe S. Increasing the number of midwives is necessary but not sufficient: using global data to support the case for investment in both midwife availability and the enabling work environment in low-and middle-income countries. Hum Resour Health. 2024;22:54.
123. O'Brien AP, McNeil KA, Fletcher R, Conrad A, Wilson AJ, Jones D, Chan SW. New fathers' perinatal depression and anxiety—treatment options: an integrative review. Am J Mens Health. 2017;11:863–76.
124. O'Reilly E, Buchanan K, Bayes S. Emotional safety in maternity care: an evolutionary concept analysis. Midwifery. 2024;140:104220.
125. Olde E, van der Hart O, Kleber R, Van Son M. Posttraumatic stress following childbirth: a review. Clin Psychol Rev. 2006;26:1–16.
126. Ollas-Skogster D, Korja R, Yada A, Mainela-Arnold E, Karlsson H, Bridgett DJ, et al. Maternal emotional availability supports child communicative development regardless of child temperament—findings from the FinnBrain birth cohort study. Infancy. 2025;30:e12649.
127. Ormsby SM, Keedle H, Dahlen HG. Women's reflections on induction of labour and birthing interventions and what they would do differently next time: a content analysis. Midwifery. 2024;140:104201.
128. Oyetunji A, Chandra P. Postpartum stress and infant outcome: a review of current literature. Psychiatry Res. 2020;284:112769.
129. Öz T, Seven ZD, İrevül G. The relationship between postpartum depression and maternal attachment in Primiparous women. J Mod Nurs Pract Res. 2024;4:12.
130. Paiz JC, de Jezus Castro SM, Giugliani ERJ, dos Santos Ahne SM, Aqua CBD, Giugliani C. Association between mistreatment of women during childbirth and symptoms suggestive of postpartum depression. BMC Pregnancy Childbirth. 2022;22:664.
131. Parfitt YM, Ayers S. The effect of post-natal symptoms of post-traumatic stress and depression on the couple's relationship and parent–baby bond. J Reprod Infant Psychol. 2009;27:127–42.
132. Parfitt Y, Pike A, Ayers S. Infant developmental outcomes: a family systems perspective. Infant Child Dev. 2014;23:353–73.
133. Paul IM, Downs DS, Schaefer EW, Beiler JS, Weisman CS. Postpartum anxiety and maternal-infant health outcomes. Pediatrics. 2013;131:e1218–24.
134. de Paula Eduardo JAF, de Rezende MG, Menezes PR, Del-Ben CM. Preterm birth as a risk factor for postpartum depression: a systematic review and meta-analysis. J Affect Disord. 2019;259:392–403.
135. Peipert A, Ward MJ, Miller ML. Narrative exposure therapy for a traumatic birth experience with the non-birthing parent: a single case study. Cogn Behav Pract. 2024. https://doi.org/10.1016/j.cbpra.2024.05.006.
136. Perry NB, Donzella B, Troy MF, Barnes AJ. Mother and child hair cortisol during the COVID-19 pandemic: associations among physiological stress, pandemic-related behaviors, and child emotional-behavioral health. Psychoneuroendocrinology. 2022;137:105656.
137. Power C, Weise V, Mack JT, Karl M, Garthus-Niegel S. Does parental mental health mediate the association between parents' perceived stress and parent-infant bonding during the early COVID-19 pandemic? Early Hum Dev. 2024;189:105931.
138. Prenoveau JM, Craske MG, West V, Giannakakis A, Zioga M, Lehtonen A, Davies B, Netsi E, Cardy J, Coope P, Murray L, Stein A. Maternal postnatal depression and anxiety and their association with child emotional negativity and behavior problems at two years. Dev Psychol. 2017;53:50–62.
139. Qi W, Wei Z, Lv H, Zhao J, Hu Y, Wang Y, et al. Postpartum depression and maternal-infant bonding: the mediating role of mentalizing and parenting self-efficacy. BMC Pregnancy Childbirth. 2025;25:667.

140. Quattrocchi P. Obstetric violence in the European Union: situational analysis and policy recommendations. 2024. https://air.uniud.it/handle/11390/1277404.
141. Rai S, Pathak A, Sharma I. Postpartum psychiatric disorders: early diagnosis and management. Indian J Psychiatry. 2015;57:S216–21.
142. Rastogi K, Weerts EM, Ellis JD. Oxytocin as a treatment for alcohol use disorder and heavy drinking: a narrative review. Exp Clin Psychopharmacol. 2024;32:625–38.
143. Reed R, Sharman R, Inglis C. Women's descriptions of childbirth trauma relating to care provider actions and interactions. BMC Pregnancy Childbirth. 2017;17:1–10.
144. Rehberg F, Rihm L, Göbel A, Thiel F, Büechl VC, Even M, Garthus-Niegel S. Perinatal PTSD and the mother-infant bond: a systematic review and meta-analysis. J Anxiety Disord. 2025;114:103050.
145. Reich JW, Zautra AJ, Hall JS, editors. Handbook of adult resilience. New York: Guilford Press; 2010.
146. Robinson KA, Atlas RO, Storr CL, Gaitens JM, Blanchard M, Ogbolu Y. Burnout among nurses, midwives, and physicians in maternity care exposed to traumatic childbirth events. MCN Am J Matern Child Nurs. 2024;49:332–40.
147. Rosen NO, Bailey K, Muise A. Degree and direction of sexual desire discrepancy are linked to sexual and relationship satisfaction in couples transitioning to parenthood. J Sex Res. 2018;55:214–25.
148. Rosen NO, Dawson SJ, Leonhardt ND, Vannier SA, Impett EA. Trajectories of sexual well-being among couples in the transition to parenthood. J Fam Psychol. 2021;35:523.
149. Rosen NO, Vannier SA, Johnson MD, McCarthy L, Impett EA. Unmet and exceeded expectations for sexual concerns across the transition to parenthood. J Sex Res. 2023;60:1235–46.
150. Rousseau S, Katz D, Schussheim A, Frenkel TI. Intergenerational transmission of maternal prenatal anxiety to infant fearfulness: the mediating role of mother-infant bonding. Arch Womens Ment Health. 2024;28:157–71.
151. Roy AS, Chaillet N. Relation between initiation of breastfeeding success and postpartum depression. J Obstet Gynaecol Can. 2024;46:102666.
152. Sasayama D, Owa T, Kudo T, Kaneko W, Makita M, Kuge R, et al. Postpartum maternal depression, mother-to-infant bonding, and their association with child difficulties in sixth grade. Arch Womens Mental Health. 2025:1–12. https://doi.org/10.1007/s00737-025-01585-y.
153. Snyder S. The experience of birth professionals who witness obstetric violence during childbirth. Affilia. 2024;40:304–19. https://doi.org/10.1177/08861099241293416.
154. Specht L, Freiberg A, Mojahed A, Garthus-Niegel S, Schellong J. Adrenocortical deviations and adverse clinical outcomes in children and adolescents exposed to interparental intimate partner violence: a systematic review. Neurosci Biobehav Rev. 2024;165:105866.
155. Sridhar H, Kishore MT, Chandra PS. Child developmental outcomes associated with postpartum depression and anxiety in low and middle-income countries: a systematic review. Arch Womens Ment Health. 2024;28:113–28.
156. Stadlmayr W, Chicherio R, Giovannini-Spinelli M, Amsler F. Development of the Swiss Postpartum Screening Tool (SPST) for the early detection of postpartum depression and acute stress reaction. Med Res Arch. 2025;13. https://doi.org/10.18103/mra.v13i5.6302.
157. Stoodley C, McKellar L, Ziaian T, Steen M, Fereday J, Gwilt I. The role of midwives in supporting the development of the mother-infant relationship: a scoping review. BMC Psychol. 2023;11:71.
158. Stuijfzand S, Garthus-Niegel S, Horsch A. Parental birth-related PTSD symptoms and bonding in the early postpartum period: a prospective population- based cohort study. Front Psychiat. 2020;11:570727.
159. Swift EM, Guðmundsdóttir F, Einarsdóttir K, Sigurðardóttir VL. Birth satisfaction and childbirth related PTSD among women in Iceland: a population-based study. Sex Reprod Healthc. 2024;42:101037.
160. Toprak FÜ, Erenel AŞ. The effect of kangaroo care practice after caesarean section on paternal-newborn interaction: a mixed-methods study in Turkey. Midwifery. 2022;115:103489.

161. Uncu B, Gök H. The effect of newborn massage training on maternal attachment and postpartum depression: randomized controlled trial. Nurs Health Sci. 2025;27:e70112.
162. Uvnäs-Moberg K. Why oxytocin matters, vol. 16. London: Pinter & Martin Ltd.; 2019.
163. Van Sieleghem S, Danckaerts M, Rieken R, Okkerse JM, de Jonge E, Bramer WM, Lambregtse-van den Berg MP. Childbirth related PTSD and its association with infant outcome: a systematic review. Early Hum Dev. 2022;174:105667.
164. Vega-Sanz M, Berastegui A, Sanchez-Lopez A. Perinatal posttraumatic stress disorder as a predictor of mother-child bonding quality 8 months after childbirth: a longitudinal study. BMC Pregnancy Childbirth. 2024;24:389.
165. Vega-Sanz M, Berastegui A, Sanchez-Lopez A. Longitudinal influences on maternal–infant bonding at 18 months postpartum: the predictive role of perinatal and postpartum depression and childbirth trauma. J Clin Med. 2025;14:3424.
166. Villarmea S, Kelly B. Barriers to establishing shared decision-making in childbirth: unveiling epistemic stereotypes about women in labour. J Eval Clin Pract. 2020;26:515–9.
167. Walter MH, Abele H, Plappert CF. The role of oxytocin and the effect of stress during childbirth: neurobiological basics and implications for mother and child. Front Endocrinol. 2021;12:742236.
168. Wang M, Song Q, Xu J, Hu Z, Gong Y, Lee AC, Chen Q. Continuous support during labour in childbirth: a cross-sectional study in a university teaching hospital in Shanghai, China. BMC Pregnancy Childbirth. 2018;18:1–7.
169. Wang D, Li YL, Qiu D, Xiao SY. Factors influencing paternal postpartum depression: a systematic review and meta-analysis. J Affect Disord. 2021;293:51–63.
170. Wang Z, Liu J, Shuai H, Cai Z, Fu X, Liu Y, et al. Mapping global prevalence of depression among postpartum women. Transl Psychiatry. 2021;11:543.
171. Wang Y, Lu H, Zhang F, Gu J. Path analysis of the factors associated with postpartum depression symptoms in postpartum women. J Psychiatr Res. 2025;182:195–203.
172. Weber AM, Burkett K, Voos KC. Care of the parents. In: Fanaroff AA, Fanaroff JM, editors. Klaus and Fanaroff's care of the high-risk neonate. 8th ed. Philadelphia: Elsevier; 2025. p. 143–58.
173. Webb R, Uddin N, Constantinou G, Cheyne H, Ayers S. Prevalence of Birth Trauma and Childbirth-Related Post-Traumatic Stress Disorder in UK Women: Results from the International Survey of Childbirth-Related Trauma. Women's Reproductive Health. 2025;25:1–2.
174. Wheeler A, Farrington S, Sweeting F, Brown A, Mayers A. Perceived pressures and mental health of breastfeeding mothers: a qualitative descriptive study. Healthcare. 2024;12:1794.
175. World Health Organization (2018). World Health Organization recommendations: Intrapartum care for a positive childbirth experience. https://www.who.int/reproductivehealth/intrapartum-care/en/.
176. Yalley AA, Jarašiūnaitė-Fedosejeva G, Kömürcü-Akik B, de Abreu L. Addressing obstetric violence: a scoping review of interventions in healthcare and their impact on maternal care quality. Front Public Health. 2024;12:1388858.
177. Yalnız Dilcen H, Ada G, Bulut E. Development and psychometric analysis of the traumatic childbirth perception scale in men. Curr Psychol. 2025;44:6481–94. https://doi.org/10.1007/s12144-025-07612-6.
178. Yildiz PD, Ayers S, Phillips L. The prevalence of posttraumatic stress disorder in pregnancy and after birth: a systematic review and meta-analysis. J Affect Disord. 2017;208:634–45.
179. Zhang K, He L, Li Z, Ding R, Han X, Chen B, et al. Bridging neurobiological insights and clinical biomarkers in postpartum depression: a narrative review. Int J Mol Sci. 2024;25:8835.
180. Zhang Y, Liu X, Liu M, Li M, Chen P, Yan G, et al. Multidimensional influencing factors of postpartum depression based on the perspective of the entire reproductive cycle: evidence from western province of China. Soc Psychiatry Psychiatr Epidemiol. 2024;59:2041–8.
181. Zhao XH, Zhang ZH. Risk factors for postpartum depression: an evidence-based systematic review of systematic reviews and meta-analyses. Asian J Psychiatr. 2020;53:102353.
182. Zhou L, Tang L, Zhou C, Wen SW, Krewski D, Xie RH. Association of maternal postpartum depression symptoms with infant neurodevelopment and gut microbiota. Front Psychol. 2024;15:1385229.

Maternity Care Providers' Perceptions of Childbirth and Baby Behaviour

5.1 Introduction to the Study

This chapter explores whether health professionals and doulas who observe, support and care for mother and baby during and after childbirth perceive any connections between the birth experience and early mother and baby behaviour, and—if they think there's a link—what they consider to be the reasons behind this. Do they observe differences in baby behaviour based on how they're born? And, if so, are these differences solely due to the physical birth experience, or do the mother's perceptions of the birth matter, too?

An adapted version of this study was published in 2019 in the journal *Midwifery*:

Power, C., Williams, C., & Brown, A. (2019). Does childbirth experience affect infant behaviour? Exploring the perceptions of maternity care providers. *Midwifery, 78*, 131–139.

To carry out this study, I interviewed a total of 18 health professionals and doulas who were currently working with mothers and babies during and after childbirth in the South-West regions of England and Wales. Face-to-face interviews with open-ended questions, designed not to lead the participants, were chosen as the most fitting way to collect the rich, in-depth data needed to gain some initial insights into whether and, if so, how the birth experience might affect the baby. As with all three studies presented in the book, the study was designed following the ethical standards outlined in the 1964 Declaration of Helsinki [24] and the British Psychological Society's [8] Code of Ethics and Conduct. This meant that all participants felt assured that their data would be stored and used in a way that respected their confidentiality and anonymity, and they had the right to withdraw at any point if they changed their minds. Doctors were not included as, in the UK, their role in childbirth is generally only required if there are complications. Although, in hindsight, I would have liked to also interview obstetricians, paediatricians and neonatologists, three types of participants were chosen based on the extended time they spend with mothers and babies during and after childbirth and the diverse range of mothers and babies they oversee. These were 11 midwives (6 hospital-based and five working in the community), four health visitors (who care for mother and baby postnatally) and three doulas (who offer emotional support to mother and baby from pregnancy through childbirth to the early postnatal period). The average time maternity care providers had spent practising within the UK's National Health Service (NHS) was approximately 15 years, with a range of 1–26 years.

The maternity care providers were asked two main questions. First, whether they thought a baby's behaviour was related to how they were born and, if so, how. Second, whether they believed the mother's birth experience might affect her feelings and behaviour towards the baby. The open-ended nature of the questions allowed midwives, health visitors and doulas to speak for as long as they wanted in as much detail as they wished, fully exploring their perceptions and beliefs about childbirth and baby behaviour. The interviews took place in cottage hospitals, health centres, midwives' homes or their local café. They often evolved into conversations as I asked many follow-up questions, building on their initial responses. After the interviews had all taken place, the recordings were transcribed and coded thematically and reflexively according to the patterns or "themes" that arose in the data [6]. For those unfamiliar with qualitative thematic analysis, it may be helpful to think of the overarching themes as trees standing side by side in a wood, with their roots intertwined. The themes can be likened to branches and the subthemes to twigs or offshoots of the larger branches.

All participants were assigned a pseudonym in place of their real names, and any references to hospitals or midwife-led units were also removed to ensure confidentiality and anonymity. Themes were chosen for their connection to the research questions, their perceived importance to the participant, their prevalence in the data, or how frequently they arose. I remain bowled over and forever grateful for the insights and wisdom given so openly and honestly by these midwives, health visitors and doulas. Without a doubt, their experiences and observations based on caring for thousands of women from all walks of life provided truly invaluable insights into how the mother and baby pair might be affected by their shared birth experience.

5.2 What the Interviews Uncovered About Birth, Bonding and Baby Behaviour

The interviews were recorded and transcribed verbatim, meaning that the excerpts of the conversations shared here are written exactly as they were spoken. The results were divided into two main sections or "overarching themes" [6]:

1. **The baby's response to childbirth**—*direct* birth impacts on baby behaviour.
2. **The mother's response to childbirth**—the perceived impact of mothers' physical and psychological birth experiences on how they feel and behave towards their baby, and how this *indirectly* affects the baby, as expressed through early baby behaviour.

5.2.1 The Baby's Response to Childbirth

The first part of the study aimed to determine whether midwives, health visitors and doulas believed baby behaviour is directly affected by their birth. To begin, the 18 maternity care providers were asked: :

In your opinion, how, if at all, do you think a baby's behaviour may be influenced by his or her experience of being born?

Two main themes emerged in response to the perceptions of health professionals and doulas regarding how childbirth may directly impact baby behaviour: *The Physical Birth Process* and *Early Postnatal Moments*. Figure 5.1 presents a summary of the themes and subthemes before we discuss each one in turn. Maternity care providers' quotes are included throughout the chapter to illustrate the interesting and insightful points they made.

Introduction to the Findings
All but one of the 18 maternity care providers believed that the physical birth experience influences early infant behaviour and the baby's developing temperament. An easy, straightforward birth with no complications or interventions was said to encourage an "easy, settled and soothable" baby behavioural style, whereas more challenging births were thought to produce babies prone to "irritable, tense, fussy, needy and unsettled" behaviour who are difficult to soothe. However, this relationship between childbirth and baby behaviour was perceived as complex. The physical birth experience could impact the baby's behaviour, but an unsettled baby may also influence the way family members interact and bond with them.

> The birth does affect the baby and then of course it does have, you know, an effect on the physical and mental wellbeing and the stability of the family as well so that affects how the baby's being cared for and how, you know, they generally attach and bond with that newborn. (Health Visitor Ruth)

The birth itself, however, was considered only one of many influential factors affecting baby behaviour postnatally.

> I think it's easy to assume that the birth experience a baby goes through has a huge impact on its temperament or its behaviour after that point, or its feelings when actually it's one of many elements, I think. (Midwife Rebecca)

The Physical Birth Process
The physical experience of being born was widely believed to affect newborn babies' behaviour. This included any complications that may arise or medical interventions that take place, but also the mother's and baby's intricately intertwined hormonal states and pain relief used during labour.

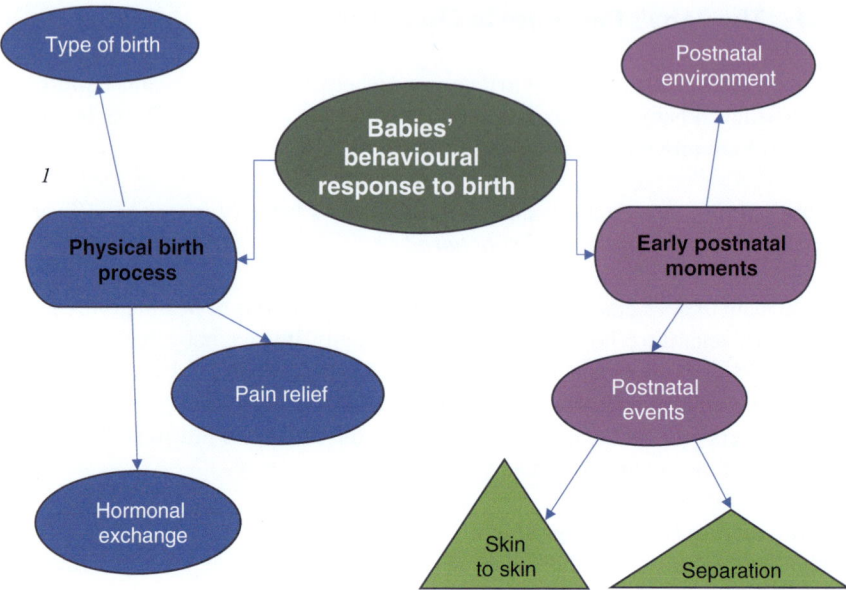

Fig. 5.1 The baby's response to childbirth

Figure key

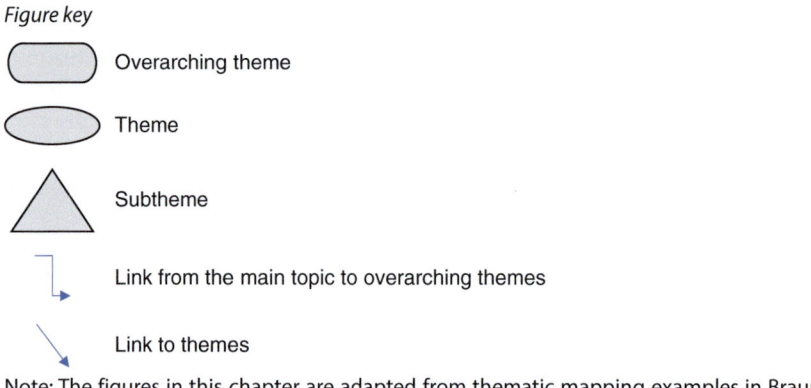

Note: The figures in this chapter are adapted from thematic mapping examples in Braun and Clarke's [6] book on Thematic Analysis and from a paper by Byrne [10]

Type of Birth

Most participants felt that the predictability of giving birth "naturally" in the way the body was designed to do was likely to create more settled newborn behaviour.

> I think there's something about the natural experience of the progression of labour, I think, which is somehow a bit more predictable for a baby. (Health Visitor Debbie)

Waterbirths were perceived as a gentle way to be born, with a calming effect on the baby as they emerge into the world.

5.2 What the Interviews Uncovered About Birth, Bonding and Baby Behaviour

> A lot of the time you do see babies that are born, particularly in water, they do seem very settled. It's almost like they haven't realised that they've been born. (Midwife Jane)

In contrast, medical interventions—in particular, instrumental births using forceps or ventouse—were considered to have a negative impact on baby behaviour due to the pain and discomfort they caused during and after the birth.

> There are obvious cases where if the baby's been pulled out by forceps and had a shoulder dystocia on the way, and come out with literally birth trauma, you know, a massive bruise on its face and a palsy and a broken clavicle, then clearly that baby is going to be uncomfortable and probably fractious and probably not feed well. In those cases, clearly the birth experience that a baby goes through affects what it then goes on to experience and how it then behaves. (Midwife Rebecca)

While some maternity care providers thought these physical birth impacts might only last a few days, others felt they could take much longer to recover from. Sensitive caregiving was considered helpful in this scenario, and giving the baby lots of gentle skin-to-skin care may help to mitigate some of the impacts of a traumatic birth.

> Some effects will continue for a long time afterwards, I think, in terms of trauma… Holding them, picking them up and touching them when they have a headache, or they've been pulled out and they've got obvious bruising—they can find that very painful. They don't want to be handled or feed but actually sometimes they just need to be with their mum or their dad skin to skin, and that can be in itself very soothing. (Midwife Sally)

Babies who were born by *elective* caesarean section were said to be calmer, as this was generally not a traumatic experience. However, some argued that being "whipped out" so abruptly could make adjusting to the outside world more difficult. In contrast to these planned caesareans, long, arduous labours followed by an *emergency* caesarean section were seen as traumatic for the baby.

> When you're looking at complications, interventions such as ventouse delivery, forceps delivery, and Caesarean sections, heart dips and so forth, you know, trauma in the last couple of minutes of the delivery, obviously that is going to have some sort of impact on the way the baby is. (Health Visitor Ruth)

The position of a baby in the womb was considered to influence physical outcomes. Midwife Rebecca explained how babies who are "malpositioned" may experience a more prolonged labour, sometimes resulting in an instrumental delivery. Even when this didn't occur, babies could still enter the world with pain and discomfort due to their positioning in the womb before birth.

> So, whether you know, even if the baby's not had an instrumental delivery, it can perhaps, you know, it can be in a slightly awkward position in pregnancy or birth. It means it comes out and has a bit of a neck ache and a bit of a headache…. (Midwife Rebecca)

Babies were said to be more likely to have "difficult" early behaviour following a long or complicated labour and birth. However, Health Visitor Emma noted that faster births may come with their own set of problems.

> It seems to be more of the quick delivery ones that seem to sort of arrive in a state of shock... because they sometimes perhaps are a little bit more fretful, and sometimes perhaps a little bit more difficult to feed. (Health Visitor Emma)

Hormonal Exchange

Midwife Sally spoke about the mysterious hormonal "dance" that takes place between mother and baby during pregnancy and labour—a mother-baby interaction which scientists acknowledge, yet still do not completely understand. Sally felt that mothers and babies experiencing a challenging, speedy or surgical birth (by caesarean section) might lack the opportunity to "build up" the natural birthing hormones conducive to positive outcomes.

> It's like a dance between the mums and babies, both of them, but if the baby hasn't had any of that, you know, the hormones or any of the adrenaline, any of the head moulding or anything else that happens in the process of birth, and it's just whipped out, then I think it could affect them. (Midwife Sally)

The midwives, health visitors and doulas all spoke about how birth hormones, such as oxytocin, play a central role in positive mother and baby outcomes. Although a certain amount of adrenaline is needed for the birth itself, releasing too many stress hormones such as cortisol during a challenging labour was thought to dysregulate newborn baby behaviour.

> We know that cortisol is passed through into the bloodstream of the baby because obviously the baby's still inside, and whatever the birth experience, if there's been a trauma of sorts, then the adults will be experiencing stress, and babies are very much in tune with stress and stressors. (Health Visitor Ruth)

Pain Relief

Midwives, health visitors and doulas all spoke about the positive and negative aspects of pharmacological pain relief. Some mentioned that babies were more likely to be sleepy, irritable and difficult to feed after using pethidine during labour.

> Things like pethidine for pain control, you know, they're quite strong opiates... those babies can be quite difficult to attach onto the breast, for instance, they're quite sluggish, you know, because of the effects of the drugs, so there are definite physical effects that can affect a baby's attachment and behaviour. (Health Visitor Ruth)

One midwife, joking that her collegial nickname was "No Pethidine Suzie", mentioned the psychological impacts of a fretful baby. She firmly believed that if babies are born with pethidine in their system and refuse to breastfeed, this could be a source of great distress for both mother and baby.

> The baby's sleepy and uninterested or just irritable after the birth... Nowadays, everyone ends up expressing and syringe feeding the babies, which is disempowering for the mothers and their ability to breastfeed... The mothers may get really distressed if they feel they can't feed their baby, and the baby picks up on their distress, and so the baby gets distressed. (Midwife Suzie)

To sum up this theme of the physical birth process, although one midwife didn't see any direct connections between the mother's physical birth experience and baby behaviour, there was a consensus among the 17 other maternity care providers that birth may have a profound physiological impact on the baby.

Early Postnatal Moments
The second central theme within this section, regarding the impacts of childbirth on baby behaviour, relates to the postnatal environment, postnatal occurrences and how the mother and baby initially respond to one another. Important events, including skin-to-skin care, bonding, breastfeeding and what happens when mother and baby are separated, were all spoken about at length.

Postnatal Environment
Alongside reflecting their mother's mood, midwives, health visitors and doulas all believed the newborn baby responds to their birth environment as soon as they are born. Whether the atmosphere is calm and relaxed or tense and dramatic, they seem to react and behave accordingly.

> I think we underestimate how much they pick up on atmosphere, you know, and how raised voices and the environment generally raised, bright lights and, you know, stressful environment; I think they clearly, very clearly respond incredibly to a calmer environment, dimmed lights, not too much noise. (Midwife Rebecca)

Postnatal Events
As we saw in earlier chapters, skin-to-skin care and separation are two mutually opposing events that make a significant difference to the wellbeing of mother and baby during the early postnatal period. If a separation of mother and baby occurs, for whatever reason, it makes skin-to-skin care very difficult, if not impossible. This can have multiple short- and long-term consequences for the mother-baby pair and their ability to feel relaxed and safe (see Chap. 3). It could also affect the bonding process that is so essential to positive infant outcomes.

Skin-to-Skin
Early skin-to-skin contact between mother and baby was considered fundamental to achieving positive outcomes, as it calms and soothes both mother and baby after the birth process, while facilitating the first steps towards successful bonding and breastfeeding. This close and special time with the baby was also believed to help mothers process and recover from the birth, particularly if they are struggling with depression or coming to terms with difficult events that may have occurred.

> The mothers who are battling with postnatal depression, with detachment, distance from babies, I always make sure with them, you know, I'm saying, 'You do skin to skin as often as you can' because in my head I think if I can get some oxytocin going somewhere, you know, maybe that mothering instinct to want to hold, to nurture, love, care for, protect, will kick in and override all of that cortisol and whatever else is swimming around her brain. (Health Visitor Emma)

Separation

Unfortunately, however, mothers and babies are still frequently separated during the early hours post-birth, sometimes for medical reasons, or sometimes to relieve a mother so she can catch up on some sleep if she is not coping well with the busy, noisy hospital environment. Midwife Annie talked about how sad it was to see a newborn baby "*in a fish bowl*" across the room from his mother, who lay helpless in a hospital bed, while Doula Rachel quoted a mother she had cared for saying, "Everyone held my baby before me".

> The idea is that babies always stay in the same place as the mothers while they're in hospital, but again if, maybe not because of the trauma, maybe not because of the birth itself, I think because of the hospital environment which is quite a sort of noisy, disruptive environment, you find a lot of mums do end up having babies taken away at night. So sometimes babies will come out and stay with the midwives overnight for one or two hours, which does give the mother time to sleep, but it's still a separation. (Midwife Adele)

Maternity care providers acknowledged that babies want to remain close to their mother and that this eases their transition from the warmth and comfort of the womb to the cold, harsh exterior world of intense lights, sounds and vibrations. Separation from their mother was said to make babies fractious and sometimes extremely distressed.

> The baby hasn't read the book (laughs)… so they're going to want to sleep with you and want to feed every hour and a half and they're not going to want to be put down. (Health Visitor Emma)

5.2.2 The Mother's Response to Childbirth

While the first part of the study explored how childbirth might *directly* impact baby behaviour, the second part sought to understand how mothers' childbirth experiences may *indirectly* influence their babies' behavioural style. In this section, we therefore explore what maternity care providers had to say about how the birth experience—as well as how mothers perceive it and try to recover from it during the postnatal period—can influence mothers' feelings and behaviour towards their baby and subsequently how the baby responds.

5.2 What the Interviews Uncovered About Birth, Bonding and Baby Behaviour

The second interview question was:

In your opinion, how, if at all, do you think a mother's experience of childbirth affects her feelings and behaviour towards her baby?

Maternity care providers' responses to this question generated four new themes: *childbirth experience, mothers' expectations and postnatal perceptions, relationships and why they matter* and *postnatal maternal wellbeing*. Once again, each theme and subtheme is described with quotes to illustrate the experiences, perceptions, attitudes and beliefs of midwives, health visitors and doulas. See Fig. 5.2 for a summary of the themes and subthemes for this section.

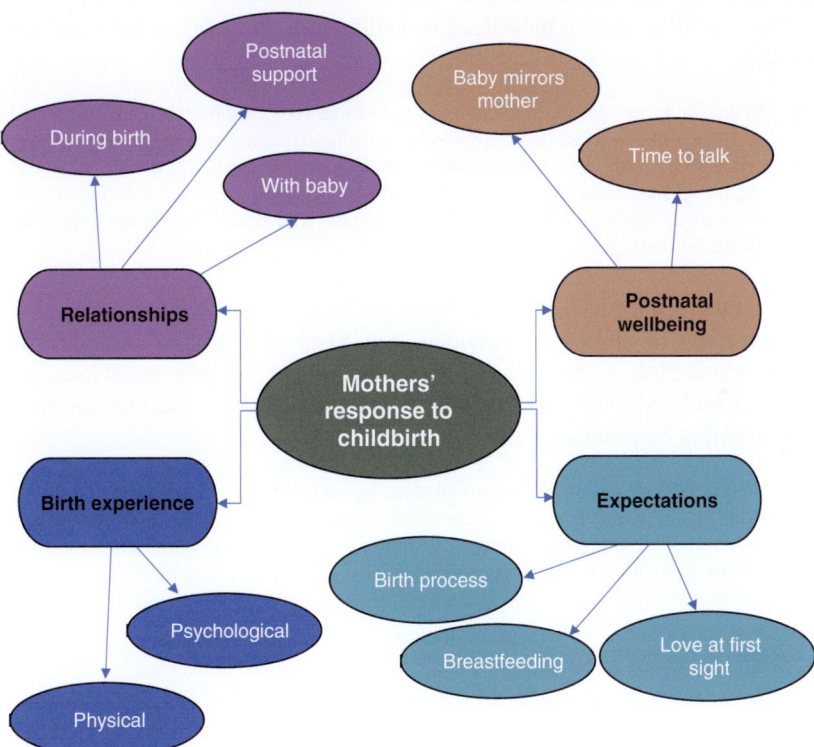

Fig. 5.2 The mother's response to childbirth

Figure key

◯ Theme

◯ Subtheme

↳ Link from main topic to overarching themes

↘ Link to themes

Birth Experience

All 18 participants believed the mother's physical and psychological birth experience could influence the way she perceives and interacts with her baby and the way the baby responds to the mother's behaviour.

Physical Birth Experience

Health professionals believed the mother's feelings and behaviour towards the baby could be affected by physiological birth variables (such as stress hormones and pain), and therefore that the physical birth experience may influence how she cares for the baby afterwards. Midwives talked about how obstetric interventions increase the mother's sense of pain and exhaustion, with a knock-on effect on mother-baby interactions and feeding decisions. A very long or medicalised birth may therefore have a negative impact on breastfeeding and bonding behaviours between mother and baby.

> If birth does involve a lot of intervention or has been a very long or exhausting process, I think women will often find themselves too physically exhausted to interact with the baby as much as they would have liked to and I witness that a lot, especially after a Caesarean section, the physical exhaustion can be quite sort of detrimental and they can be much more likely to want the midwife to take the baby, or more likely to bottle-feed as well rather than breastfeed. (Midwife Adele)

The mother's hormonal state was known to be a significant factor in the physiological aspects of childbirth. Oxytocin was associated with a straightforward, uncomplicated birth. Alongside directly calming effects on baby behaviour, oxytocin was considered important for mother-infant bonding and facilitating sensitive maternal caring by promoting "motherly love".

> Oxytocin is probably far more important than we really think… It's actually extremely important for the fourth trimester (after birth) where oxytocin is needed for mother and child bonding, promoting breastfeeding, promoting motherly love, which is ultimately a survival mechanism for the baby. (Doula Rachel)

Psychological Birth Experience

Psychological aspects of childbirth were also believed to affect bonding and breastfeeding. If these important mother-baby behaviours didn't go according to plan, this could lead to self-blame, shame and guilt, contributing to feelings of remorse, helplessness, grief, resentment, depression or even trauma. Midwives explained how mothers often experience these kinds of negative emotions following a difficult birth. However, they also mentioned the importance of the mother's *perceptions* of birth, and how a spontaneous birth, especially if exceptionally speedy, could also feel like an assault on the system. Health professionals described these women as "trying to cope", sometimes in "isolation" as they battled with their emotions, experiencing "sadness" and at times "desperation". They spoke in detail about the extreme vulnerability of new mothers and how negative emotional states during the postnatal period could disrupt mother-baby interactions and bonding.

Health professionals also noted the impact that childbirth can have on women's sense of self, including their body image and trust in their body to function as it was designed to. They suggested these feelings might affect the mother's self-esteem and confidence, and consequently her ability to care for the baby.

> I think if they've had a difficult birth then it might knock their confidence, inevitably, so their faith in their body, their ability to maybe breastfeed, and their ability to care for the baby. (Midwife Sally)

Positive birth experiences were spoken of in terms of empowerment, confidence and control. Mothers who were properly consulted before interventions and given enough space to make informed decisions in collaboration with their midwife were said to fare well emotionally, even after a complicated birth. This type of experience was thought to increase the mother's confidence, which in turn facilitated caring for and bonding with the baby.

> I think if women have a positive birth experience, then they're more likely to feel really good and empowered, so I think they'll probably feel more confident about their ability as a mother to start with. (Midwife Sally)

Doula Alice also spoke poignantly about how when mothers feel fully involved in their own birth experience, it is the sense of empowerment this brings that enables them to become mothers.

> If she's felt involved and empowered in her birth, she takes the baby into her life. (Doula Alice)

However, birth experiences did not seem to affect everyone in the same way. Certain women were seen as more resilient than others. The ability to cope with giving birth and becoming a mother was believed to depend on mothers' support networks and how well they were emotionally supported during and after childbirth. Mothers who were more resilient could override any complications they faced, "stoically" giving birth and caring for their baby regardless of how traumatic the birth appeared from a midwife's perspective.

> I always think that women who seem to do really well, and carry on doing really well, are just like the ones who just accept everything they have to do. They have to give birth to their child, and so they feel confident in their ability and they just do it, and it just seems to flow. They seem to deal with everything quite well really. (Midwife Annie)

Expectations and Postnatal Perceptions
Pre-birth expectations and postnatal perceptions of childbirth were considered important indicators of how mothers might perceive their babies and how well they interacted with them. Where there were consistent disparities between expectations and reality, a mother could experience a whole range of negative emotions, including "disappointment, grief, guilt and trauma". This could have negative consequences for the mother-baby relationship.

> There are times when women can be quite taken by surprise by the trauma of birth and can find themselves in a bit of a place they didn't expect to be. (Midwife Adele)

Expectations were linked to a range of perinatal factors, including the birth itself, breastfeeding and becoming a mother. Health professionals discussed the impact of modern media, including social media, and its significant role in forming misconceptions about childbirth, mothering and baby behaviour, such as feeding and sleeping. As the general media and social media often build false expectations for mothers before birth, these influences were considered largely responsible for mothers' negative perceptions when faced with the reality of their birth, breastfeeding and mothering experiences. However, one of the midwives who was interviewed here (Adele) recently wanted to update her views on social media, explaining how it can be a useful resource for networking, asking questions and peer support.

> It has all changed so quickly, and these days I certainly refer people to social media resources because it's one place women can so easily find good information and supportive communities. Not as good as IRL (in real life)—but a start. (Midwife Adele)

Birth Process Expectations

How mothers felt before childbirth, including their expectations around the birth, were thought to determine how they felt postnatally. A positive birth experience that matched the mother's pre-birth expectations could be very empowering. Meanwhile, a negative birth experience that failed to live up to expectations was said to leave mothers feeling disillusioned and distressed. This could then affect how well they were able to bond with and care for their baby.

> I often think the preconceived ideas about how birth will go ... heavily influence the experience ... that also then has a huge influence on the parenting journey—how that is shaped and formed at the very early stages. (Health Visitor Emma)

Breastfeeding Expectations

Mothers' expectations around breastfeeding their baby also mattered. Midwife Suzie explained how mothers felt like a failure when they struggled to breastfeed their baby, particularly if they had expected it to come naturally or others had told them it was easy. This, said Suzie, could affect a mother's feelings towards her baby and lead to a loss of confidence in her ability to mother. Hospital protocols and other external pressures may exacerbate the problem, encouraging mothers to breastfeed before they're ready, or to push through and persevere even when the baby was still too "drugged up" and sleepy to feed.

> They used to be allowed to go 24 hours before feeding and now they say 6 hours, but if the baby's drugged up for the first 6 hours and not interested, there's pressure on the mum to feed and then she gets upset with her baby. (Midwife Suzie)

Love at First Sight

Sometimes, unrealistically high expectations of their baby to be "a good baby" and themselves to be good mothers were thought to stem from family and friends as well as from general cultural attitudes and the media. Health Visitor Emma made impressions of flicking through a Next Baby Clothing catalogue as she explained what she meant by the "Next Baby Syndrome".

> I think (mothers) expect everything to be easy. I often call this the 'Next Baby Syndrome'— that's the way I look at it—you know, they flick through the 'Next' directory and see them all sitting there beautifully in their little clothes and peacefully and … It ain't like that! (Health Visitor Emma)

Expectations of themselves as perfect "earth mothers" were also said to dominate, and this phenomenon included mothers assuming they would simply fall in love with their baby at first sight. Health visitors and doulas (who both see more of mother and baby *after* childbirth) believed that the concept of "instant love" placed a huge burden of pressure on the mother. This might lead to feeling a failure when the love didn't happen immediately, especially if the mother and baby had a challenging birth experience and were still in pain or undergoing the after-effects of pharmacological pain relief or other medications such as antibiotics following a caesarean section or wound infection.

> A lot of mums will say they expected to instantly fall in love with their babies and they didn't, and they feel really guilty about that… but generally, it's a relationship that builds and develops over time. (Health Visitor Julie)

Other aspects of mothering were also seen to affect the mother's feelings and behaviour towards the baby. If the pre-birth expectations were different from a harsher reality that may involve depression or birth trauma, loss of identity and disruptions to sleep as well as to marital or social life as it was before, this could lead to acute disappointment.

> In the real world, having a baby can be one of the most traumatic experiences. I think, you know, with modern life, people expect it to be happy and, you know, the most fantastic thing that's ever going to happen to them, and the reality sometimes can be very, very far from that. (Health Visitor Ruth)

Relationships and Why They Matter

Midwives, health visitors and doulas all believed in the vital importance of positive relationships for mother and baby wellbeing. Midwives and doulas perceived their role of supporting mothers through childbirth as pivotal to mothers' experiences and how they felt post-birth. They believed this to be the case regardless of birth mode and that a mother's perceptions of the birth are centred around how well she was cared for during and after childbirth. The mothers' relationships after childbirth were perceived to influence their feelings and behaviour towards the baby as well as their confidence, self-esteem and general attitude towards themselves. When mothers felt well-supported by those around them (e.g. partner, family, friends and health professionals), they were more likely to feel empowered to care for their babies. In contrast, a mother lacking this support system could more easily feel disempowered and detached from the baby. Being properly informed and consulted by health professionals during childbirth was deemed crucial to how the mother felt postnatally.

> She will be more traumatised by her experience if she feels unsupported or ill-informed. (Midwife Suzie)

Furthermore, health professionals felt that 'individualised and sensitive care' was preferable to the one-size-fits-all approach to maternity care that was reportedly practised on large maternity wards. Professional and social support was believed to be an absolute necessity for mothers' psychological wellbeing, particularly if overcoming any birth trauma.

Relationships During Childbirth

It was considered of paramount importance that mothers received adequate emotional support from both their partner and midwife during childbirth. Providing this this type of care enabled better birth experiences with a positive knock-on effect on maternal behaviour and the baby's response. The only real area of disagreement among maternity care providers was about which person in the room was *most* essential to these positive psychosocial outcomes—the partner or the midwife. Some emphasised the partner's role ("They approached it like a team"), while others considered it imperative to have continuous professional support throughout the birth.

> Without the support, it's very hard for women to have a really good experience. I do think it's a really pivotal thing to feeling confident as a parent… A birth isn't just creating a baby but creating a mother as well. (Midwife Annie)

Postnatal Support

Maternity care providers talked about how the social and emotional support given post-birth was as necessary to a mother's mental and emotional state as it had been during childbirth.

> Support that she gets postnatally from her partner, from her family, can all have a massive influence. (Midwife Pippa)

Postnatal care and support from health professionals were described in terms of protecting mothers' space and offering practical guidance. Although midwives felt they were ideally placed to support mothers and babies after childbirth, they bemoaned the fact that this was not always possible on busy postnatal wards. This meant that the early postnatal support they saw as so "essential" could sometimes get deferred until mothers were home and connected with their local health visitor (although UK health visitors have also been in steep decline since government austerity measures and redeployment during the pandemic).

> If there was some way that women were, I don't know, allowed to have more peace on the ward, or there were more midwives at the bedside to make sure babies are feeding and settling properly. (Midwife Adele)

After reading this chapter, Midwife Adele (one of the original participants) mentioned the advantages of peer support—new parents supporting one another—and how this could be better facilitated these days, especially as resources, including midwives being given enough time to spend with mothers, are becoming ever more stretched.

> I do think peer networks are the key for a lot of women. It's such a shame we don't facilitate that as much as we used to. (Midwife Adele)

Relationship with the Baby

Maternity care providers spoke in detail about mothers' relationships with their babies. They believed that the birth experience consciously or subconsciously affects the mother's feelings about her baby. Positive experiences were thought to promote bonding and attachment, and it was observed that the way mother and baby respond to one another post-birth is a good measure of a successful birth outcome. Reciprocal responsiveness between mother and baby was considered of the utmost importance to the baby's wellbeing and development, with the birth experience providing an important backdrop to this.

> Birth experience is vital, absolutely vital, pivotal, to that transition then into parenthood, you know getting that secure attachment early on. (Midwife Sally)

A negative birth experience involving pain, trauma and complications might damage these natural bonding processes and disturb the mother's transition into parenthood.

> How can you feel connected to a baby that's caused you lots of pain and that's brought up issues for you… if you just feel disempowered, abused, mistreated? (Midwife Annie)

Similarly, it was felt that the baby's distress could disrupt bonding and attachment between mother and baby if the newborn was uncomfortable or in pain after a challenging ventouse or forceps birth. Mothers may struggle to cope with a crying baby, and midwives reported how they often became distressed in response to their baby's distress. Although most midwives and health visitors associated challenging birth experiences with disruptions to mother-baby interactions, Midwife Adele considered the possibility that they might facilitate rather than deter bonding.

> I'm just wondering, maybe does a traumatic birth sometimes make the mother more—a bigger attachment because—I think it can make them sort of more keen to bond with the baby, more tactile and more attentive. (Midwife Adele)

Doula Beth mentioned how, with the right kind of support, mothers could bond with their babies no matter what kind of birth experience they had.

> I don't think it's necessarily that if she has a bad experience she doesn't bond with her baby, but it's about the care and support she receives during her birth and afterwards that actually affects her. If she's supported well, then there's no reason that she shouldn't bond with her baby properly. (Doula Beth)

Maternal Postnatal Wellbeing and the Baby

The maternity care providers all seemed to agree that how the mother feels during the postnatal period can affect how well she copes with the task of parenting and how the baby responds behaviourally. As we saw earlier, midwives and doulas noted the potential impacts of the physical birth experience, interventions and pain relief medications on baby behaviour. However, several health visitors (who see more of mothers and their babies after childbirth) remarked on how the baby could be *even more* affected by their mother's *emotional* postnatal state. These health professionals perceived maternal stress as contagious, observing how the baby responds to its mother's distress by exhibiting signs of distress, perhaps refusing or finding it very difficult to feed, sleep or settle.

> Babies are looking to mum for safety and security, and then if she's not that safety net, babies will think, 'If they're stressed, I need to be stressed'. (Health Visitor Emma)

Baby Mirrors Mother

Several health visitors discussed the baby's sensitivity to their mother's mood and emotional state during the postnatal period. When a baby senses a stressful environment, they may not be able to relax and feel safe. The health visitors spoke about the impacts of mothers' stress and anxiety levels on the baby, potentially affecting bonding and breastfeeding.

> You can see the baby mirroring how the mother's feeling, and we see it often, so there's this baby that's basically living on his nerves—very twitched, very insecure, hates being put down, very rarely settles, almost on alert, you know, not quite sure what's gonna come next. And even in the mums who haven't had a hugely traumatic birth, if their anxiety levels are high after, and they've just got general worries, concerns, anxieties, even that you can see in a baby's behaviour. (Health Visitor Emma)

Newborn babies were recognised as social beings who actively seek out contact and interactions with their caregivers. Health visitors also observed how, when mothers feel too stressed, anxious or depressed to engage with their baby, the baby may become quiet and withdrawn, again mirroring their mother's mood and behaviour.

> Mums who are, you know, postnatally depressed, and not able to give the non-verbal contact to the baby, we know that those babies shut down quite quickly… A lot of people are oblivious to the fact that babies are very attentive to communication and stimulation in the

early months. People can be very naive as regards to the fact that, you know, they kind of think that the baby just eats and sleeps.... (Health Visitor Ruth)

These babies were said to require a lot of extra comforting and nurturing, though their mothers may not be in a fit state to provide the level of care they so desperately need.

Yeah, if it's been a difficult birth, you often see the mothers ... it maybe takes a while to become in tune with the baby. (Health Visitor Debbie)

Several health professionals were concerned that this situation could affect the very earliest days, influencing how mothers bond with their babies.

I do worry about this idea that... her pain, her discomfort, her thoughts, her feelings about this whole process that's just gone on, and (she) is then handed this little baby who's completely dependent on her and can just struggle with tuning in to what that baby needs because all of her wants and needs are all-consuming almost. So, I do feel that it does impact hugely on that early days' relationship. (Health Visitor Emma)

Time to Talk

Midwives, health visitors and doulas discussed mothers' opportunities for debriefing after the birth and how this could be of enormous benefit, especially after a difficult birth experience. They felt that mothers need to be able to revisit their notes and understand why certain decisions were made, especially if they feel traumatised in response to the birth. It was firmly believed that this debriefing process could help mothers recover and cope better with their babies. However, given the mixed research on the benefits of this, health professionals should have specialised trauma-informed training in order to debrief parents after childbirth in a way that is not re-traumatising. Although there's always a risk of re-traumatising by talking about the trauma, women with post-traumatic symptoms generally seem to appreciate being given the opportunity to discuss their birth with a midwife [4]. In fact, a recent large-scale study of over 2.5 thousand women found that, overall, they valued being heard rather than "dismissed" and appreciated having the opportunity to "validate" their feelings after childbirth [2]. Qualitative studies have also demonstrated how postnatal debriefing can make women feel valued and enable them to make sense of their birth experiences [12].

Health Visitor Julie spoke wistfully about a previous debriefing service that no longer existed in her area since the government cuts to mental health services.

It was a way of getting rid of all this negative emotion. (Health Visitor Julie)

Health Visitor Emma believed that having time to talk and grieve might help prevent the development of postnatal depression and other mood disorders.

I do worry about how we diagnose postnatal depression as the answer is, 'Let's use some pills to sort you out' whereas sometimes I think almost debriefing, and allowing mothers to just talk about the experience, and allow them to grieve the experience they didn't have.... (Health Visitor Emma)

In some areas where I interviewed midwives and health visitors, such as West Wales, debriefing services do still exist, albeit with some waiting lists, and women are referred to these services if they feel the need to discuss their birth experience with a health professional. In this study, however, many mothers were said to get overlooked, slip through the net and not get the care or attention they so desperately need postnatally. Sometimes, rather than being encouraged to talk and process their emotions around the birth, Doula Rachel had observed mothers being "silenced" by health professionals, who could be adamant that all the best options had been taken, and there was no point mulling over different possible scenarios after a traumatic birth.

Doula Rachel spoke about the wider social and cultural pressures within society to simply "be grateful" for a live baby, regardless of how damaging and traumatic the experience may have been. She felt this would certainly affect the early formation of a positive mother-baby relationship.

> I would say that it's actually very difficult to know exactly how mothers feel because they're not going to tell you for fear of being branded a bad mother… 'But you've got a healthy baby, you should be grateful'… I think that when you hold all of that inside, it becomes inevitable that it will change your relationship with your child. (Doula Rachel)

5.2.3 Chapter Summary, Conclusions and New Insights

The 18 interviews with midwives, health visitors and doulas presented here highlight how baby behaviour appears to be influenced by the mother's birth experience, both directly (via physical factors such as interventions, pain relief and hormones) and indirectly (by influencing the way a mother perceives and interacts with her baby). Calm, resilient mothers were associated with calmer babies, while less resilient mothers required more support. Regardless of birth mode (including caesarean sections), calm, well-supported birth experiences were perceived to encourage settled newborn behaviour. At the same time, a nurturing postnatal environment was considered beneficial for both mother and baby.

Positive perceptions of the birth experience helped mothers feel empowered and confident in their ability to care for their babies. Conversely, if they had experienced physical and emotional distress during childbirth, this was believed to affect them postnatally and influence their feelings and behaviour towards the baby. Babies were observed to mirror their mother's mood, withdrawing and shutting down if she was depressed or being on high alert and "nervy" if she was anxious and stressed. Stressed, anxious or distressed mothers were therefore much more likely to have a crying, fussing and generally unsettled newborn baby born already on full alert to the slightest signal of stress or "danger". It was said that some of these negative birth impacts could be mediated (or reduced) by providing consistent emotional support to mothers throughout childbirth and into the postnatal period.

Midwives also emphasised the importance of calm birthing and postnatal environments to allow mothers and babies time and space to connect through holding, breastfeeding and bonding. Encouraging skin-to-skin contact between the pair was believed to facilitate breastfeeding and bonding, thereby promoting the release of oxytocin and soothing both mother and baby after a difficult birth experience. As we know, however, breastfeeding can be a contentious issue. Previous research has highlighted the essential role of oxytocin in breastfeeding and mother-baby bonding in addition to highlighting breastfeeding as a protective factor in perinatal mental health [22]. Furthermore, there is a significant link between mothers who desperately wanted to breastfeed (but do not manage this for whatever reason) and postnatal depression [5]. When all goes well, breastfeeding can lead to a calming physiological response [20]. Therefore, those who manage to breastfeed successfully tend to have lower cortisol levels, heart rate and blood pressure compared to non-breastfeeding mothers [13]. When breastfeeding is established successfully, it can also benefit the mother-baby relationship and infant development [21], facilitating bonding [15] and helping to protect the baby from high-risk parenting [14]. Despite all this evidence, however, health professionals also need to maintain an awareness that pressurising rather than encouraging and supporting women to breastfeed may cause feelings of guilt and shame [17], possibly triggering or worsening depressive symptoms [3].

Staffing shortages and austerity-driven funding cuts in maternity services have limited the time midwives can dedicate to nurturing women postnatally [16], and midwives appeared to struggle to provide the care they want to within such an overstretched maternity care system. Consequently, the need for quiet, nurturing environments remains unmet in many busy maternity wards, risking birth trauma and disrupting the natural biological processes so vital for mother and baby wellbeing. Separation of mothers and babies in hospitals was also mentioned as a significant challenge, disrupting immediate skin-to-skin care and its associated benefits. Despite extensive evidence and recommendations by UNICEF and the World Health Organisation [23], only 74% of full-term babies in England experience skin-to-skin contact within an hour of birth [19].

Health professionals and doulas consistently highlighted the crucial role of the mothers' relationships with their midwives, partners and babies. A health visitor I met at a birth conference once told me, "We care for the mothers so they can care for their babies". This support was seen as pivotal in shaping mothers' perceptions of childbirth and their postnatal experience. Ensuring personalised, respectful and woman-centred maternity care that nurtures empowerment and control during childbirth was recommended as a way to promote the mother's wellbeing, as ultimately, this will also benefit the baby [18]. Without adequate support, mothers may feel stressed or overwhelmed when faced with a new baby who needs lots of care and attention, and the stress contagion—where maternal stress influences the baby—was noted as a key factor in shaping baby behaviour. However, while many studies have identified correlations between mother and baby cortisol levels [7], further research is still needed in this area [9].

The partner's role was also highlighted as significant in mediating the mother-baby bonding process. Strong partner support could alleviate maternal distress or depression and positively influence reciprocal mother-baby interactions, laying the groundwork for secure attachment [11]. There is also new evidence that relationship satisfaction between the parents helps to mitigate the effects of a traumatic birth, improving post-traumatic stress outcomes [1].

Midwives and health visitors emphasised that the mother's neurohormonal state *post-birth* is just as critical as during childbirth. Protecting endogenous oxytocin and reducing cortisol levels were of paramount importance for the long-term health of both mother and baby, whose hormonal states are deeply interconnected. Providing safe, respectful, person-centred care tailored to individual circumstances was believed to be essential for creating a nurturing environment. This includes offering emotional support, clear communication and consistent care throughout the perinatal period, all of which would help enable mothers and babies to thrive.

References

1. Alves S, Pratas M, Sousa M, Fidalgo D, Morais A, Jongenelen I, Costa R. Prenatal couple relationship satisfaction, romantic attachment, and childbirth-related posttraumatic stress symptoms. Journal of Reproductive and Infant Psychology. 2025:1–17.
2. Bannister L, Hammond A, Dahlen HG, Keedle H. A content analysis of women's experiences of debriefing following childbirth: the Birth Experience Study (BESt). Midwifery. 2025;104421
3. Baron-Cohen KL, Fearon P, Feldman R, Hardiman P, Zagoory-Sharon O, Meins E, Fonagy P. Intranasal oxytocin increases breast milk oxytocin, but has a reduced effect in depressed mothers: a randomized controlled trial. Psychoneuroendocrinology. 2025;107374. https://www.sciencedirect.com/science/article/abs/pii/S0306453025000976
4. Baxter J. Postnatal debriefing: women's need to talk after birth. British Journal of Midwifery. 2019;27(9):563–71.
5. Borra C, Iacovou M, Sevilla A. New evidence on breastfeeding and postpartum depression: the importance of understanding women's intentions. Maternal and Child Health Journal. 2015;19:897–907.
6. Braun V, Clarke V. One size fits all? What counts as quality practice in (reflexive) thematic analysis? Qualitative Research in Psychology. 2021;18(3):328–52.
7. Brennan PA, Pargas R, Walker EF, Green P, Jeffrey Newport D, Stowe Z. Maternal depression and infant cortisol: influences of timing, comorbidity and treatment. Journal of Child Psychology and Psychiatry. 2008;49(10):1099–107.
8. British Psychological Society. BPS code of human research ethics; 2021. Available at: https://explore.bps.org.uk/binary/bpsworks/06096a55b82ca73a/9787a5959b2bfdff7ed2a43ad5b3f333a5278925cfd667b1b2e64b5387c91b92/inf180_2021.pdf. Accessed 15.12.24.
9. Bruinhof N, Beijers R, Lustermans H, de Weerth C. Mother–infant stress contagion? Effects of an acute maternal stressor on maternal caregiving behavior and infant cortisol and crying. Journal of Child Psychology and Psychiatry. 2025; https://acamh.onlinelibrary.wiley.com/doi/pdf/10.1111/jcpp.14119
10. Byrne D. A worked example of Braun and Clarke's approach to reflexive thematic analysis. Quality & quantity. 2022;56(3):1391–412.
11. Curci SG, Frangos MP, Torres-Aguirre K, Clifford BN, Luecken LJ. Postpartum depressive symptoms and mother–infant dyadic reciprocity: the moderating role of partner support. Developmental Psychology. 2025; https://doi.org/10.1037/dev0001860.
12. Demirci AD, Oruc M, Kabukcuoglu K. "I need to make sense of my birth experience": a descriptive qualitative study of postnatal women's opinions and expectations about postnatal debriefing. Midwifery. 2024;131:103955.

References

13. Ebina S, Kashiwakura I. Influence of breastfeeding on maternal blood pressure at one month postpartum. International Journal of Women's Health. 2012:333–9.
14. Feldman R. Sensitive periods in human social development: new insights from research on oxytocin, synchrony, and high-risk parenting. Development and Psychopathology. 2015;27(2):369–95.
15. Feldman R, Gordon I, Zagoory-Sharon O. Maternal and paternal plasma, salivary, and urinary oxytocin and parent–infant synchrony: considering stress and affiliation components of human bonding. Developmental Science. 2011;14(4):752–61.
16. Hunter L, Magill-Cuerden J, McCourt C. 'Oh no, no, no, we haven't got time to be doing that': challenges encountered introducing a breast-feeding support intervention on a postnatal ward. Midwifery. 2015;31(8):798–804.
17. Jackson L, De Pascalis L, Harrold J, Fallon V. Guilt, shame, and postpartum infant feeding outcomes: a systematic review. Maternal & Child Nutrition. 2021;17(3):e13141.
18. Leinweber J, Fontein-Kuipers Y, Karlsdottir SI, Ekström-Bergström A, Nilsson C, Stramrood C, Thomson G. Developing a woman-centered, inclusive definition of positive childbirth experiences: a discussion paper. Birth. 2023;50(2):362–83.
19. NHS England. NHS Maternity Statistics, England 2021–22: skin-to-skin contact; 2022. https://digital.nhs.uk/data-and-information/publications/statistical/nhs-maternity-statistics/2021-22
20. Ohmura N, Okuma L, Truzzi A, Esposito G, Kuroda KO. Maternal physiological calming responses to infant suckling at the breast. The Journal of Physiological Sciences. 2023;73(1):3.
21. Sanefuji M, Senju A, Shimono M, Ogawa M, Sonoda Y, Torio M, Ohga S. Breast feeding and infant development in a cohort with sibling pair analysis: the Japan Environment and Children's Study. BMJ Open. 2021;11(8):e043202.
22. Wang Z, Liu J, Shuai H, Cai Z, Fu X, Liu Y, Yang BX. Mapping global prevalence of depression among postpartum women. Translational Psychiatry. 2021;11(1):543.
23. WHO Immediate KMC Study Group. Immediate "kangaroo mother care" and survival of infants with low birth weight. New England Journal of Medicine. 2021;384(21):2028–38.
24. World Medical Association. World Medical Association Declaration of Helsinki: ethical principles for medical research involving human subjects. JAMA. 2013;310(20):2191–4.

Mothers' Childbirth Experiences and Perceptions of Their Baby's Behaviour

6

There is nothing either good or bad, but thinking makes it so.
(William Shakespeare: Hamlet, Act 2, Scene 2)

6.1 Introduction to Mothers' Perceptions of Childbirth and Baby Behaviour

The second of the two qualitative studies sought to discover what mothers think about their childbirth experience and baby's behaviour during the first year of life. Did mothers recognise the possibility of a connection between the birth and their baby's behaviour and temperament, or were they oblivious to this possibility? If they did see a connection, what did they attribute this to? Did the events that occurred during childbirth (e.g. induction or emergency caesarean) affect the way they perceived the birth and their baby, and did the care and support they received during and after childbirth make a difference to their perceptions?

These questions were explored by interviewing 22 healthy mothers with healthy full-term babies aged 0–12 months from South-West regions of the UK (from Bristol to West Wales). The study aimed to begin unravelling the mystery of the apparent connection between childbirth experience and baby behaviour (as recognised by midwives, health visitors and doulas in the previous chapter) and find out a little more about what could be influencing this link. In other words, what could be the driving forces or "mechanisms" behind the relationship that maternity care providers perceived between childbirth experience and baby behaviour, and why do midwives and health visitors think that mothers' psychological and emotional states during and after childbirth are so crucial to their babies? What might lessen the baby's stress response to childbirth? We know that mothers who experience childbirth as traumatic are more likely to suffer from postnatal distress and other mood disorders [5, 29]. We also know that a mother's negative postnatal mood affects her baby's emotionality, behaviour and development [30, 33, 52]. However, there are still many missing pieces to this jigsaw puzzle, and it seems important to try and figure out how and why the birth experience and its impacts on the mother might also affect the baby.

Mothers were given ample space to talk about whatever they wished concerning the birth experience and their baby's behaviour. After taking some basic background details (e.g. the baby's current age and the mother's age and education), I asked them to tell me their birth story. This was followed by two open-ended questions:

1. *"How have you found your baby's behaviour since birth?"*
2. *"Do you think your baby's behaviour was at all affected by the birth?"*

All interviewees were offered coffee and cake as recompense for an hour of their time; therefore, most of the interviews took place in cafes, although a few mothers chose to be interviewed at home, and one asked for a telephone interview as her baby was currently unwell. Mothers who reported a traumatic birth experience were encouraged to share this information with their health visitor or doctor and offered contact details for the Birth Trauma Association.

In a similar way to the health professional interviews in the previous chapter, after the interviews had taken place, they were transcribed and coded thematically according to perceived patterns in the data [11]. While every birth story differed from the one before, recurring patterns eventually began to appear. These were arranged into themes to tell an intricate, detailed, and intimate tale about mothers' subjective experiences of childbirth and the early postnatal days before commenting on their baby's behaviour and, finally, stating whether they thought the two were connected in any way. In telling this narrative, I was mindful of staying close to the data and not allowing my own experiences to colour my interpretation of mothers' spoken words. With this in mind, following Sandelowski's [57, 58] methods of qualitative description, mothers' own choices of language are used here to explore their interpretations of childbirth events and the meanings they attributed to these.

An adapted version of this study can be found in the journal *PLoS One*:

Power, C., Williams, C., & Brown, A. (2023). Does a mother's childbirth experience influence her perceptions of her baby's behaviour? A qualitative interview study. *PLoS One, 18*(4), e0284183.

6.2 Outline of Childbirth Experiences and Baby Behaviour

The 22 mothers who took part were aged between 21 and 37, and their babies were 1–41 weeks old. All the mothers were white British, and nearly 70% had higher education. Approximately two-thirds of mothers were married; the others were cohabiting, and 64% of the babies were firstborn. Nine women had a spontaneous physiological birth, and of these, seven babies were born in a birthing pool. There were three planned and eight unplanned inductions or accelerations of labour. Two women initially had planned caesarean births, although one of these was moved forward due to reduced foetal movement, making it an "emergency" section. Babies generally seemed more settled after a straightforward birth that went as expected. This included *planned* inductions and *planned* caesarean sections. Overall, therefore, mothers and babies seemed to fare better when there were no *unexpected* complications or interventions, and babies were reported as much more *unsettled* after unpredictable, complicated, challenging or very medicalised births.

Baby behaviour according to the type of birth and overall birth experience is colour-coded in the figures below. Figure 6.1 illustrates the number of settled, mixed behaviour or unsettled babies depending on whether the birth was physiological (without any interventions) or had medical interventions. For this study, choosing to have an epidural was not counted as a medical intervention but as requested pain relief (although it was often used during medical interventions).

As you can see here, of the nine physiological births, seven babies were described by their mothers as settled, two as mixed and none as unsettled, whereas, for medical births, this pattern was reversed. Six of the 13 babies born after a medical intervention were unsettled, and four exhibited a more mixed behavioural style. Notably, the three described as settled in this group were born by planned caesarean section or planned induction. Thus, babies born within a calm, predictable environment were all perceived as calm and settled in their behaviour.

Figure 6.2 illustrates the number of settled, mixed-behaviour or unsettled babies depending on mothers' *perceptions* of the birth.

Although this is a fairly small qualitative sample and therefore no statistical analysis of the data was carried out, it is noteworthy that *no* mothers who experienced spontaneous physiological childbirth (see Fig. 6.1) or who had positive perceptions of their birth experience (see Fig. 6.2) reported any unsettled baby behaviours. Despite these stark figures, only 10 mothers believed their baby's behaviour might be linked to the birth. Several mothers were unsure about whether the birth could have affected their baby, while some said this concept had never occurred to them, so they hadn't thought about it (see Fig. 6.3).

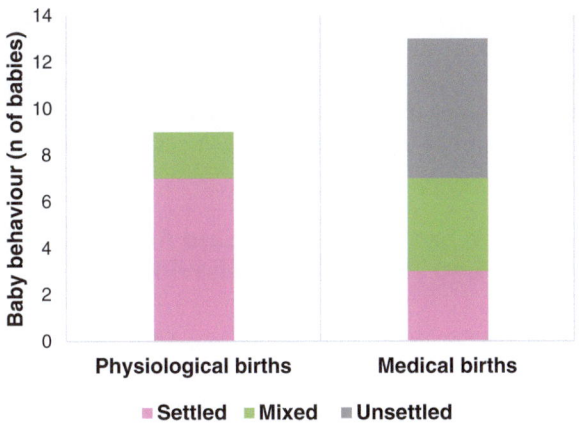

Fig. 6.1 Type of birth and baby behaviour. *Note*: The graphs in this chapter were created by Spoorthy Deepak

Fig. 6.2 Overall birth experience and baby behaviour

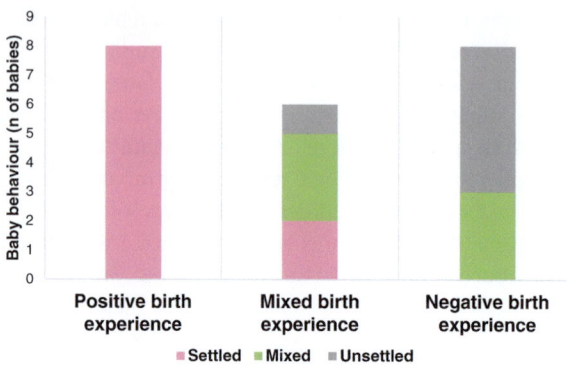

Fig. 6.3 Did the birth affect your baby?

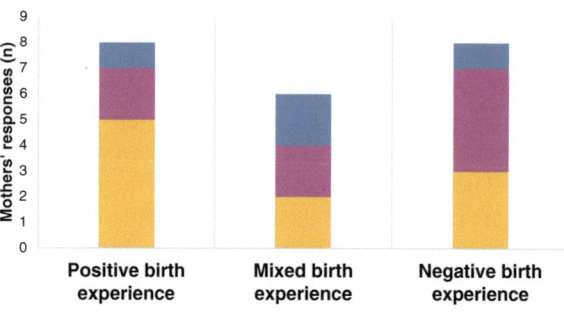

As illustrated in Fig. 6.3, mothers who had a positive experience were more likely to believe there was a link between the birth and their baby's behaviour than those who had a negative experience—where they were more likely to say "no". It is possible (though by no means certain) that this was due to feelings of guilt and shame attached to the nature of the birth, or dissociation and denial after a difficult birth experience [62]. Such emotions could be very damaging to mother and baby during the postnatal period, potentially affecting the mother's mental health and her early relationship with the baby [17]. In these circumstances, it is perfectly understandable that—whether consciously or subconsciously—mothers may wish to avoid blaming their baby's unsettled temperament on how the birth went, especially if they felt like they had somehow "failed" at giving birth.

6.3 What the Mothers Said About Their Birth Experience and Their Baby's Behaviour

Tucked away in quiet corners of cosy cafes between Southwest England and West Wales, mothers spoke to me at length about their births over multiple teas, coffees and cakes. It was perhaps not the healthiest time of my life because, of course, I felt

6.3 What the Mothers Said About Their Birth Experience and Their Baby's Behaviour

I had to join them in this indulgence, but it was well worth the effort of having these cafe sessions to gather such incredible stories of joy, distress, empowerment, stoicism, bravery and strength. Mothers spoke, sometimes euphorically and occasionally in grim detail, about what had happened to them and their babies during and after childbirth, explaining how it had made them feel and how it had affected them or may have affected their babies. Childbirth experiences varied dramatically. While some mothers had felt very well cared for, emotionally supported, joyful, proud and empowered, others had felt very let down, coerced, abandoned and afraid. Mothers also spoke about the immediate postnatal period. This was either in hospital if something was amiss (which for some was experienced as sheer torment) or at home if the birth had gone smoothly and mother and baby were healthy. Nine childbirth themes emerged from the birth stories and are organised under two overarching headings: *Physical Birth Experience* and *Psychological Birth Experience* (see the thematic map in Fig. 6.4 for a summary).

The first overarching theme, *Physical Birth Experience,* as the name suggests, relates to mothers' physical birth experiences; for example, their perceptions of the birthing environment or birthplace and their experiences with pain relief. The second overarching theme, *Psychological Birth Experience*, relates to mothers' emotional states, expectations and perceived support. Physical birth experiences were very much interwoven with psychological birth experiences. Notably, *all* mothers who had a *challenging* birth and *negative* postnatal perceptions had experienced *unplanned and unwanted interventions*, with a proportion of these feeling coerced. Conversely, 75% of mothers who felt they had a positive birth experience had given birth spontaneously. The other 25% of mothers with positive experiences had either had a planned induction or planned caesarean, indicating that mothers and babies may do better when they've been part of the decision-making process and either not required or *accepted and agreed to* the need for an intervention. However, as can be seen in the birth event details provided alongside mothers' names below, one seemingly simple intervention often led to another; and for some mothers, this seemed to spiral out of control, often resulting in a physically and emotionally traumatic birth experience.

6.3.1 Physical Birth Experience

The overarching theme *Physical Birth Experience* encompasses birth mode and other birth events (such as induction or acceleration), birthplace, pain intensity and pain relief, how mothers perceived these experiences and how they were affected. As it was impossible to completely separate the physical experience from the psychological one, mothers' emotional responses to supposedly "objective" factors are at times included. The themes are presented here using direct quotes from the interviews that seemed to best represent mothers' experiences, perceptions and feelings around the given topic. To provide readers with a more comprehensive understanding of the birth experiences each mother had, basic details such as birth mode and significant birth events are listed after their names. The type of pain relief used

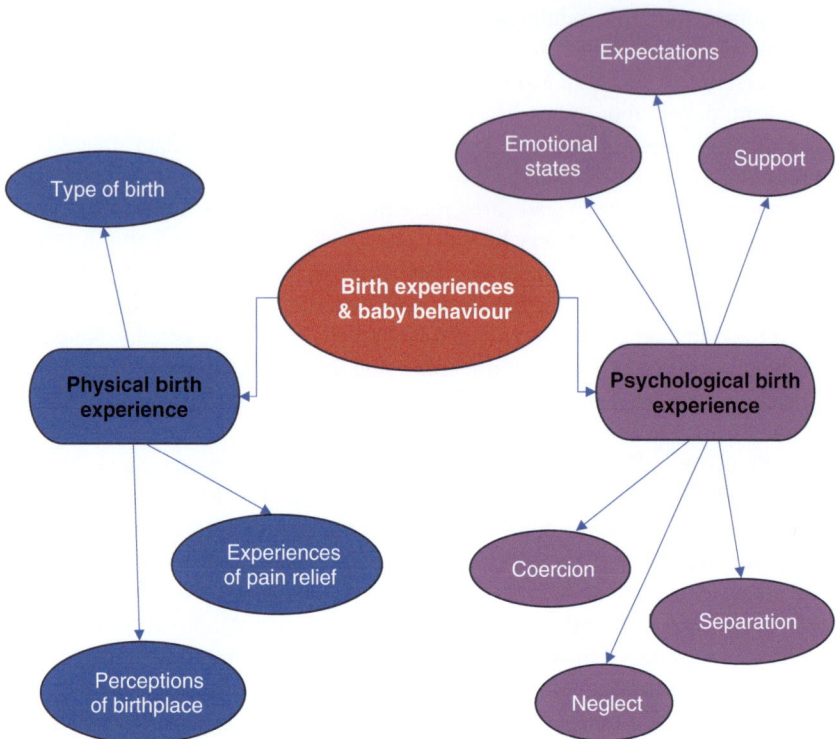

Fig. 6.4 An overview of birth mothers' experiences and their baby's behaviour

Figure key

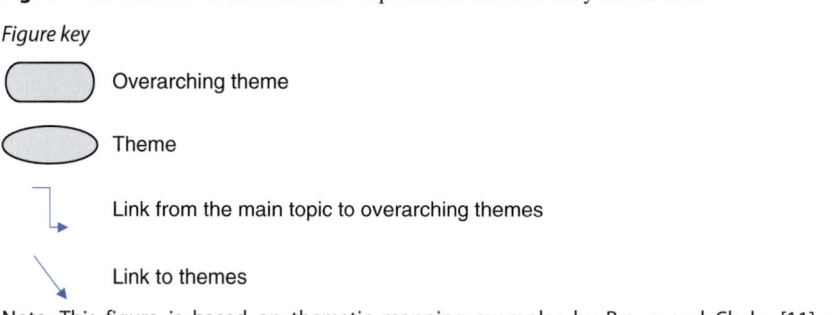

Note: This figure is based on thematic mapping examples by Braun and Clarke [11] and Byrne [15]

during labour is added to this list within the pain relief theme. Mothers', babies' and partners' names have all been changed to protect their confidentiality and anonymity.

Physical Birth Experience was arranged into three main themes: *Type of birth*, *Perceptions of birthplace* and *Experiences of pain relief* (including natural methods). Within these themes were multiple subthemes (e.g. the mother's and baby's responses to different types of pain relief).

6.3 What the Mothers Said About Their Birth Experience and Their Baby's Behaviour

Type of Birth

The type of birth mothers experienced influenced how they perceived the birth. For example, some mothers reported feeling very empowered after a spontaneous physiological labour and birth. This tended to enhance their feelings of self-confidence and ability to cope with and enjoy caring for their baby post-birth. Mothers who had a spontaneous birth often revelled in the marvel of it unfolding, almost without any conscious effort. Emily was one such mother.

> It was very much my body did it, and like I enjoyed feeling it. (Emily: spontaneous hospital birth)

In contrast to Emily's positive experience, Kate compared giving birth to being a player on a football pitch as she was loudly cheered on to do Valsalva pushing, which is a non-evidence-based type of pushing where midwives or obstetricians take control of labour and birth away from the mother to direct her through contractions during the second ("pushing") stage [34].

> It was like football sidelines. 'Go on, PUSH!' I wish they hadn't 'cause my bottom took a while to recover—3 months of piles and bruising. (Kate: home to hospital transfer, acceleration)

Millie, on the other hand, was excited about her spontaneous home waterbirth, which happened so quickly that the baby arrived before midwives and paramedics could get there.

> It sort of burns a bit but it's not pain… 'cause you can feel something happening… It just happened. I couldn't stop it… My birth was incredible! I'm very lucky… I got in the pool and little Keegan was born fifteen minutes later. (Millie: home waterbirth; accidental free birth)

Millie also commented on how the birth experience may have contributed to her baby's calm and settled temperament.

> It was a very calm birth, and he was pretty calm coming out… he was very settled. (Millie: home waterbirth; accidental free birth)

Others were not so lucky. Even mothers who had a spontaneous birth could struggle with the birth experience and the way they felt during and after it. Alex was dismissed as not being "in established labour" until it was too late for pain relief. The birth then happened very quickly, and she felt this had affected her ability to manage her "feisty" baby postnatally.

> I don't think I had a traumatic birth, but… being told nothing was happening and thinking, I can't cope with it if that's the case…. (Alex: MLU waterbirth)

Alex described how she found her baby's early "colicky" behaviour difficult to cope with. She realised that part of this may have been due to experiencing a slow labour without any pain relief, which had led to a difficult emotional aftermath for both her and the baby.

> I think I found her quite difficult because I was a little bit shell-shocked after the birth… in the early days… I mean we did have some days in the early days where she was really hard to console for no reason other than maybe feeling a bit colicky…. (Alex: MLU waterbirth)

Although Tessa eventually managed to give birth after a long process of labour acceleration, she underwent extreme measures to get her labour going, which were initially ineffectual.

> I had the sweep, and it stopped all my contractions… Yeah, everything stopped after the sweep… but nothing was really happening as fast as we needed it to and the (hormone) dose was going up and up and up and up. (Tessa: hospital transfer, acceleration)

Tessa's experience of her labour stalling is not uncommon after arrival at a hospital or having interventions. It's part of an instinctive protective mechanism caused by hormonal activity (the release of stress hormones known as catecholamines) when exposed to extreme uncertainty or fear. After all, it would never have been safe to give birth in the mouth of a cave if a tiger had been spotted prowling about, so our bodies are designed to shut down all but their most essential activities when experiencing extreme fear or uncertainty. Although Tessa came away from her challenging birth experience physically unscathed, she wondered whether her emotional state during childbirth had affected the baby, especially as she had felt unsupported by both the midwife *and* her partner.

> Yeah, I think in the early days, I do think umm…(pause) it's really hard to say. I don't know whether she was affected, or I was affected… It was just a bit on edge that birth… just a bit on edge. (Tessa: hospital transfer, acceleration)

Labour could be long and arduous; babies could become stuck and need help to be born. Obstetric interventions such as induction or acceleration (especially if unplanned) often led to fear, increased pain, and maternal or neonatal distress, sometimes leaving the mother feeling helpless and physically or emotionally out of control.

> I didn't progress at all… then they gave me the top up (synthetic oxytocin) … It just overstimulated my uterus… absolute agony. (Tara: induction, acceleration, neonatal distress, NICU)

Despite some challenging birth outcomes involving neonatal distress and the baby's admission to the Neonatal Intensive Care Unit (NICU), Tara didn't think there was any connection between her birth experience and the baby's slightly hyperactive temperament (*a busy bod*). While confessing there had been a few feeding issues and sickness during the early weeks post-birth, her baby seemed to have settled into easier feeding and sleeping routines over time.

> She's a really contented happy baby… She's really active… She wants to do everything; she wants to be in everything. She's just so content, she just plays by herself… I don't think it's anything to do with that (the birth) 'cause while I was pregnant, she was quite a busy bod then. I think it was just in her nature. (Tara: induction, acceleration, neonatal distress, NICU)

6.3 What the Mothers Said About Their Birth Experience and Their Baby's Behaviour

Whether mothers perceived a connection or not, those with a challenging birth experience more often reported unsettled baby behaviour during the first few weeks.

> There were about five or six doctors in there and midwives... it was quite distracting, and I was starting to panic—I thought well what? You keep talking about theatre... I desperately didn't want to have another section... And they were gonna do an epidural. I was begging for it! (laughs). I don't wanna feel anything ever again! (Anna: induction, episiotomy, cervical tear, postpartum haemorrhage, infection, blood transfusion)

Anna tried to laugh off her challenging birth experience where she had suffered internal and external tears followed by a postpartum haemorrhage, infection and an unsettled newborn. She simply put this down to hunger as the baby settled soon after transferring to bottle feeding.

> The first 3 weeks, she screamed a lot; yeah, it was constant all-day screaming. She really wasn't contented at all. But she did sleep, you know—she woke up once during the night. (Anna: induction, episiotomy, cervical tear, postpartum haemorrhage, infection, blood transfusion)

In contrast to Anna's blasé attitude regarding her traumatic birth experience and the baby's behaviour, Ava attributed her baby's breastfeeding problems to his neck and head injury during the emergency forceps delivery, causing him to suffer residual pain and distress.

> I put it (breastfeeding problems) down to the fact that, because he was forceps... when I was trying to put him on the boob, I was pressing the back of his head and neck, not realising... So I felt really upset that I was really useless and couldn't do it. (Ava: hospital transfer, acceleration, episiotomy, forceps)

As we saw in earlier chapters, birth physiology is intricately linked to birth psychology and previous studies testing umbilical cord cortisol levels demonstrate how babies are as likely to feel distressed after an assisted birth as their mothers [23, 32, 61]. Babies respond to their mother's raised cortisol levels during childbirth due to their exposure to the stress hormones via the placenta [31]. This impacts the baby's immature stress response system, known as the hypothalamic-pituitary-adrenal (HPA) axis [8], while also affecting their immune system, epigenome, and microbiome (see Chap. 3). Together, these changes to the baby's delicate internal systems can mean a newborn who is more susceptible to excessive crying and fussing during the first weeks and months and one who develops higher infant stress reactivity and fearfulness [50], more difficult child behaviour and poorer future physical and mental health [21, 28, 63]. Most mothers in our study, however, wouldn't have known about how these birth-related factors can be linked to their baby's behaviour. Instead, they were more likely to see difficult early infant temperament through the lens of physical issues such as breastfeeding, pain and discomfort.

Tilly, who had an emergency caesarean section, said the early postnatal moments had seemed easier to begin with but became more challenging afterwards when she had struggled with the pain and felt unwell.

> I had a really easy and pleasant few hours with her whereas a lot of mums are taken off for stitches or in another room, or in lots of pain. I didn't have that, but then I think the day after, when most people start to feel a lot better, I felt so much worse. (Tilly: emergency caesarean section [CS], internal haemorrhage, morphine)

Despite her own suffering post-birth, Tilly thought her baby had benefitted from having a calm atmosphere during the birth. The initially planned caesarean section had been brought forward, becoming an 'emergency' caesarean due to reduced foetal movements.

> Yes. There was a calm mummy and a calm daddy and a happy atmosphere. No pain, no upset, cuddles straight away, music in the background… She didn't have any of the trauma of birth, and just immediately, she had all my love and attention… and all Ed's love and attention. And even when I was in pain the next day, she got so many cuddles from Ed and his parents… So her character is calm, happy and interested. (Tilly: emergency CS, internal haemorrhage, morphine)

Mothers who had planned inductions or planned caesarean sections tended to view their birth much more positively than those who had unplanned interventions. However, mothers could find even planned interventions difficult if they felt unprepared and therefore unequipped to deal with them. Sara, for example, struggled with the physical sensations of her planned caesarean section.

> I went in (theatre)… it wasn't an enjoyable experience (laughs)… The baby was out in 6 or 7 minutes, it's the sewing up that takes time… I didn't feel any pain, but I feel like I wasn't prepared enough for how much I might feel, 'cause you can feel each layer dragging back… horrible… but as soon as they showed me the baby, I said, 'Oh forget it', you know, it was fine (laughs). It was rather nice…. (Sara: planned CS, postpartum infection)

Although she tried to put on a brave face and laugh it off, Sara had a challenging time both during birth and postnatally as she had a very painful postpartum infection, combined with feeling neglected on the postnatal ward and going hours without any pain relief, even with a serious wound infection. The baby initially had a lot of trouble breastfeeding. Despite these experiences, Sara didn't perceive the birth as having unsettled her baby, though she did express her relief that he hadn't suffered an adverse physical reaction to the antibiotics.

> I couldn't breastfeed, which I wanted to do, but he wasn't latching on, and I was in agony anyway, so I was expressing… I don't know. He stayed sort of calm like when he was born, so I don't think so really—obviously, things could have gone wrong, but they didn't for him. I was worried the antibiotics would affect him, but they didn't. No thrush…. (Sara: planned CS, postpartum infection)

6.3 What the Mothers Said About Their Birth Experience and Their Baby's Behaviour

Perceptions of Birthplace

Mothers spoke at length about how the birth environment had made them feel. Perceptions of their chosen or unchosen birthplace were very personal and varied enormously between mothers. While some preferred the comforting and perhaps more "homely" or "more natural" surroundings of a midwife-led unit, others had wanted to be in hospital for such a momentous event and found this very reassuring.

> I really felt I needed just to know that people were with me if anything happened… It was brilliant. (Emily: physiological hospital birth)

Mothers who'd chosen to give birth to their baby in a hospital seemed to feel much happier about their birth experience than those who had chosen to give birth elsewhere but then got transferred to a hospital. Some mothers, such as Tessa, who longed to give birth in a midwife-led unit (MLU), had their dreams thwarted at the last minute. Tessa explained in detail how cheated and disappointed she and her husband had felt to lose any prospect of having the nice MLU experience they'd been planning.

> So she said, 'Oo, we'll just send you upstairs for monitoring and then you can come back down'. And I knew as soon as she said monitoring that we wouldn't come back down… That's (the hospital) where we wanted to avoid being… It's just we were so spoilt with Fiona (first baby) with the MLU 'cause that was really big, it had a pool there, a changing light and a double bed, you know, and the care was—midwives were, you know really nice…. (Tessa: hospital transfer, acceleration)

Mothers like Ava felt fear creeping in when birth events suddenly spiralled out of their control, especially if they felt pressured or coerced or experienced an in-labour transfer. Transfers from a chosen setting (home or MLU) to a hospital during labour could lead to a sense of panic and distress.

> I had planned a pool birth in the midwife-led (unit), but when I went back, they sent me up a floor (to the hospital) … I was absolutely devastated that I couldn't go down… I'd laminated me' birth plan! (Ava, hospital transfer, acceleration, episiotomy, forceps)

In some hospitals and midwife-led units, the maternity services seemed to be very stretched. Women were sometimes left alone with their partner for long stretches of advanced labour (see the theme "Neglected" in Sect. 6.3.2). In spite of our knowledge about the mother's and baby's stress response systems working in unison during childbirth, and decades of recommendations about the importance of respectful, continuous one-to-one maternity care for all women in established labour [46], unfortunately, we still don't seem to have a maternity care system that adequately supports and nurtures mothers and babies. Inconsistent care was also experienced in hospital postnatal wards due to perceived staff shortages, causing significant distress for all the mothers it affected. Sara had a painful wound infection after her caesarean, yet was expected to get out of bed and look after herself though she was barely able to walk.

They'd come in and wake everyone up screaming, 'Breakfast!' and you'd have to go and help yourself. It was a bit of a nightmare. I thought I was never gonna get out of there (laughs)… You've just gotta get on with it. But they don't bring anything to you, you've gotta go out into the corridor and help yourself…. (Sara: planned CS, postpartum infection)

While this type of negative experience was fairly common for hospital births, many mothers who gave birth in midwife-led units praised the quality of care they had received both during childbirth and postnatally.

It was a fantastic experience really… The midwife care was brilliant, and the facilities there are great… So the midwife caught her and then just passed her over to me (laughs), and then Sam cut the cord. (Bethan: MLU, waterbirth)

Bethan believed this positive birth experience may have contributed to her baby's calm, easy temperament.

Pretty much everything that's around her that has helped her to feel safe and secure and calm. And yeah, maybe that started off with having a well and truly sort of straightforward arrival. (Bethan: MLU, waterbirth)

Two of the 22 births were homebirths. Both took place in birthing pools and went smoothly, avoiding interventions and negating the need for any pain relief but water. The homebirths were reportedly calm, positive experiences in the comfort of mothers' own homes. However, the midwife for baby Keegan's birth got stuck in early morning traffic and didn't manage to arrive in time for the birth.

Yeah, it felt very calm in the house, really calm… I was in bed until pretty much he was coming down… I was very relaxed… it wasn't even too painful. (Millie: home waterbirth; accidental free birth)

Millie felt that as she was so relaxed during the homebirth, this may have benefitted Keegan's temperament as he was a very relaxed baby, settling easily into family life.

I think that a waterbirth is definitely a relaxing way, definitely relaxing for me, so it must have some impact on them. (Millie: home waterbirth; accidental free birth)

Experiences of Pain Relief

Mothers felt they were affected not only by the type of pain relief they chose to use during labour but also by being deprived of pain relief when they had felt they really needed it. This could impact their overall birth experience, at times turning what might have been a straightforward birth into one of "agony". Martha had a particularly traumatic experience involving being in intense pain and not being heard.

They kept saying they couldn't check because of the pessary, and they wouldn't give me any pain relief 'cause they just thought I was really whingey. (Martha: hospital induction, third-degree tear; baby born without pain relief)

Sara, who was in pain after the birth with a postnatal infection around her caesarean section wound, had a difficult time accessing regular and consistent pain relief after the birth.

> They told me I would need regular pain relief… one day I had to wait 15 hours. (Sara: planned CS, postpartum infection)

Gas and Air

Mothers' experiences of using pharmacological and natural forms of pain relief varied. While some mothers managed to cope solely with breathing techniques or by relaxing in a birthing pool, others ended up using whatever pain relief methods they could get hold of to try and alleviate their pain and distress. Although Entonox ("gas and air") did not suit everyone, making some mothers feel dizzy, sick or disorientated, many enjoyed its mildly analgesic effects. However, these benefits might have been difficult to distinguish from other forms of pain relief that were being used simultaneously, such as water.

> I went back in the pool, and they gave me gas and air. It was great, amazing… What I felt after that was not pain, like I didn't feel any pain with gas and air. (Amanda: MLU waterbirth, Entonox, pethidine, NICU)

For some, the positive effects of gas and air included relaxation, light-headedness and the ability to laugh it seemed to give them.

> I loved it, it was fantastic after nine months of sobriety (laughs); it was really great. (Bethan: MLU, waterbirth, Entonox)

Although others didn't feel it helped them very much, Entonox was considered to have fewer side effects than pethidine or epidural, meaning mothers like Sophia felt they were still in control and therefore could more easily trust, let go and enjoy the experience.

> I didn't feel the gas and air did much, it just made me focus on the breathing… it was lovely being able to be with it and just enjoy it rather than being out of it on pethidine. (Sophia: planned induction, Entonox)

Epidural

Some mothers like Kate below, who had set out on their birth journey fully intending to have a "natural" birth and avoid all pharmacological medication, were pleasantly surprised and experienced an overwhelming sense of relief when their epidural finally released them from hours of ever-increasing agony. This could mean the trauma of intense and unbearable pain was finally over.

> When I got into the room, I was delirious, crying a lot, really not good… Once they'd put the epidural in my back, the rest of the experience was just amazing… for 8 hours, I just sat there… and really enjoyed it. Then they said, 'I think you should push', and I pushed for ten minutes…. (Kate: home to hospital transfer, acceleration, hypnobirthing, epidural)

Kate didn't think the birth or the epidural had impacted her baby, although she felt the baby may have been affected by her stress hormones during the early stages of labour *before* she had any pain relief.

> I don't think so, but I don't know. She had a pretty easy coming into the world. Whether my stress hormones in the earlier part of labour got through, I don't know… but she didn't get distressed, no. (Kate: home to hospital transfer, acceleration, hypnobirthing, epidural)

Kate had also used hypnobirthing to prepare for childbirth, and anecdotally at least, this may produce a calmer baby. Mothers who attend a course in hypnobirthing are expected to practise frequently during their pregnancy and, ideally, they spend a period of relaxation every day. In theory, therefore, they should release fewer of the stress hormones that can affect the baby.

Ava also changed her mind about wanting an epidural after an upsetting hospital transfer and many hours of seemingly fruitless labour.

> At 16 hours when they told me I was just 3cm I completely lost the plot, and I said, 'Can I have an epidural?' My husband was like, 'It's not in the birth plan', and I was like, 'I don't care about the birth plan!' (laughs). (Ava: hospital transfer, acceleration, epidural, episiotomy, forceps)

However, epidural analgesia didn't suit everyone. Issy, for instance, experienced it as traumatic because it meant she was unable to move, instead having to remain on the bed.

> I didn't want an epidural 'cause that scared me more than childbirth… and then within 2 hours, I begged them for an epidural… Then obviously with that you can't really stand up at all, and I think it was the sitting down which was the most traumatic and painful part of it because you could feel the pressure a lot more… I didn't find it helped at all. (Issy: induction, forceps, pethidine, epidural, NICU—neonatal infection)

Pethidine

In spite of some of the recommendations above for epidural analgesia, no one in this sample of 22 mothers had a positive experience with pethidine. Those who did have pethidine tended to be neutral or even outright negative about their experiences. Emily, in particular, spoke fervently about managing to avoid pethidine after a 'horrible' experience with her first baby.

> I hated it… I hallucinated and everything, it was horrible, really horrible… and I think that really aided towards my not coping with Ryan (first baby). (Emily: physiological hospital birth, Entonox)

6.3 What the Mothers Said About Their Birth Experience and Their Baby's Behaviour

In the best-case scenarios, it seemed to simply relax the mother while not reducing painful sensations, aligning with previous research highlighting pethidine's ineffectiveness as a form of pain relief [4].

> It (pethidine) just made me sleepy, really, really sleepy. I can't say that it really took away much pain, but it just made me just completely relaxed.... (Anna: induction, Entonox, pethidine, local anaesthetic, episiotomy, cervical tear, postpartum haemorrhage, infection, blood transfusion)

In other cases, such as Meg and Amanda, pethidine made mothers feel out of control, heightening the sudden shock of pain as it could feel like an unexpected 'stab in the dark', *increasing* perceptions of a traumatic birth experience rather than reducing them as it was supposed to.

> I didn't really think much of that (pethidine) because it just made me feel like I wasn't there, had no control, but I still had pain. (Meg: hospital waterbirth, Entonox, pethidine)

> I think I went into transition phase whilst I was asleep. I woke up and just screamed like blue murder… you know, like one of those really like… blood-curdling screams…. (Amanda: MLU waterbirth, Entonox, pethidine, NICU)

Although not everybody made a link between pethidine and baby behaviour, a couple of mothers felt their baby may have been affected, at least during the early postnatal days. Meg thought her baby had slept too much, making it difficult to breastfeed.

> No, the only thing that I was worried about in the beginning was she slept loads and loads and loads, and I was worried that it was something to do with the pethidine. She slept like a ridiculous amount in the beginning, and they had to say like, 'Have you fed your baby? Wake her up!'. (Meg: hospital waterbirth, Entonox, pethidine)

These findings are consistent with prior research highlighting the effects of pethidine on reduced alertness and excessive sleepiness in the newborn, potentially leading to breastfeeding problems, disturbances in newborn temperature, and infant crying [35, 47, 54]. Moreover, in-labour medications can affect early suckling behaviours [12], and babies are more likely to need assisted birth or a visit to NICU after an epidural, further complicating the mother and baby's difficulties establishing breastfeeding [1]. Indeed, several mothers reported issues with initiating breastfeeding after a combination of synthetic oxytocin, pethidine and/or epidural, which perhaps isn't too surprising given how these substances tend to block endogenous oxytocin—the powerful birth, bonding and breastfeeding hormone (see Chap. 3 for details).

Issy felt that pethidine may have affected her baby's difficult early temperament, as she had exhibited "clingy" and unsettled behaviours from the beginning.

> She's definitely a more clingy baby than my first. She does not like to be put down, she doesn't lie down, she's quite sicky… She won't settle away from me. My mum thinks it's all the chemicals she had. (Issy: induction, forceps, pethidine, epidural, NICU—neonatal infection, antibiotics)

While it's possible that the antibiotics Issy's baby had for the infection may also have upset their delicate digestive system, Issy found the only way to get her baby to settle was to sleep together. This provided some respite from sleeplessness.

> I co-sleep with this one which I never did with my first, mostly because it's the only way I can get some rest. (Issy: induction, forceps, pethidine, epidural, NICU—neonatal infection, antibiotics)

Natural Forms of Pain Relief

In contrast to the negative impacts of opiates like pethidine, certain non-pharmacological forms of pain relief could help mothers cope better with their labour pains, with the added benefit of no side effects. The evening before going into labour, Tessa had learned some hypnobirthing techniques, which she found useful when she was suddenly transferred to the hospital after a midwife discovered meconium in her waters.

> She did some hypnobirthing work with me. It was really good that it was the night before, so I thought of the things she said to make me not worry 'cause there wasn't much reassurance coming from the midwife and um and Ben was like all on edge. (Tessa: hospital transfer, acceleration)

Natural methods of relaxation and positive mental programming such as hypnobirthing, however, did not always provide as much pain relief as expected, occasionally leading to acute disappointment. Nevertheless, mothers were resourceful, and sometimes a specific technique from their hypnobirthing or pregnancy yoga course could be applied during labour with beneficial results, even if the method itself hadn't helped.

> The only thing I really took away from the hypnobirthing was the breathing. The breathing got me through. (Kate: home to hospital transfer, acceleration, hypnobirthing, epidural)

Waterbirths were often experienced as calming and relaxing, although this feeling wasn't always sustained. Some mothers felt the need to get out of the water to keep their focus, while others, like Alison, had a sudden urge to push.

> The first contractions in the pool were so blissful, then the novelty wore off... very quickly I needed to push. (Alison: home waterbirth)

Alison went on to describe her baby's behaviour as "easy" and believed this was linked to his calm birth experience.

> Oh, he's been so calm and content and he's been very easy... He is generally very happy, smiles a lot, is very good at being passed around... very calm. (Alison, home waterbirth)

As you can see from mothers' quotes, when physical problems occurred during childbirth, this seemed to impact their mental and emotional wellbeing. It potentially also influenced the baby's behaviour post-birth, although not all mothers perceived any connection between the birth and their baby's behaviour. The next section explores *psychological* aspects of childbirth in greater depth.

6.3.2 Psychological Birth Experience

Mothers' psychological birth experiences were interwoven with their physical birth experiences. Given the well-known links between birth physiology and maternal psychology [20], the possible pathway between childbirth experience and baby behaviour might also be explained through the mother's subjective emotional experience of childbirth and her subsequent psychological state postnatally. For example, if a mother feels stressed or scared during childbirth, her cortisol (stress hormone) production will rise sharply, increasing perceptions of pain and trauma. Maternal cortisol travels directly through the placenta to the baby, meaning they become physiologically stressed too. In addition to these in-labour effects, if a mother isn't well-supported and cared for postnatally, especially after a difficult birth experience, excess cortisol may continue passing on to the baby through breastmilk. As mentioned, this could affect infant behaviour and wellbeing as it increases the baby's stress response, including their response to fear [48].

Overall, the more subjective and psychological elements of the childbirth experience seemed to have a greater ongoing impact on the wellbeing and behaviour of mother and baby than actual physical events. When arranging the emotional and psychological aspects of childbirth that mothers spoke about into themes, the most dominant were: *emotional states during childbirth*, *expectations*, *support*, *health professional authority* (or *coercion*), *neglect* and *separation* (from partner and/or baby). Mothers' birth stories could be positive, negative or traumatic. Once again, they're presented using direct quotes from the mothers themselves to illustrate the various points of interest.

Emotional States During Childbirth
Mothers frequently talked about their emotional states during childbirth. Aligning with previous studies on mothers' recall of birth experience, the feelings they had during that vulnerable time seemed to remain with them for a long time afterwards. Birth experiences that induce negative emotional states could lead to the potentially long-term impacts of birth trauma, and such experiences can affect mothers both physically and mentally, with adverse impacts on their parenting capacity, self-identity and bonding with their child [42]. Conversely, birth experiences that bring mothers long-term satisfaction seemed to make them feel as if they'd accomplished something worthwhile, generating greater confidence and self-esteem [59].

Several mothers in this sample, such as Amanda, seemed to actively enjoy giving birth to their baby.

I didn't feel any pain, so I was just going with it. I was enjoying it, in the moment... I was still screaming and stuff, but it was more like an animal instinct like... not in pain... All this bit I remember like it was the best thing I've ever done. It was amazing like. The whole like established labour and actually getting him out was amazing. (Amanda: MLU waterbirth, NICU)

However, things didn't go smoothly for them all, and if labour wasn't progressing "normally", this could result in mothers feeling scared of potential upcoming interventions. Tessa was particularly terrified at the prospect of having a surgical birth.

So maximum dosage (of synthetic oxytocin) and the surgeon was ready behind the curtain—they were polishing their cutlery.... (Tessa: hospital transfer, acceleration)

Meanwhile, Emily interpreted her fear of childbirth in quite an unusual way. After a difficult first birth experience, she was hoping for the second one to go better, and yet seemed content to relinquish all control to the hospital staff, highlighting that one size never fits all.

I phoned my mum and I said, 'I'm so scared I feel really calm'. You know when they tell you to write a birth plan, they tell you to prepare yourself, pack your bags, everything... I suddenly felt like everything was out of my control, and it almost relaxed me completely... because I no longer could control it, I think, if that makes any sense. (Emily: physiological hospital birth)

Expectations

Mothers tended to be more accepting of what had happened and to perceive their birth positively if they'd felt well-prepared beforehand. This was especially true for those who experienced *planned* interventions (such as a pre-scheduled induction or caesarean section) as they knew what to expect and had prepared for it mentally and emotionally.

Well, I had to be induced because of my diabetes so we went into hospital on the Saturday... A little cut and the head popped out. It was lovely. (Sophia: planned induction)

Sophia believed the baby had picked up on her relaxed state before and during the birth.

I suppose having a chilled out relaxed-ish birth might help—I wasn't stressed out at all. It helps the baby not feeling any stresses from the mum. Yeah, he's a very chilled out little boy. (Sophia: planned induction)

Sometimes, however, high expectations of having a natural or easy birth could lead to mothers feeling acutely disappointed afterwards.

... because I used to be super fit and healthy and run half marathons and I thought, yeah, I can do this. I thought I'm the sort of person who's got a body that can deliver a child... Wrong way round! (Tilly: emergency caesarean, internal haemorrhage, morphine)

6.3 What the Mothers Said About Their Birth Experience and Their Baby's Behaviour

As we saw earlier, an unexpected hospital transfer from home or a midwife-led unit could be very distressing for a labouring mother, especially if the hospital seemed unprepared.

> When we got there, the bed wasn't there. I was on the floor on all fours at reception. It was 32 degrees that day. The hospital was unbearably hot, so they had all the windows open. When they showed me to the delivery suite, they had building works going on outside the window. That really distressed me. I was kind of holding myself together until that point, but I just started crying. (Kate: home to hospital transfer with midwife, acceleration)

Mothers who weren't expecting to have to stay in hospital afterwards also struggled to cope with the change of plans if they or their baby now required specialist medical treatment.

> That was the worst week, well five days, of my life. It really traumatised me, that stay in hospital… which is really hard because when you speak to some people they say, 'Oh we loved it, you know, the support we got from the midwives…' I said quite often, 'This is worse than prison. In prison you get an Xbox, and you get a TV, and you don't have a baby that's waking you up every half an hour'. (Amanda: MLU waterbirth, NICU)

Although Amanda's baby was born in a birthing pool, which generally represents a scene of serenity, she felt he may have been affected by her very long labour, combined with his medical issues after birth.

> I think so… Yeah… I think his difficulties feeding were affected by the birth… the length of it… I felt like he would have suffered for quite a long time… being squashed and stuff, because it was going on for so long… Yeah, I can't really put my finger on why it would have affected him but I'm sure it would…. (Amanda MLU waterbirth, NICU)

Mothers like Ava, who had an unexpectedly challenging birth involving trauma, could experience conflicting emotions postnatally, making it difficult to bond with their baby.

> And I think as a result of that as well I didn't feel I could bond with him at all well… We really struggled with him the first couple of weeks. 'Have I done the right thing having a baby?' All this jazz. (Ava: hospital transfer, acceleration, episiotomy, forceps)

In contrast, when mothers' prenatal expectations of childbirth were met, they seemed to fare well and feel good about themselves, the birth and their baby.

> I found both births really empowering… quite euphoric. They gave me a sense of achievement. (Jenny: physiological hospital birth)

Notwithstanding this positive experience and a contented, settled baby, Jenny didn't link her baby's easy-going temperament to the birth.

> Sleep was good. He'd sleep for 5–6 hours at a time… he's quite a content little baby…as long as he's fed, he will self-soothe, let me leave the room, go to anybody… No, I don't think so… I think 'cause I didn't have a traumatic birth… but I think if I had experienced trauma it may have affected him. (Jenny: physiological hospital birth)

On the whole, unmet birth expectations negatively influenced mothers' postnatal mood and the way they perceived the birth and early postnatal period while they grappled with learning how to care for their new baby [6, 22]. Some mothers with unmet expectations felt a deep sense of failure and disappointment around the birth, occasionally affecting their ability to bond with the baby. Although all births are different and largely unpredictable, and it's very difficult to prepare mothers for every possible eventuality without filling them with unnecessary fear, attending antenatal classes could prepare mothers better for the reality of childbirth and early parenting, and face-to-face antenatal classes providing unbiased trustworthy information about childbirth and parenthood might reduce some of the mystery, anxiety and fear around childbirth. This is known to improve the overall birth experience, boosting confidence and empowering both mothers and their partners while better preparing them for the parenting journey ahead [60]. It's also imperative that all parents have easy access to clear and consistent information after the baby is born, as well as postnatal help and support when it's needed [45].

Support

Getting the right support during and after childbirth was linked to women feeling positive postnatally. Those who received the appropriate physical and emotional support during and after childbirth felt as if they'd been well cared for, enhancing their perceptions of the birth experience.

> She (midwife) was brilliant… She really looked after me afterwards… She even washed me… Yeah, she was very, very special. (Emily: physiological hospital birth)

Being well-supported could also benefit a mother's postnatal mood and perceptions of the baby. Emily believed there could be a link between her positive postnatal emotional state and the baby's temperament.

> He's really happy; he's really placid as well… Um, well yeah and particularly my um emotions I suppose... like I felt confident and calm and happy...and I still do. (Emily: physiological hospital birth)

Partners often played an active role in supporting the mother during labour.

> My husband was doing all the things he'd learnt… supporting me, um, rubbing my back, making sure I was drinking. He also did some of the things he wasn't taught to do, which was, um, get lots of kidney dishes because I was vomiting a lot (laughs). (Susan: physiological hospital birth)

Susan thought the smooth, straightforward birth without any need for medication had contributed to her baby's alert and responsive behaviour postnatally, which she felt had facilitated bonding.

> We didn't really have any drugs, so she came out as alert as she was going to be. It was quite nice to know that we could bond straight away, and she was a hundred per cent rather than dosed up on pethidine or something. (Susan: physiological hospital birth)

6.3 What the Mothers Said About Their Birth Experience and Their Baby's Behaviour

Postnatally, midwives played a key role in settling new mothers and babies, often helping mothers like Kate to establish breastfeeding, particularly if they were finding this difficult or challenging.

> I was lying to the midwife, saying she was latching on 'cause I was so desperate to go home… then this lovely Columbian midwife saved the day. She literally grabbed my boob and flung it in her (baby's) mouth (laughs). So that's how it's done! (Kate: home to hospital transfer, acceleration)

Ensuring that mothers didn't feel judged while supporting them was vital.

> She's just amazing (health visitor)—I call her the boob whisperer 'cause… She calmed me more than anything… She just chilled me out, and I didn't feel like she was judging me because I can't do it. (Ava: hospital transfer, acceleration, episiotomy, forceps)

Sadly, some mothers experienced a distinct lack of support at a time when they needed it most, and a light-hearted approach from health professionals could be misconstrued as carelessness.

> So, we went upstairs to the hospital into this tiny little room with a crazy old midwife… She put all the sort of bleepers on the belly and stuff just to make sure everything was alright, but some of the things weren't working and stuff and… Every time she came in, she would wipe her nose on her sleeve, or she was eating something… So, I don't know, she was just trying to be light-hearted, but it didn't inspire confidence. (Tessa, hospital transfer, acceleration)

Unfortunately, Tessa's partner didn't manage to plug the gap in health professional support for his labouring wife. This led to her feeling very alone during labour and birth.

> I walked around, but there was no bars and nothing to hold onto, so I grabbed hold of my thighs to balance, and like I held onto my thighs, and the room was so small, and when I was walking around, Ben then went on the bed, and he fell asleep on the (single) bed, and I felt like totally on my own … I just felt all on my own. And then the midwife would come in and check the reading on the machines and time it, and they would just sort of pop in and out, pop in and out, you know. (Tessa: hospital transfer, acceleration)

Tessa's lack of support from her partner and midwife at such a crucial time had negatively impacted her perceptions of any physical and psychological safety during and after childbirth. Despite these feelings, however, she managed to console the newborn baby by keeping her close during the postnatal period.

> I did just cuddle her and mollycoddle her for a long time… She was contented on me… So yeah, we were quite stuck… I didn't really let others in as much to hold her and carry her round and things when she was a tiny baby 'cause I just felt like she just needed to be back in the womb (laughs). (Tessa: hospital transfer, acceleration)

Tessa wasn't the only mother who responded to their baby's needs during the postnatal period by keeping them close. Others were also willing to mother in a new way if it might help their baby become more settled and content over time. The developmental psychologist Dieter Wolke, who designed the "Mother and Baby Scales" [68, 69] used in the following two chapters, has found that this kind of sensitive maternal caregiving for the baby helps the newborn in their initial 'behavioural organisation' after birth [66]. More recent research indicates that when mothers are sensitive to their baby's distress, it can also help babies overcome negative emotionality and promote attachment [39, 40].

Health Professional Authority (Coercion)

Comments about health professionals exerting their power and authority arose surprisingly often. This theme describes women being coerced or told what to do during childbirth, often leading to an acute loss of control in their situation or surroundings. "Lack of control" is commonly cited as the most significant factor in a traumatic birth, followed closely by 'intense pain' [37]. In the current study, loss of control frequently occurred around hospital transfers and unwanted interventions such as continuous electronic foetal monitoring, which, unfortunately, is still standard hospital practice in spite of limited evidence to support its routine use in low-risk pregnancies. Indeed, as highlighted by a well-cited Cochrane review, it appears to increase caesarean section and assisted birth rates without increasing safety [3].

In our study, several mothers talked about how they had felt coerced into agreeing to unwanted medical interventions for the baby's "safety". This could lead to regrets around the birth, which may have coloured the early postnatal days of parenting, bonding, and how mothers perceived their babies.

> If the doctors decide this is the way they want you to do it, it's very hard not to. If something then happened… I'd never forgive myself. (Issy: induction, forceps, NICU—neonatal infection)

Coercion seemed to happen when parents weren't given adequate information or enough time and opportunity to participate in an unbiased discussion with their healthcare providers that would enable them to make *informed choices* about their baby's birth. Such potentially life-changing decisions should be made by parents based on *unbiased* scientific evidence, rather than by hospital staff based on a fear of litigation, as they often seem to be. A nationwide Swiss study of over 6000 women shows that "informal coercion" could be at least partially responsible for some of the rise in obstetric interventions we are seeing across developed countries. Alongside hospital transfer and emergency caesarean section, such coercion reduces mothers' birth satisfaction and increases the risk of developing postnatal depression [49]. Allowing mothers' autonomy during childbirth is therefore an essential aspect of good maternity care as it increases birth satisfaction and the likelihood of a positive birth experience [24].

In addition to coercion, some mothers were treated or spoken to unkindly by the health professionals attending them during childbirth.

> And then everything I didn't want to happen happened, which was, I didn't want to have stirrups or anything like that, and the next thing was they took the gas and air away and said

6.3 What the Mothers Said About Their Birth Experience and Their Baby's Behaviour

> I wasn't pushing hard enough.... (Rachael: hospital induction, third-degree tear, postpartum haemorrhage)

Somewhat surprisingly, although Rachael acknowledged that her baby wasn't happy after his birth, she didn't connect this in any way to her traumatic birth experience.

> No, not directly, I don't think. If he'd been born naturally premature, we may have got a bit more support... Looking back, there wasn't a time when he wasn't crying... He'd feed little and often 'cause he was so uncomfortable as well... He wasn't sleeping, and nor was I.... (Rachael: hospital induction, third-degree tear, postpartum haemorrhage)

When women's sense of privacy and self-control was violated, this could lead to deep and lasting psychological distress, which stayed with mothers like Abigail long after the birth of their baby.

> It was traumatic, horrific... first they did an internal examination... I felt... kind of exposed, my private bits being examined by a stranger... I spent the whole night in absolute agony... like someone ripping my insides apart.... They broke my waters – they didn't ask. Suddenly, there was stuff coming out of me. I didn't know what was happening ... They were telling me, 'Keep your legs open, keep your legs open', though my natural instinct was to curl up in foetal position to protect myself. (Abigail: overnight hospital induction)

Abigail experienced much of this trauma alone, as the hospital staff had sent her partner home to sleep during her night induction. Breaking the waters (amniotic sac) without the mother's permission is classed as obstetric violence as it breaks the code of respectful maternity care, which should always ensure mothers' physical *and psychological* safety [18]. This experience may have had some negative physiological and psychological repercussions for the mother and baby, although Abigail didn't perceive her baby's difficult, easily distressed behavioural style to be in any way connected to her upsetting and challenging birth experience.

> He's very angry when he's changed or bathed... he screams his head off. Feeding... was a battle. It feels like the hardest job I've ever had. (Abigail: overnight hospital induction)

Issy also had a negative experience of painful vaginal examinations though she was more forthright about her discomfort and disapproval than Abigail.

> I don't think my husband was there yet. The doctor did an examination. It was horrific—really uncomfortable... I just told her to get out. (Issy: induction, forceps, NICU—neonatal infection)

Mothers were frequently told they were 'not allowed' to do something—even, in Susan's case, to bring their partner into the bathroom while she had a bath due to its position in a patient-only zone. Thankfully, the midwife managed to work around the strict hospital protocols.

> She suggested I had a bath, but I was very reluctant because Robin couldn't come with me, and as I said, I'd been basically sleeping or passing out. And I wasn't overly keen on the idea of being in a bath when I could barely stay conscious... I agreed to a bath in the end...

> I think I did (pass out) for a little bit... They left me on my own in the bath... But, um, I'd taken my phone in with me, and I was about to be sick, so I called Robin and told him I was going to be sick and um, one of the midwives let him in and um, she let him stay. She kind of sneaked him in. (Susan: physiological hospital birth)

In other cases, such as Ava's, a health professional's authoritative tone could leave mothers feeling 'devastated' about a change in their birth plan on which they'd not been consulted.

> And I said, 'Well I'm having a waterbirth', and he (Dr) said, 'Oh no you're not, you've gone over 24 hours now'... so I lost the plot and burst out crying.... (Ava: hospital transfer, acceleration, episiotomy, forceps)

Labouring mothers could also be made to feel they *had* to do something they didn't want to, such as continuous electronic foetal monitoring. This could be experienced as restrictive to natural in-labour movement and very uncomfortable. However, mothers didn't always feel they had a choice or that they'd been adequately consulted for this standard, non-evidence-based intervention.

> I wanted to do it on all fours... I kept saying I needed the toilet just so I could get the straps taken off me. It's horrendous pain. I don't understand why they don't just put them on you intermittently to see if the baby's alright... you're trying to move around attached to the ruddy machine... 'cause I was connected to all the machines, I wasn't really allowed to move.... (Ava: hospital transfer, acceleration, episiotomy, forceps)

Neglect

Although labouring mothers clearly need unwavering physical and emotional support throughout labour and birth, staff shortages and the busyness of modern maternity wards could mean that midwifery care was, at best, intermittent and, at worst, downright neglectful. Mothers who felt abandoned or neglected could become frightened about what might happen to them and their babies. Martha had requested pain relief with increasing urgency but wasn't listened to or granted any until it was too late, and the baby was being born.

> Yeah, we kept getting left a lot in the room on our own with nobody – it was quite scary... The pain was like getting worse and worse. I was getting really dizzy and sick, but they told me they couldn't give me any pain relief because what would I be like if I was in proper labour? But at this point nobody checked me at all... to see if I was in labour or not.... (Martha: hospital induction, third-degree tear)

Inspite of having such a frightening birth experience, Martha still managed to feel sympathy for the overworked hospital staff.

> The midwives actually in the labour bit were lovely. They were just really short staffed I think, otherwise they would have probably checked more and done more. (Martha: hospital induction, third-degree tear)

However, Martha's postnatal experiences weren't much better.

6.3 What the Mothers Said About Their Birth Experience and Their Baby's Behaviour

> They brought me out of theatre, and he (the father) stayed with us for an hour, but then he wasn't allowed down to the ward… I couldn't move in the bed, so every time he (the baby) cried, I'd have to ring the buzzer; it was horrible. (Martha: hospital induction, third-degree tear)

Although Martha had such traumatic birth and postnatal experiences, she didn't see any connection between this and her baby seeming very unsettled and in pain.

> The first few weeks. he was just constantly sick, constantly in pain and screaming…. jittery. He does it all the time, it's like he's startled and his hands sort of shake. (Martha: hospital induction, third-degree tear)

Other mothers who felt neglected were also sympathetic towards the over-stretched midwives. They experienced conflicting emotions as they attempted to balance an awareness of how 'rushed off their feet' the midwives must be with their own and their baby's acute distress. Unfortunately, the mother's and baby's most basic essential needs were often left unmet, as was the case for poor Tilly, who couldn't even reach her baby when he was hungry or needed comforting.

> The antenatal care was good, but the postnatal care… I was left in dirty sheets, I had to shower myself, and at times I had to sit on the floor in the shower because I couldn't stand up… One night I was left with a drip in one arm but the baby over the other side…. (Tilly: emergency caesarean, internal haemorrhage, morphine)

Given the amount of distress experienced by some of these mothers, and the outcomes of this for them and their babies, it seems clear that partners should always be allowed to remain during childbirth and postnatally, not only as a source of solace and comfort for the mother, but also to advocate for her rights and help care for the baby. Unfortunately, this was not the case during the Covid-19 pandemic, when partners were often banned from accompanying mothers into hospitals or midwife-led units for essential maternity care. These emotionally barbaric rules were the cause of much distress among parents while hampering health professionals from forming supportive, caring relationships with families [55]. When looking at the implementation of enforced isolation and separation between parents (or sometimes between mothers and their babies), and the potential impacts of such a violation of human rights on the mother's mental health, it's possible these healthcare decisions could still be affecting the parents and babies who experienced them.

Separation

When the women in this study were separated from their partner or baby, this presented another source of distress, impacting mothers' perceptions of the birth and their newborn babies' wellbeing and behaviour. Separation of mother and baby may occur if either has urgent medical needs or if doctors feel the need to conduct further medical checks on them. It often happens when a baby's whisked off to the NICU, where the mother and baby's intrinsic physiological and emotional need to remain together may be abandoned in favour of urgent medical attention. Although we've known for decades that this kind of separation can cause extreme distress for both the mother and the newborn baby [19], many hospitals continue to separate the pair during this crucial time. To help overcome the problem, scientists [26, 27] have emphasised the vital importance of providing a quiet and comfortable space within busy neonatal intensive care units. This would allow mothers to spend time with their babies, enabling emotional closeness and bonding to take place.

Although the mothers in this study were interviewed pre-pandemic, women could be abruptly separated from their partners—especially during night inductions when staff would simply send them home 'to sleep'. The long, dark night alone in pain could then feel like an eternity.

> The worst was when they took my husband away from me—it may not have been very long—it felt like a very long time… I was just on my own, honestly, it's horrible… I think your partner should be with you… I was quite lonely… I didn't sleep…. (Issy: induction, forceps, NICU—neonatal infection)

Separation from an emotionally close and trusted person, like a partner, seemed to have a huge impact on a mother's psyche and ability to relax into labour, which may not have been conducive to efficient labour progression. Partners were sometimes whisked away *after* the birth as well. This was more likely to happen following birth complications, where mothers were taken off to be stitched, or when the father was escorted out of the theatre holding the baby if the baby required more medical checks while the mother rested after giving birth. Kate commented on how abandoned she felt when unexpectedly left alone after the busy chaos of the birth scene.

> Then I was left on my own in that room for 2 hours. It was strange after all that, and all the people, suddenly completely alone. (Kate: home to hospital transfer, acceleration)

Separation from a partner, baby or both could make new mothers like Amanda feel quite distraught.

> I was taken… to have a shower and he went with his dad to NICU… I suddenly panicked—Where's my husband and my baby? (Amanda: MLU waterbirth, NICU)

Amanda thought her baby's behaviour may have been disturbed by all the stress around his birth as well as by the separation post-birth. She also felt he may have been affected by her negative postnatal physiological and mental state.

> I think so yeah… I know it definitely affected me (laughs), and that in turn probably affects him as well—and that I was just so tired—but I can't specifically say what… I think his difficulties feeding were affected by the birth... and also, he was taken away from me straight away…. (Amanda: MLU waterbirth, NICU)

In addition, Amanda acknowledged how having constant tests performed on her baby in the NICU for the first 5 days may have upset his wellbeing during the early postnatal period.

He was waking a lot in the night to feed. And then, probably from about two months old, he's been a really laid-back baby. He's been really calm… (In NICU) They were doing obs. every half hour, which was very disruptive for him… he'd scream and cry… He didn't have a very nice start. (Amanda: MLU waterbirth, NICU)

Sometimes, for a mother like Issy, seeing their new baby in the room but not being able to hold or even touch them could feel just as cruel.

They took her away straight away, and I didn't see her—she was in a corner—it was a shame. I wanted to be attached, but she was over in the corner with the paediatrician. (Issy: induction, pethidine, epidural, forceps, NICU—neonatal infection)

Issy went on to struggle with her baby and put some of the issues with the baby down to how the birth had made her feel postnatally. She also felt that what had occurred during labour and birth—including separation from her partner and subsequent isolation during a night induction, coercion into unwanted interventions, intensive pain relief medication and a forceps delivery—may have had a negative impact on her own and the baby's wellbeing.

Part of me wonders if her behaviour's been affected by my reaction to the birth, if that makes sense… she is very different to the first in terms of her neediness…. (Issy)

Concluding Concepts

Consistent with prior research, mothers in this study who experienced obstetric complications and unplanned interventions more often reported feelings of intense pain, distress and fear during childbirth than those who gave birth more easily. These mothers were also more likely to experience difficulties with infant feeding and sleeping in addition to a more challenging adjustment to motherhood and bonding with their baby. In contrast, those who gave birth spontaneously without the need for medical interventions often talked about feelings of joy and elation along with a sense of empowerment after the birth. Moreover, they tended to bond with their babies more easily and reported more settled, calm and content baby behaviour. This may be directly due to the physical birth experience itself being easier for the mother and baby, but it could also be the result of positive maternal mood and its associated release of beneficial birth hormones, including prolactin, endorphins and oxytocin.

These "happy" hormones are highly conducive to easier birthing, bonding and breastfeeding and a positive maternal mood [13, 14, 25], all of which facilitate a calmer, more content and settled baby. As we saw in Chap. 4, mother-baby oxytocin levels correspond with one another, being *lower* in both mother and baby if the mother is depressed post-birth [7]. A recent study demonstrates how the postnatal moods of mother and baby bidirectionally covary throughout the day, indicating that the pair are intricately bound together, not just for essential physical tasks such as breastfeeding, but also in their expression of fluctuating positive or negative physiological states [36]. Put simply, a happy mother means a happy baby, while a depressed mother, unfortunately, seems much more likely to have an unsettled and fretful baby.

Negative birth experiences could also stem from mothers' unmet expectations, unexpected birth events, whether they were well-supported and how they were treated during and after childbirth. Consistent with an abundance of previous research evidence on the importance of positive interactions with health professionals and high-quality continuous support during childbirth [10, 38, 51], how well mothers felt cared for during this momentous life event seemed to make a substantial difference to their postnatal mood, how they perceived the birth, and how they described their baby's physiological wellbeing and behaviour. Those who had received good emotional and physical support felt immense gratitude towards the health professionals and partners (as well as doulas, friends or family) who had supported them. Professional postnatal support was especially appreciated by mothers who had struggled to initiate breastfeeding successfully. But these positive experiences of appropriate care were not shared by all. Some mothers felt neglected by health professionals during or after childbirth, negatively impacting their overall birth experience.

Sadly, the neglect or mistreatment of women during childbirth is still all too common. A seminal review defined in-labour "mistreatments" as awareness of staff shortages, not being "allowed" to bring one's partner into the bathroom, painful vaginal examinations, feeling neglected or inadequately supported, health professionals refusing to provide adequate pain relief, feeling that birth choices have been disrespected and a lack of informed consent [9]. While these issues go directly against the World Health Organization's [64] recommendations and the NICE [46] intrapartum care guidelines for healthy mothers and babies, each mistreatment on this list was reported at some point by a mother in this study. I found it quite astonishing that more than a couple of decades after my first birth experience, women were still being treated like this. The research evidence today shows quite clearly how mothers and babies are being negatively impacted by birth trauma, perhaps for a lifetime. Given the fact that every single one of us experiences being born, and approximately half of us experience giving birth, positive childbirth experiences ought to be made a priority.

The interviews with mothers also found that postnatal events affected the mother and baby. When things went wrong (e.g. the baby had to spend time in NICU or the mother experienced a postpartum haemorrhage or wound infection), this seemed to knock the mother's early confidence in coping with and caring for their baby, who was more likely to be unsettled following separation from their mother. Aligning with prior research [1, 41], many mothers struggled to breastfeed after pethidine, an epidural or a caesarean section. In contrast, those with a straightforward, spontaneous birth and immediate skin-to-skin time with their baby were more likely to describe successful breastfeeding behaviours. When struggling mothers received breastfeeding support in the postnatal ward, this could help to heal a negative birth experience, increase natural skin-to-skin contact between mother and baby and encourage bonding.

As described in earlier chapters, mother and baby release and mutually exchange the powerful birth, breastfeeding and bonding hormone oxytocin during intimate skin-to-skin time. This encourages instinctive newborn behaviours such as the 'breast crawl' [65], decreases neonatal crying [44] and improves the baby's self-regulation and ability to soothe themselves [66]. Skin-to-skin contact naturally improves breastfeeding outcomes [43], partly by increasing maternal self-efficacy and breastfeeding confidence [2]. When the mothers in our study were well-supported, encouraged to maintain proximity with their baby through skin-to-skin care and to persevere with breastfeeding after a challenging birth, this seemed mutually restorative for mother and baby, with some mothers reporting how their babies became calmer and easier to handle in time [16, 56]. Equally, if mothers chose to quit breastfeeding and convert to bottle feeding, especially after a difficult birth or postnatal experience that may have involved mother-baby separation and the hormonal disruptions that go with this, it was vital for these mothers to receive non-judgemental support for their decision.

Although many mothers didn't perceive any connection between their birth experience and their baby's behaviour, the results of this qualitative interview study support the concept that something appears to be happening. Regardless of birth mode, how mothers experienced childbirth and how well cared for they felt during and after birth seemed to affect how well they coped with early motherhood and how they perceived their baby's early temperament and behaviour. Less than half of the mothers saw a connection between childbirth and baby behaviour, yet the data show some apparent trends; it appears that the birth experience might affect how mothers feel about themselves and cope with their baby after childbirth, as well as how the baby behaves. Regardless of whether this was true, the findings further emphasise the importance of continuous, empathic care, where mothers are listened to and involved in the decision-making process regarding their baby's birth. The following two chapters aim to shed more light on the picture by presenting the findings of an extensive online survey of over a thousand mothers that examined multiple physical and psychological perinatal variables in relation to mothers' perceptions of their babies' behaviours.

References

1. Adams J, Frawley J, Steel A, Broom A, Sibbritt D. Use of pharmacological and non-pharmacological labour pain management techniques and their relationship to maternal and infant birth outcomes: examination of a nationally representative sample of 1835 pregnant women. Midwifery. 2015;31(4):458–63.
2. Aghdas K, Talat K, Sepideh B. Effect of immediate and continuous mother–infant skin-to-skin contact on breastfeeding self-efficacy of primiparous women: a randomised control trial. Women Birth. 2014;27(1):37–40.
3. Alfirevic Z, Gyte GM, Cuthbert A, Devane D. Continuous cardiotocography (CTG) as a form of electronic fetal monitoring (EFM) for fetal assessment during labour. Cochrane Database Syst Rev. 2017;(2). https://www.cochranelibrary.com/cdsr/doi/10.1002/14651858.CD006066.pub3/pdf/full.

4. Anderson D. A review of systemic opioids commonly used for labor pain relief. J Midwifery Womens Health. 2011;56(3):222–39.
5. Ayers S, Bond R, Bertullies S, Wijma K. The aetiology of post-traumatic stress following childbirth: a meta-analysis and theoretical framework. Psychol Med. 2016;46(6):1121–34.
6. Ayers S, Pickering AD. Women's expectations and experience of birth. Psychol Health. 2005;20(1):79–92.
7. Baron-Cohen KL, Fearon P, Meins E, Feldman R, Hardiman P, Rosan C, Fonagy P. Maternal mind-mindedness and infant oxytocin are interrelated and negatively associated with postnatal depression. Dev Psychopathol. 2024:1–12.
8. Beijers R, Buitelaar JK, de Weerth C. Mechanisms underlying the effects of prenatal psychosocial stress on child outcomes: beyond the HPA axis. Eur Child Adolesc Psychiatry. 2014;23(10):943–56.
9. Bohren MA, Vogel JP, Hunter EC, Lutsiv O, Makh SK, Souza JP, Aguiar C, Coneglian FS, Araújo Diniz AL, Tunçalp O, Javadi D, Oladapo OT, Khosla R, Hindin MJ, Gülmezoglu AM. The mistreatment of women during childbirth in health facilities globally: a mixed-methods systematic review. PLoS Med. 2015;12(6):e1001847.
10. Bohren MA, Hofmeyr GJ, Sakala C, Fukuzawa RK, Cuthbert A. Continuous support for women during childbirth. Cochrane Database Syst Rev. 2017;(7):CD003766.
11. Braun V, Clarke V. One size fits all? What counts as quality practice in (reflexive) thematic analysis? Qual Res Psychol. 2021;18(3):328–52.
12. Brimdyr K, Cadwell K, Widström AM, Svensson K, Phillips R. The effect of labor medications on normal newborn behavior in the first hour after birth: a prospective cohort study. Early Hum Dev. 2019;132:30–6.
13. Buckley SJ. Executive summary of hormonal physiology of childbearing: evidence and implications for women, babies, and maternity care. J Perinat Educ. 2015;24(3):145–53.
14. Buckley S, Uvnäs-Moberg K. Nature and consequences of oxytocin and other neurohormones in the perinatal period. In: Downe S, Byrom S, editors. Squaring the circle: normal birth research, theory and practice in a technological age. London: Pinter and Martin; 2019. p. 19–31.
15. Byrne D. A worked example of Braun and Clarke's approach to reflexive thematic analysis. Qual Quant. 2022;56(3):1391–412.
16. Bystrova K, Ivanova V, Edhborg M, Matthieson AS, Ransjo-Arvidson AB, Mukhamedrakhimov R, Uvnäs-Moberg K, Widstrom AM. Early contact versus separation: effects on mother-infant interaction one year later. Birth. 2009;36(2):97–109.
17. Caldwell J, Meredith P, Whittingham K, Ziviani J. Shame and guilt in the postnatal period: a systematic review. J Reprod Infant Psychol. 2021;39(1):67–85.
18. Cantor AG, Jungbauer RM, Skelly AC, Hart EL, Jorda K, Davis-O'Reilly C, et al. Respectful maternity care: dissemination and implementation of perinatal safety culture to improve equitable maternal healthcare delivery and outcomes. NIH National Library of Medicine; 2024. Available at: https://www.ncbi.nlm.nih.gov/books/NBK599318/. Accessed 17 Aug 2024.
19. Christensson K, Cabrera T, Christensson E, Uvnäs-Moberg K, Winberg J. Separation distress call in the human neonate in the absence of maternal body contact. Acta Paediatr. 1995;84(5):468–73.
20. Dahan O, Zibenberg A, Goldberg A. Birthing consciousness and the flow experience during physiological childbirth. Midwifery. 2024;138:104151.
21. Dahlen HG, Kennedy HP, Anderson CM, Bell AF, Clark A, Foureur M, Ohm JE, Shearman AM, Taylor JY, Wright ML, Downe S. The EPIIC hypothesis: intrapartum effects on the neonatal epigenome and consequent health outcomes. Med Hypotheses. 2013;80(5):656–62.
22. Danehchin N, Javadifar N, Iravani M, Dastoorpoor M. Service quality gap of care during childbirth and postpartum and its relationship with childbirth satisfaction. J Health Sci Surveill Syst. 2023;11(1):63–9.
23. Douglas PS, Hill PS. A neurobiological model for cry-fuss problems in the first three to four months of life. Med Hypotheses. 2013;81(5):816–22.

24. Ďuríčeková B, Škodová Z, Bašková M. Satisfaction with childbirth and level of autonomy of women during the childbirth. Cent Eur J Nurs Midwifery. 2024;15(4):2060–8.
25. Feldman R, Weller A, Zagoory-Sharon O, Levine A. Evidence for a neuroendocrinological foundation of human affiliation: plasma oxytocin levels across pregnancy and the postpartum period predict mother-infant bonding. Psychol Sci. 2007;18(11):965–70.
26. Flacking R, Lehtonen L, Thomson G, Axelin A, Ahlqvist S, Moran VH, Ewald U, Dykes F, SCENE Group. Closeness and separation in neonatal intensive care. Acta Paediatr. 2012;101(10):1032–7.
27. Flacking R, Thomson G, Axelin A. Pathways to emotional closeness in neonatal units–a cross-national qualitative study. BMC Pregnancy Childbirth. 2016;16(1):1–8.
28. Foster JA, Neufeld KAM. Gut–brain axis: how the microbiome influences anxiety and depression. Trends Neurosci. 2013;36(5):305–12.
29. Garthus-Niegel S, von Soest T, Vollrath ME, Eberhard-Gran M. The impact of subjective birth experiences on post-traumatic stress symptoms: a longitudinal study. Arch Womens Ment Health. 2013;16(1):1–10.
30. Garthus-Niegel S, Ayers S, Martini J, von Soest T, Eberhard-Gran M. The impact of postpartum post-traumatic stress disorder symptoms on child development: a population-based, 2-year follow-up study. Psychol Med. 2017;47(1):161.
31. Gitau R, Cameron A, Fisk NM, Glover V. Fetal exposure to maternal cortisol. Lancet. 1998;352(9129):707–8.
32. Gitau R, Menson E, Pickles V, Fisk NM, Glover V, MacLachlan N. Umbilical cortisol levels as an indicator of the fetal stress response to assisted vaginal delivery. Eur J Obstet Gynecol Reprod Biol. 2001;98(1):14–7.
33. Granat A, Gadassi R, Gilboa-Schechtman E, Feldman R. Maternal depression and anxiety, social synchrony, and infant regulation of negative and positive emotions. Emotion. 2017;17(1):11.27.
34. Hamilton C. Using the Valsalva technique during the second stage of labour. Br J Midwifery. 2016;24(2):90–4.
35. Hemati Z, Abdollahi M, Broumand S, Delaram M, Namnabati M, Kiani D. Association between newborns' breastfeeding behaviors in the first two hours after birth and drugs used for their mothers in labor. Iran J Child Neurol. 2018;12(2):33.
36. Hibel LC, Liu S, Boyer C. Mother-infant covariation of positive and negative emotions across the day. Infant Child Dev. 2024;34:e2562.
37. Hollander MH, van Hastenberg E, van Dillen J, Van Pampus MG, de Miranda E, Stramrood CA. Preventing traumatic childbirth experiences: 2192 women's perceptions and views. Arch Womens Ment Health. 2017;20(4):515–23.
38. Horsch A, Garthus-Niegel S. Posttraumatic stress disorder following childbirth. In: Childbirth, vulnerability and law. Routledge; 2019. p. 49–66.
39. Leerkes EM, Zhou N. Maternal sensitivity to distress and attachment outcomes: interactions with sensitivity to nondistress and infant temperament. J Fam Psychol. 2018;32(6):753.
40. Letourneau N, Tryphonopoulos P, Giesbrecht G, Dennis CL, Bhogal S, Watson B. Narrative and meta-analytic review of interventions aiming to improve maternal–child attachment security. Infant Ment Health J. 2015;36(4):366–87.
41. Li L, Wan W, Zhu C. Breastfeeding after a cesarean section: a literature review. Midwifery. 2021;103:103117.
42. Molloy E, Biggerstaff DL, Sidebotham P. A phenomenological exploration of parenting after birth trauma: mothers perceptions of the first year. Women Birth. 2021;34(3):278–87.
43. Moore ER, Anderson GC. Randomized controlled trial of very early mother-infant skin-to-skin contact and breastfeeding status. J Midwifery Womens Health. 2007;52(2):116–25.
44. Moore ER, Bergman N, Anderson GC, Medley N. Early skin-to-skin contact for mothers and their healthy newborn infants. Cochrane Database Syst Rev. 2016;(11):CD003519.
45. National Institute for Health and Care Research (NIHR). First-time mothers need clear and consistent information about the care they can expect after giving birth. 2024. https://evidence.

nihr.ac.uk/alert/first-time-mothers-need-clear-and-consistent-information-about-the-care-they-can-expect-after-giving-birth/.
46. NICE. Intrapartum care (NICE guideline [NG235]). 2023. Available at: https://www.nice.org.uk/guidance/ng235/chapter/Recommendations#care-throughout-labour-in-all-birth-settings. Accessed 31.12.24.
47. Nissen E, Lilja G, Matthiesen AS, Ransjö-Arvidsson AB, Uvnäs-Moberg K, Widstrom AM. Effects of maternal pethidine on infants' developing breast feeding behaviour. Acta Paediatr. 1995;84(2):140–5.
48. Nolvi S, Uusitupa HM, Bridgett DJ, Pesonen H, Aatsinki AK, Kataja EL, Korja R, Karlsson H, Karlsson L. Human milk cortisol concentration predicts experimentally induced infant fear reactivity: moderation by infant sex. Dev Sci. 2018;21(4):e12625.
49. Oelhafen S, Trachsel M, Monteverde S, Raio L, Cignacco E. Informal coercion during childbirth: risk factors and prevalence estimates from a nationwide survey of women in Switzerland. BMC Pregnancy Childbirth. 2021;21(1):369.
50. Ostlund BD, Conradt E, Crowell SE, Tyrka AR, Marsit CJ, Lester BM. Prenatal stress, fearfulness, and the epigenome: exploratory analysis of sex differences in DNA methylation of the glucocorticoid receptor gene. Front Behav Neurosci. 2016;10:147.
51. Patterson J, Hollins Martin C, Karatzias T. PTSD post-childbirth: a systematic review of women's and midwives' subjective experiences of care provider interaction. J Reprod Infant Psychol. 2019;37(1):56–83.
52. Prenoveau JM, Craske MG, West V, Giannakakis A, Zioga M, Lehtonen A, et al. Maternal postnatal depression and anxiety and their association with child emotional negativity and behavior problems at two years. Dev Psychol. 2017;53(1):50–62.
53. Power C, Williams C, Brown A. Does a mother's childbirth experience influence her perceptions of her baby's behaviour? A qualitative interview study. PLoS One. 2023;18(4):e0284183.
54. Ransjö-Arvidson AB, Matthiesen AS, Lilja G, Nissen E, Widström AM, Uvnäs-Moberg K. Maternal analgesia during labor disturbs newborn behavior: effects on breastfeeding, temperature, and crying. Birth. 2001;28(1):5–12.
55. Redhead CA, Silverio SA, Payne E, Greenfield M, Barnett SM, Chiumento A, et al. A consensus statement on child and family health during the COVID-19 pandemic and recommendations for post-pandemic recovery and re-build. Front Child Adolesc Psychiatry. 2025;4:1520291.
56. Redshaw M, Hennegan J, Kruske S. Holding the baby: early mother–infant contact after childbirth and outcomes. Midwifery. 2014;30(5):e177–87.
57. Sandelowski M. Focus on research methods-whatever happened to qualitative description? Res Nurs Health. 2000;23(4):334–40.
58. Sandelowski M. What's in a name? Qualitative description revisited. Res Nurs Health. 2010;33(1):77–84.
59. Simkin P. Just another day in a woman's life? Women's long-term perceptions of their first birth experience. Part I. Birth. 1991;18(4):203–10.
60. Spiby H, Stewart J, Watts K, Hughes AJ, Slade P. The importance of face to face, group antenatal education classes for first time mothers: a qualitative study. Midwifery. 2022;109:103295.
61. Taylor A, Fisk NM, Glover V. Mode of delivery and subsequent stress response. Lancet. 2000;355(9198):120.
62. Thomson GM, Downe S. Changing the future to change the past: women's experiences of a positive birth following a traumatic birth experience. J Reprod Infant Psychol. 2010;28(1):102–12.
63. Vaiserman AM. Epigenetic programming by early-life stress: evidence from human populations. Dev Dyn. 2015;244(3):254–65.
64. WHO. World Health Organization recommendations: intrapartum care for a positive childbirth experience. 2018. Available at: https://www.who.int/publications/i/item/9789241550215. Accessed 31.12.24.

65. Widström AM, Lilja G, Aaltomaa-Michalias P, Dahllöf A, Lintula M, Nissen E. Newborn behaviour to locate the breast when skin-to-skin: a possible method for enabling early self-regulation. Acta Paediatr. 2011;100(1):79–85.
66. Widström AM, Brimdyr K, Svensson K, Cadwell K, Nissen E. Skin-to-skin contact the first hour after birth, underlying implications and clinical practice. Acta Paediatr. 2019;108(7):1192–204.
67. Wolke D. Parents' perceptions as guides for conducting NBAS clinical sessions. In: Brazelton TB, Nugent JK, editors. Neonatal behavioral assessment scale. 3rd ed. London: Mac Keith Press; 1995. p. 117–25.
68. Wolke D, James-Roberts I. Multi-method measurement of the early parent-infant system with easy and difficult newborns. Psychobiol Early Dev. 1987;46:49–70.
69. Wolke D, James-Roberts I. Mother and baby scales (MABS). Appendix 2. In: Brazelton TB, Nugent JK, editors. Neonatal behavioral assessment scale. 3rd ed. London: Mac Keith Press; 1987. p. 135–7.

Physical and Psychological Experiences of Childbirth and Baby Behaviour

A Survey of a Thousand Mothers: Part One

7

7.1 Introduction to the Survey

This chapter presents the first part of the findings from an online survey of mothers with babies aged up to 6 months old. It was designed to answer the following questions:

1. Which childbirth and perinatal factors are *related* to early infant behaviour?
2. Which childbirth and perinatal factors *contribute most* to early infant behaviour?

Because of the large volume of data collected and analysed for this study (which included over 150 questions), Chap. 7 will cover the first research question, and Chap. 8 will address the second. In these two chapters, I have tried to make the numerical findings more accessible for busy midwives (including student midwives) and other practising health professionals. If numerical findings bore you, feel free to focus on the qualitative chapters in this book and go straight to the conclusions in these two chapters. However, there are some diagrams that might be helpful to examine along the way, which I hope will clarify some of the complex, interconnected statistical relationships between all the different variables.

The questionnaire designed for this study was based on prior research evidence regarding the potential impacts of childbirth on baby behaviour and temperament (as discussed in Chaps. 3 and 4). It was created on SurveyMonkey and shared through UK-based online parent-child discussion forums, such as Mumsnet and Netmums, as well as social media platforms like Twitter and Facebook, and collegial networks across several UK universities. It initially attracted over a thousand women who identified as "mothers of a baby up to 6 months of age" (maximum 30 weeks). A streamlined version of the survey results, including the result tables and figures, is available in the journal *Frontiers in Psychology*, published on March 14th, coinciding with International Women's Day [38]. This was part of a special edition titled "From Childbearing to Childrearing: Parental Mental Health and

Infant Development", led by an expert panel of clinical psychologists specialising in perinatal mental health [33].

As we saw in the previous chapters, rising levels of childbirth interventions have become a major global concern in recent years, due to growing evidence that the harm caused by current levels of intervention now outweighs the intended benefits [55]. Of particular concern are the increasing rates of maternal and neonatal morbidity and mortality associated with the "overuse" of medical interventions as well as the added potential for long-term impacts on mothers' and infants' physical and mental health [14, 41]. While interventions such as inductions and caesarean sections were originally designed to save lives and protect the physical wellbeing of mothers and babies, *unnecessary* interventions may disrupt the natural progression of spontaneous, physiological labour and birth, thereby increasing the risk of further interventions and complications [50].

Furthermore, a medicalised birth experience may interfere with instinctive maternal and neonatal behaviours that facilitate mother-infant bonding and breastfeeding post-birth [51], potentially affecting long-term mother and baby health outcomes. In addition to these physical outcomes, obstetric interventions increase the risk of the mother developing postnatal depression or childbirth-related post-traumatic stress disorder (PTSD), especially if the care she receives during and after childbirth is less than optimal [2, 23]. As discussed in Chap. 4, the mother's state of mental health is all-important to her baby, and postnatal mood disturbances such as these could have detrimental impacts on the baby's short- and longer-term wellbeing. However, the relationships between postnatal distress, symptoms of PTSD and baby behaviour have not been widely studied, so there is still a lot that remains undiscovered about these complex, interwoven relationships.

When researching this topic before carrying out the studies, an indirect pathway between childbirth experiences and baby behaviour via postnatal maternal mood was conceivable. Given that postnatal mood disorders are highly comorbid, the well-established and widely used 10-item questionnaire known as the Edinburgh Postnatal Depression Scale [9] was included in the study. At the point of designing the survey, two reliable, validated instruments for measuring symptoms of post-traumatic stress following childbirth and the mother's satisfaction with her birth experience had not yet been designed. These were the City Birth Trauma Scale, known as City BiTS [3], and the Birth Satisfaction Scale-Revised [29], both of which should be included in further research examining the outcomes of mothers' childbirth experiences. Until a decade or so ago, however, there was little awareness around the significance of the mother's subjective birth experience, her perceptions of a traumatic birth, and the potential implications of this for parent-infant bonding and baby behaviour.

Even now, the research evidence for mother-and-baby outcomes of birth trauma is somewhat mixed and inconclusive. As the survey was designed and launched before the interviews took place, the questionnaire for this study didn't include any questions about mothers' bonding with their baby, although this topic emerged prominently in the interviews. Nor did the survey ask mothers about all the symptoms of birth trauma, such as hyper-arousal or dissociation. However, it *did* ask the mothers to state how much they agreed or disagreed with multiple statements concerning physical and psychological aspects of their pregnancy, birth and postnatal experiences, including their feelings about the birth and their experiences of postnatal wellbeing, euphoria, depression or distress. This last variable, which I named "postnatal distress", is very closely linked to post-traumatic stress symptoms [46], enabling us to establish under what circumstances mothers tended to experience this primary symptom of PTSD [38].

Professor Ruth Feldman [13], whose high-profile lab has extensively researched parent-infant relationships and the development of "biobehavioural synchrony" between healthy, well-adjusted parent-infant pairs, found that postnatal depression can disrupt mother-baby interactions. This sometimes severe postnatal mood disorder also reduces the mother's confidence in caring for the baby, which has been linked to early infant regulatory problems [30]. These disruptions to the mother and baby's functioning could hinder the building of a lasting positive relationship between mother and baby, negatively affecting the baby's wellbeing and behaviour. In addition, the mother's mental health issues could be exacerbated by unsettled early infant behaviour [6], which might further impact mother-baby relationships and infant temperament development. This cyclical effect may initially stem from the influence of obstetric complications on the intricately interlinked mother-baby stress response systems [10, 12]. However, despite earlier suggestions regarding the potential physical and physiological impacts of childbirth on mother and baby (see Chap. 3), research investigating how childbirth experiences might directly or *indirectly* influence early baby behaviour is sparse. The study presented here was inspired by Taylor et al.'s [47] original suggestion that a mother's *psychological reaction* to childbirth complications and interventions might mediate the baby's crying and stress response, meaning that if the mother's response to a challenging birth experience is calm, the baby's might be too.

7.2 How the Survey Was Carried Out

The study was a retrospective online survey designed and implemented in accordance with the ethical standards outlined in the 1964 Declaration of Helsinki [56] and the British Psychological Society's [5] Code of Ethics and Conduct. The survey asked mothers of babies aged 6 months or less about their physical and psychological childbirth experiences, postnatal mood and baby's behaviour. Established in June 2014 and running for nearly 3 years until March 2017, the survey didn't inquire about gender identity, as this wasn't generally considered in the way it is today (please refer to the asterisked paragraph in Chap. 1 regarding intentions of inclusivity). Mothers could choose to participate if they were over the age of 18, had a baby aged 0–30 weeks from a "singleton" pregnancy (i.e. not twins or triplets), lived in the UK and had no major physical or mental health issues. They were asked *not* to participate if they or their baby had any major health problems, had been born prematurely (less than 37 weeks' gestation at birth) or had a low birth weight (less than 5.5 lb), as these births may all have significantly different outcomes [48]. Following a study brief and electronic consent, participating mothers completed standard questions about their baby's characteristics (such as gestational age and birth weight) and their own age, education, income and ethnicity before proceeding with the rest of the questionnaire. This information was tested so that variables correlating with baby behaviour could be "controlled for" throughout the study, ensuring they would not skew the results.

The questions about mothers' childbirth experiences and the wider perinatal period broadly fell into two categories: physical (objective) and psychological (subjective).

Physical (Objective) Factors
Questions about the physical aspects of pregnancy, birth and the postnatal period included pre- and postnatal complications (such as infection or urinary retention), birthplace, how labour commenced (e.g. induction or spontaneous), how labour progressed (e.g. acceleration or spontaneous), the timings for each stage of labour, birth interventions (such as continuous electronic foetal monitoring), birth mode, pain ratings and pain relief methods. Mothers were also asked about complications directly affecting the baby (such as foetal distress, meconium in the waters or resuscitation), how the baby was born, whether they had immediate skin-to-skin contact and how they were initially and currently fed. The newborn's Apgar score [1]—a well-known measure of the baby's physiological state immediately post-birth—was reported by the mothers who knew what Apgar scores their babies had been given at 1 and 5 minutes post-birth. Alongside this standard medical scale, a few brief questions explored mothers' perceptions of their baby's behaviour and general wellbeing during the first 24 hours.

Psychological (Subjective) Factors
At the time of designing and launching the survey, no measurement scale concerned with childbirth experiences covered the entire perinatal period with the required depth and breadth for the current study. Consequently, mothers were asked to respond to multiple statements about how they had *felt* physically and emotionally during pregnancy, childbirth and the postnatal period (e.g. how well, happy, alert, relaxed, afraid, vulnerable, neglected or cared for they had felt). These subjective measures of pregnancy, birth and postnatal experiences were based on the research literature around women's psychological responses to childbirth and the perinatal period.

Measuring Infant Behaviour
Two primary measures were used to assess baby behaviour, wellbeing and developing infant temperament immediately post-birth and during the first 6 months afterwards:

1. The 24-Hour Baby Scale, as briefly outlined here and fully described in Power [37];
2. The Mother and Baby Scales designed by Wolke and James-Roberts [53, 54].

It's possible that a mother's initial perceptions of her newborn baby's appearance, wellbeing and behaviour could serve as a precedent for the baby's ongoing temperament development. Therefore, the 24-Hour Baby Scale was designed specially for this study to provide a simple measure of the newborn baby's physiological and behavioural state post-birth. Mothers were asked to rate their level of agreement with seven statements about their baby's appearance, physiological wellbeing and behaviour during the first 24 hours; for example, "My baby's head looked bruised and swollen", "My baby cried a lot" or "My baby appeared calm and relaxed". Applying principal components analysis to the data reduced the seven statements to two main variables, which were labelled *alert-content baby* and *cry-fuss baby*. These new variables generated by the principal components analysis are described in more detail in Sect. 7.3.

The Mother and Baby Scales, known as MABS [54], is a 63-item questionnaire that assesses the mother's confidence and self-efficacy alongside her perceptions of her baby's behaviour over the past seven-day period. This deepened the study's exploration of interrelated mother and baby outcomes due to the well-known links between postnatal mood disorders (such as anxiety or depression), maternal confidence and self-efficacy [11], the mother's interactions and relationship with her baby and the baby's behaviour and development [32, 40]. The MABS was chosen as it was one of the few measurement scales that assesses baby behaviour from birth (most baby behaviour scales only work from 3 months). The MABS has high levels of validity and reliability [52]; in other words, it consistently measures what it intends to measure, specifically baby behaviour and maternal confidence. Although the MABS was initially designed for newborn babies, it has previously been used with infants aged up to 8 months. When I met its co-designer, the UK-based, charming and enthusiastic German developmental psychologist Dieter Wolke at a conference and asked him what he thought, he was happy for the MABS to be used for babies from 0 to 6 months. The MABS questions are phrased in a simple and straightforward manner, for example: "My baby has settled quickly and easily" or "During feeds my baby has tended to fuss and cry". The MABS questionnaire is made up of eight sub-scales: alert-responsive, unsettled-irregular, overall easiness, alertness during feeds, irritability during feeds, lack of confidence in caretaking (caring for baby) or breastfeeding and global confidence (see Table 7.1).

The Mother's Personality Traits and Postnatal Wellbeing
Genetic factors play an important role in the development of a baby's personality and behaviour [31]. We also know that the mother's mood during pregnancy and postnatally can affect baby behaviour and infant development [15]. Therefore, it was essential to include short questionnaires about these factors in the survey. The mother's personality was assessed using the Ten-Item Personality Inventory (TIPI), developed by Gosling et al. [17] as a brief version of the well-known "Big Five" Personality Inventory [16]. The TIPI measures the five personality traits of extroversion, conscientiousness, openness (to new experiences), agreeableness and emotional stability.

Table 7.1 Mother and Baby Scales (MABS)

MABS sub-scale	Description of measure
General	
Alert-responsive	How alert, attentive and communicative the baby seems
Unsettled-irregular	How much the baby cries and fusses; how easy they are to settle
Lack of confidence in caretaking	How capable the mother feels when caring for her baby
Overall impressions	
Easiness	How calm, alert and settled the baby seems to be overall
Global confidence	How confident the mother feels about coping + maternal anxiety
Feeding	
Alertness during feeds	How alert the baby is during and after feeding
Irritable during feeds	Whether the baby feeds reluctantly or with difficulty or irritability
Lack of confidence in breastfeeding	If breastfeeding, whether this is problematic (e.g. due to tension, conflicting advice, technique, confidence or any childbirth impacts)

The mother's state of mental health at the time of completing the survey was assessed using the 10-item Edinburgh Postnatal Depression Scale, known as the EPDS [9]. This self-report scale assesses the mother's postnatal mood over the past week. The EPDS is quick and easy to complete, consisting of just 10 statements for the mother to respond to via multiple-choice answers about how much she agrees or disagrees with each statement, or how often she experiences that particular emotion (e.g. "I have been able to laugh and see the funny side of things" or "I have felt sad or miserable").

Another issue that could affect a baby's behaviour or influence the mother's perceptions of childbirth and her baby's behaviour is how anxious or relaxed she feels at the time of reporting these things. Therefore, the six-item short form of the "State" section of Spielberger et al.'s [45]. State-Trait Anxiety Inventory, commonly referred to as the STAI, was included to measure mothers' current anxiety levels [28]. This brief version of the STAI State contains six statements regarding the mother's current emotional state (e.g., "I feel calm/tense/content/upset"), to which the mother responds with multiple-choice answers indicating her level of agreement or disagreement with each statement.

How the Survey Results Were Analysed

To begin, correlational analyses (using Pearson's correlations to assess *similarities* between different variables) and multiple analyses of (co)variance (MANCOVAs—to evaluate *differences* in outcomes according to various variables) were used to determine which physical and psychological perinatal factors were related to early baby behaviour and maternal confidence. In Chap. 8, multiple linear regression analyses will be used to identify which perinatal variables *contribute most significantly* to positive and negative outcomes for mothers and babies while controlling for all other variables that could also be influencing the results.

7.3 The Findings: Relationships Between Childbirth Experiences and Baby Behaviour

Over a thousand mothers completed the survey, although some didn't meet all the inclusion criteria, resulting in 999 mothers aged 19–44 years included in the final study. The average age of the babies at the time of survey completion was 15 weeks, with a range of 0–30 weeks. While a diverse sample is always sought in research, public health surveys often fail to attract a diverse range of participants. In this study, the majority of participating mothers were white and well-qualified and lived in England with their partners. However, approximately 13% reported relatively low household earnings, providing some level of sociodemographic diversity.

Although there was no space to include initial "24-Hour" newborn wellbeing and behaviour in the published article [38], the survey results are presented here in relation to both measures of baby behaviour (as described above)—the 24-Hour Baby Scale [37], designed to measure the newborn baby's physiological wellbeing and behaviour, and the Mother and Baby Scales [54], designed to assess early infant behavioural style known as temperament. I'll begin with a summary of the correlations between Apgar scores, 24-Hour Baby and MABS before describing the main findings: mothers' physical (objective) and psychological (subjective) birth and perinatal experiences in relation to the baby's physiological wellbeing and behaviour, and the mother's confidence and self-efficacy. To see the full statistical results tables for 24-Hour Baby, please refer to the published thesis [37], and for MABS, the published article [38].

24-Hour Baby
Following a "principal components" analysis of seven statements asking mothers to rate their newborn baby's appearance, physiological well-being and behaviour post-birth, the 24-Hour Baby Scale was divided into two main components representing opposite newborn states. The seven statements for mothers to rate (from strongly disagree to strongly agree) were: "My baby's head looked bruised and swollen", "My baby appeared calm and relaxed", "My baby seemed irritable", "My baby was very sleepy", "My baby cried a lot", "My baby smiled" and "My baby latched onto the breast easily". The first component, *cry-fuss baby*, described a baby with a bruised or swollen head who cried excessively and appeared irritable, rather than calm or relaxed. In contrast, *alert-content baby* described the newborn as calm, relaxed, alert (i.e. *not* very sleepy), smiling, and easily latching onto the breast for breastfeeding. Notably, the 24-Hour Baby Scale correlated with the widely used Apgar score (as described above), and Apgar scores were strongly related to mothers' reports of their pregnancy, birth and postnatal experiences. This provided some validity for both the 24-Hour Baby Scale and the questions about perinatal experiences designed for this survey. Approximately half of the survey participants didn't know their baby's Apgar scores; therefore, Apgar scores were excluded from the final report. Nonetheless, it is interesting to note that Apgar scores have since been found to correlate with birth satisfaction [36], indicating how mothers' subjective experiences of childbirth could have implications not only for her own wellbeing

but also for the newborn baby's physical health. In the future, it might be interesting to further explore the significant relationships between Apgar scores and baby behaviour found in this survey.

The Mother and Baby Scales (MABS)

The MABS were the primary measure of baby behaviour for this study. Therefore, for new mothers keen to participate in the research, completing the MABS questionnaire was essential. A total of 999 mothers met all the inclusion criteria and completed the MABS. Of these, 855 completed the section on breastfeeding, indicating that a high proportion of mothers were either currently breastfeeding or had previously done so. Notably, 24-Hour Baby correlated with the Mother and Baby Scales (as illustrated in Figs. 7.1 and 7.2). Mothers' confidence and self-efficacy were also interconnected with babies' behaviour. Therefore, how the baby appears and behaves during the first 24 hours, along with how confident the mother feels postnatally, may continue to influence the baby's temperament development. In particular, cry-fuss baby corresponded with unsettled and irregular baby behaviour, and alert-content baby (which included the newborn having an easy breastfeeding latch) was related to mothers' breastfeeding confidence and to alert and responsive baby behaviours during the first 6 months.

The Venn diagram in Fig. 7.1 illustrates the overlap (or "association/correlation") between newborn behavioural style (as rated by the 24-Hour Baby Scale) and ongoing infant temperament up to 6 months (as measured by the Mother and Baby Scales, MABS). The left circle (alert-content 24-Hour Baby) describes calm, relaxed and alert baby behaviours observed during the first 24 hours post-birth, while the right circle (cry-fuss 24-Hour Baby) describes irritable, fussy or distressed newborn behaviour. The centre oval (baby behaviour 0–6 months) represents the five MABS sub-scales of early temperament traits, which correlated significantly with the newborn (24-hour) behavioural states of cry-fuss and alert-content baby.

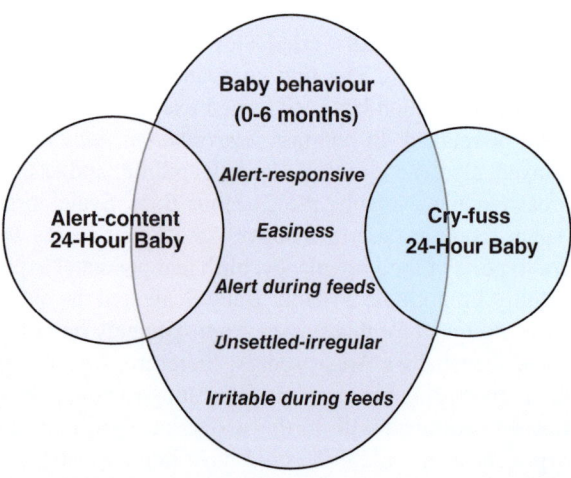

Fig. 7.1 Relationship between 24-Hour Baby and early infant behavioural style

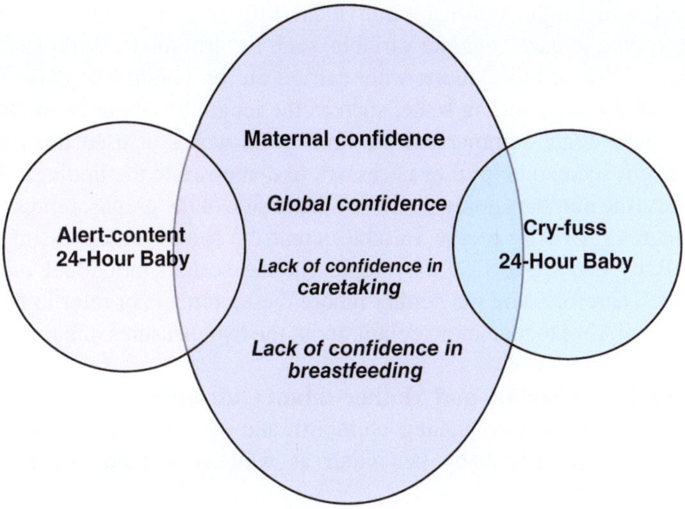

7.3 The Findings: Relationships Between Childbirth Experiences and Baby Behaviour

Fig. 7.2 Relationship between 24-Hour Baby and maternal confidence

The Venn diagram in Fig. 7.2 illustrates the relationship between how babies appear and behave within the first 24 hours after birth (as rated by the 24-Hour Baby Scale) and the mother's confidence in caring for her baby (as assessed by the Mother and Baby Scales, MABS). Once again, the left circle (alert-content 24-Hour Baby) represents babies who appeared calm, alert and easy to settle shortly after birth; the right circle (cry-fuss 24-Hour Baby) represents babies who cried excessively, were difficult to soothe or appeared distressed. The centre oval represents maternal confidence, which includes the MABS sub-scales relating to the mother's confidence and self-efficacy. Global confidence refers to a mother's overall confidence in coping; lack of confidence in caretaking measures a mother's self-perceived ability to care for her baby; and lack of confidence in breastfeeding assesses the confidence and ease mothers experience with breastfeeding, including any stress or difficulties they may encounter. These overlapping areas suggest that newborn baby behaviour is linked to how confident a mother feels in her new caregiving role.

These relationships will now be examined more closely using graphs to display the findings from the MANCOVAs (as described earlier). Although the graphs are based on numerical results, they are intended primarily as a visual aid. Before reviewing these visual results to assess the differences in mother and baby outcomes depending on various childbirth and perinatal experiences (e.g. birth mode or birthplace), it is worth noting that when interpreting multiple statistical findings based on a large sample (in this case, 999 mothers), the separate results for each individual variable may be quite small. However, while each of the perinatal variables associated with baby behaviour made only a modest contribution to the outcomes when considered alone, when taken collectively, they had a substantial impact on the mother's and baby's mood and behaviour (see Chap. 8 for diagrams illustrating the overall findings).

The graphs highlight significant individual differences in mother and baby outcomes according to each separate variable, such as birth mode, birthplace or types of pain relief. Where correlations were carried out on continuous data—i.e. variables measurable on a sliding scale, such as the length of labour or mothers' pain ratings—I have either summarised the findings in words or used illustrative diagrams where it seemed helpful or necessary to demonstrate the findings. The scoring methods (the numbers going up the left-hand side of the graphs, representing the average scores for each specific variable) could be somewhat confusing for both 24-Hour Baby and MABS as they represent the scales' individual methods of assessment. Therefore, you may either ignore these numbers or refer to Power [37] and Power et al. [38] to read more details about the two measures of baby behaviour.

Physical Perinatal Factors and Mother-Infant Outcomes

Events occurring during pregnancy, childbirth and the postnatal period correlated with newborn and early baby behaviour as well as mothers' confidence and self-efficacy.

Pregnancy and Postnatal Complications

Pregnancy and postnatal complications will inevitably impact maternal wellbeing. They may also have a physical impact on the baby (potentially causing pain or disability depending on the complication) as well as affecting them physiologically and psychologically through the mother's stress hormones. This is likely to be reflected in the baby's behaviour—the only way babies have of communicating that something is amiss [4]. Approximately 37% of mothers experienced complications during pregnancy, while 50% experienced postnatal complications—a high number by any standards. Both pregnancy and postnatal complications *negatively* correlated with alert-content newborn wellbeing and behaviour (meaning the *more* complications there were, the *less* alert and content the newborn appeared) and *positively* correlated with cry-fuss baby, meaning the newborn was more likely to cry and fuss, exhibiting more unhappy, irritable behaviours as the number of complications increased [37]. Similarly, as the number of pregnancy and postnatal complications increased, babies aged 0–6 months were more likely to be unsettled-irregular and irritable-during-feeds (negative behaviour items on the Mother and Baby Scales). At the same time, mothers reported lower confidence levels in caring for and breastfeeding their babies [38].

Birthplace

Where a mother gives birth to her baby may significantly affect how the birth proceeds, the number of interventions that occur and the type of care she receives. The Birthplace Study demonstrated that *planned* homebirths are a safe option for healthy women with low-risk pregnancies [7], as long as the plan involves NHS midwives who are plugged into the wider system should an emergency occur. Having a homebirth usually means being attended by two well-qualified midwives, which is a level of care rarely available during childbirth in a hospital or a midwife-led unit.

In the Birthplace Study, although there were no differences in overall outcomes and fewer interventions across homebirths and midwife-led units, first-time mothers

7.3 The Findings: Relationships Between Childbirth Experiences and Baby Behaviour

experienced *slightly better* perinatal outcomes (including foetal and neonatal outcomes) in obstetric settings. Some first-time mothers who've carefully considered all the physical and mental health outcomes may choose this homebirth option with a slightly increased perinatal risk to avoid the increased risks of intervention and trauma attached to a hospital birth. This is a decision that all parents living in the UK, as well as many other countries, have the right to make for themselves based on unbiased scientific information shared through conversations with a midwife who knows them well and, if they are in a higher-risk group, their obstetrician. Sadly, however, homebirths have been restricted in many areas across the UK, primarily due to a lack of adequate staffing and resources, and this postcode lottery deprives some parents of the opportunity to make an informed choice that works for them and their baby.

In this survey, mothers were asked where they had given birth and how their baby had behaved after the birth. As shown in Fig. 7.3, newborn babies exhibited significantly *fewer* cry-fuss behaviours (−0.6) and appeared *more* alert and content (+0.6) if they were born at home.

Beyond this initial 24-hour period, babies were reported as significantly *more* unsettled and irregular in their routines of feeding, sleeping and elimination (weeing and pooing) after a hospital or midwife-led unit birth (Fig. 7.4)—as illustrated by the extended orange and pink towers for unsettled-irregular baby behaviour. They were also significantly *less* alert and responsive after a hospital birth, although these differences were relatively small and are therefore more difficult to represent visually.

In addition to these differences in baby wellbeing and behaviour according to where they were born, mothers reported significantly *more* confidence in caring for and breastfeeding their baby (i.e. *less* lack of confidence in caretaking and breastfeeding) after giving birth at home or in a midwife-led unit (Fig. 7.5). As you can see from the extended lengths of the pale orange towers for Lack of confidence in caretaking (caring for their baby) and breastfeeding, mothers were significantly *less* confident (i.e. they lacked confidence) in these areas after a hospital birth.

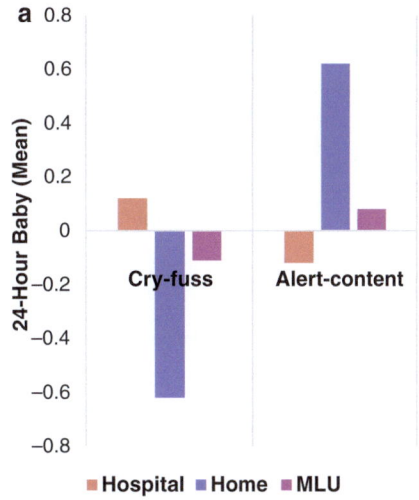

Fig. 7.3 24-Hour Baby according to birthplace. *Note:* Mean = average scores for each condition—in this case, place of birth (e.g. hospital/home). The graphs in this chapter were created by Spoorthy Deepak

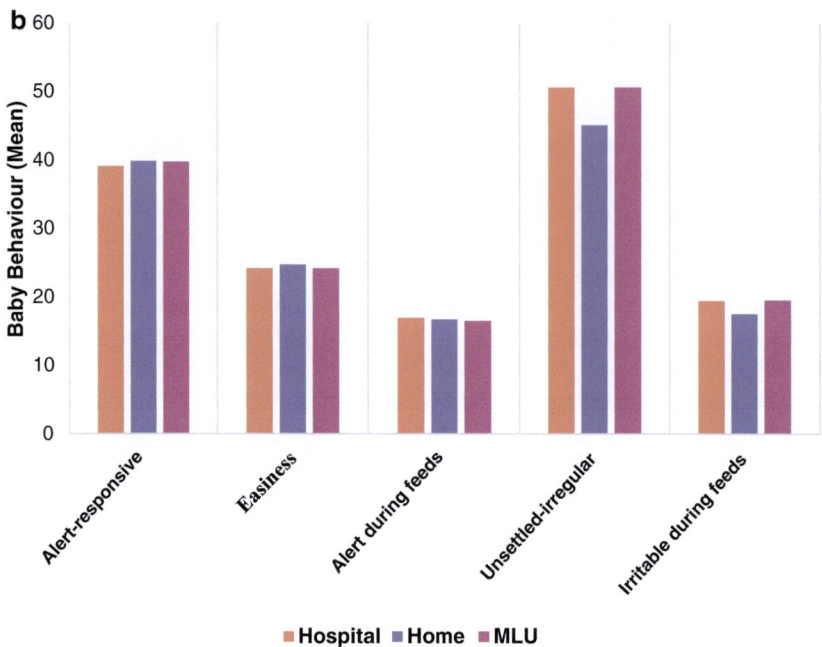

Fig. 7.4 Baby behaviour (0–6 months) according to birthplace

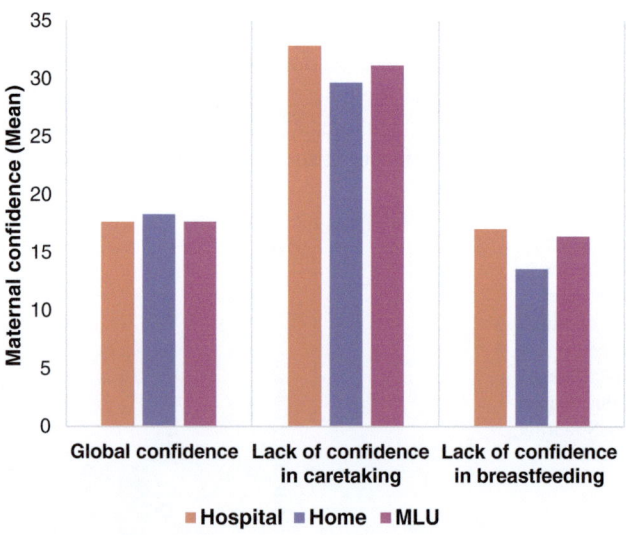

Fig. 7.5 Maternal confidence according to birthplace

7.3 The Findings: Relationships Between Childbirth Experiences and Baby Behaviour

Tearing and Episiotomy

Perineal tears can be a serious issue. If severe, they may cause pain, discomfort, bleeding or infection. There is also the potential for ongoing problems regarding partner intimacy post-birth, as tears, episiotomies and the scars they leave may all impact a woman's body image and confidence, contributing to postnatal distress while also affecting the couple's relationship and sexual wellbeing [43]. For these reasons, tears can be experienced as traumatic and debilitating after childbirth in the days, months and sometimes years that follow. However, as discovered during the nationwide birth trauma inquiry, the seriousness of this situation depends on the severity of the tear, the cause of it and the care the mother received surrounding it [49]. In the most serious cases, a perineal tear can extend to the rectum, causing later urinary and bowel incontinence in addition to a series of issues related to everyday functioning and the mother's physical and mental health (see Chap. 3).

Episiotomies (a surgical cut to the perineum), initially introduced to prevent severe tearing and facilitate birth, at one time became a common practice. Fortunately, they are now less popular, as their alleged long-term benefits (a cleaner, potentially less severe wound that is easier to stitch and heals better) have been extensively debated [20, 24]. In the current study, the overall number of tears experienced was high, with 660 mothers reporting them. Among these, five were classified as third-degree tears and 148 as fourth-degree tears. Very few women (n = 4) experienced an episiotomy; therefore, to include them in the analysis, episiotomies were grouped with other types of tear.

Newborn babies were perceived as more alert and content (+0.19) and were *less* likely to cry or fuss (−0.24) when their mother had *not* experienced a tear or episiotomy (Fig. 7.6).

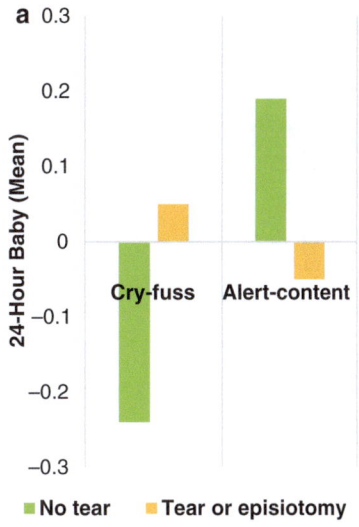

Fig. 7.6 24-Hour Baby after tear or episiotomy

This initial association appeared to disappear as ongoing infant behaviour scores were *not* significantly affected by tears and episiotomies, despite 0–6-month-old infants being *slightly* more unsettled if their mothers had experienced either (Fig. 7.7).

Importantly, mothers felt *significantly more confident*—in other words, they had *less* "Lack of Confidence" in Caretaking (caring for) and Breastfeeding their baby— if they had *not* experienced a tear or episiotomy (Fig. 7.8—note the higher yellow towers for lack of confidence in these areas).

Start of Labour

The way labour begins or is initiated can influence how a mother feels about her birth. If everything is going as planned, mothers may wish for their labour to start naturally and on time. Often, however, this is not the case. Although most babies arrive between 37 and 41 weeks, only about 5% of women go into labour spontaneously on their due date. Meanwhile, there are mixed and currently quite polarised views on how best to address the potential risks of an overdue baby (see Chap. 3). The diverse mix of opinions about this can make it difficult for parents to make an informed decision, balancing both the scientific evidence and what feels right for them and their baby. Just under half of the mothers in this study ($n = 489$) experienced spontaneous labour; the rest (over 50%) were induced in some way.

Newborn babies exhibited *fewer* crying and fussing behaviours after a spontaneous labour and birth, and *more* crying and fussing behaviours following an artificial rupture of membranes (ARM) or if their mother had experienced both a pessary and

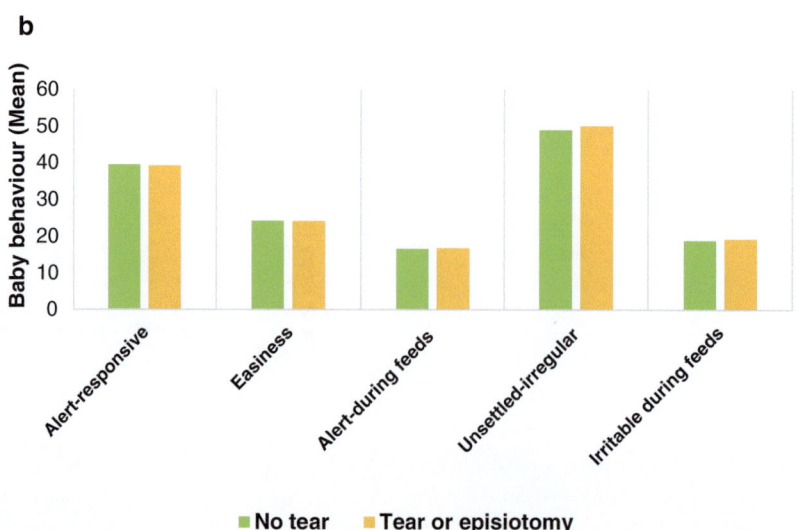

Fig. 7.7 Baby behaviour (0–6 months) after tear or episiotomy

7.3 The Findings: Relationships Between Childbirth Experiences and Baby Behaviour

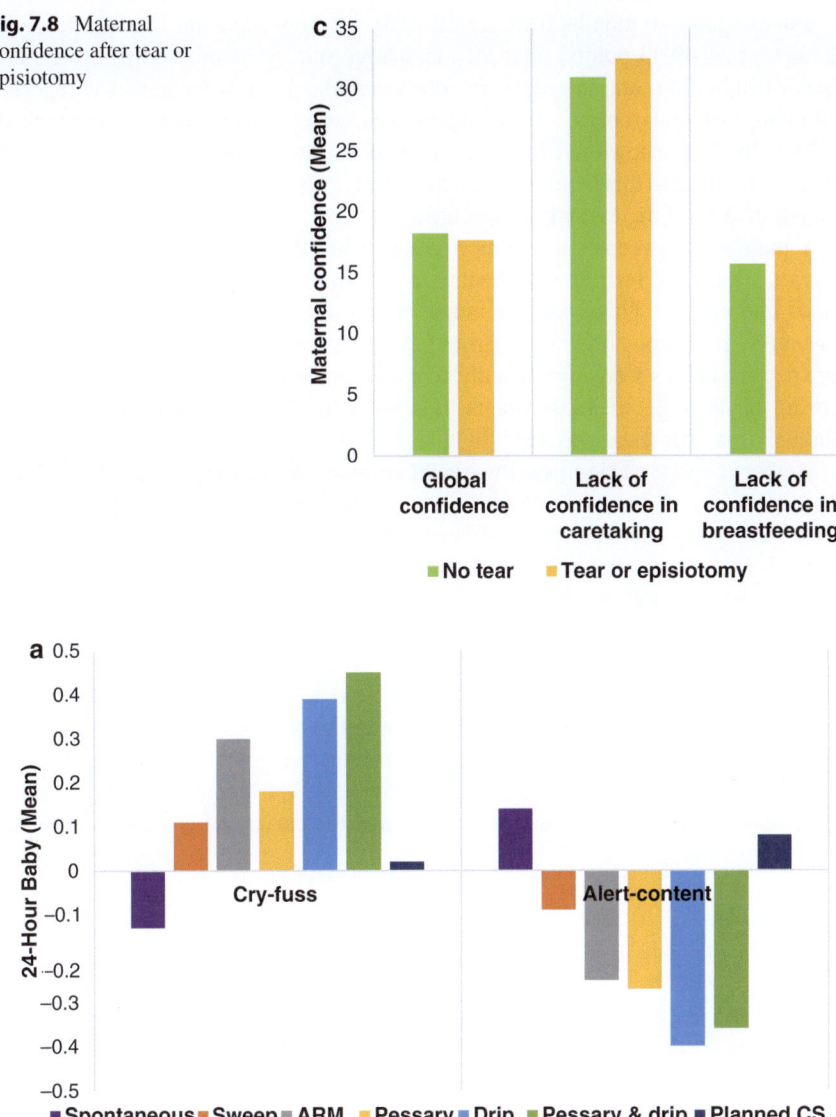

Fig. 7.8 Maternal confidence after tear or episiotomy

Fig. 7.9 24-Hour Baby according to the start of labour method

a synthetic oxytocin drip. Corresponding with this, they tended to be *more* alert and content after spontaneous birth and did *more* crying and fussing following a medically induced birth, which may have involved the artificial rupture of membranes (ARM), pessary, drip, or both pessary and drip. As you can see in Fig. 7.9, newborn babies cried *most* after having both a pessary and a drip. Notably, they did *not* appear to be distressed after *planned* caesarean sections, perhaps because this was generally a relatively calm way to be born.

Babies aged 0–6 months were significantly *less* unsettled and irregular (scoring an average of 49.43 points) after a spontaneous start to labour compared to most types of induction, and the *most* unsettled-irregular baby behaviour was reported following artificial rupture of the membranes (where they scored an average of 52.23 points). As shown in Fig. 7.10, many, if not most, young babies were unsettled and irregular in their routines to *some* extent, as is often the case with early baby behaviour. Therefore, everything is relative.

A membrane sweep is a common practice to initiate labour when the cervix appears "ripe" and birth is imminent, and 179 mothers underwent this seemingly minor intervention. Given the commonality of this practice, mothers often readily consent to it without finding it particularly invasive. Therefore, the results were unexpected: babies were significantly *less* alert and responsive following a sweep, scoring an average of 38.64 points compared to 39.35 for spontaneous births, although this difference was very slight (Fig. 7.10).

Mothers expressed significantly greater confidence in caring for and breastfeeding their baby (i.e. *less* Lack of confidence in these two areas) after a spontaneous labour compared to when they had been induced (by any method) or following a planned caesarean section (Fig. 7.11). In particular, inductions tended to have a negative impact on mothers' breastfeeding confidence. Their overall (global) confidence, however, was *not* significantly affected by the start of labour method.

Length of Labour: Duration of the Latent, Active and Pushing Stages

The duration of labour and childbirth is important to both mother and baby, as it can be a painful and challenging (as well as rewarding) event. Childbirth occurs in several stages. To begin, there is an initial "latent stage" of labour—the initial part of the "first stage", where the body warms up, and the cervix softens and dilates over

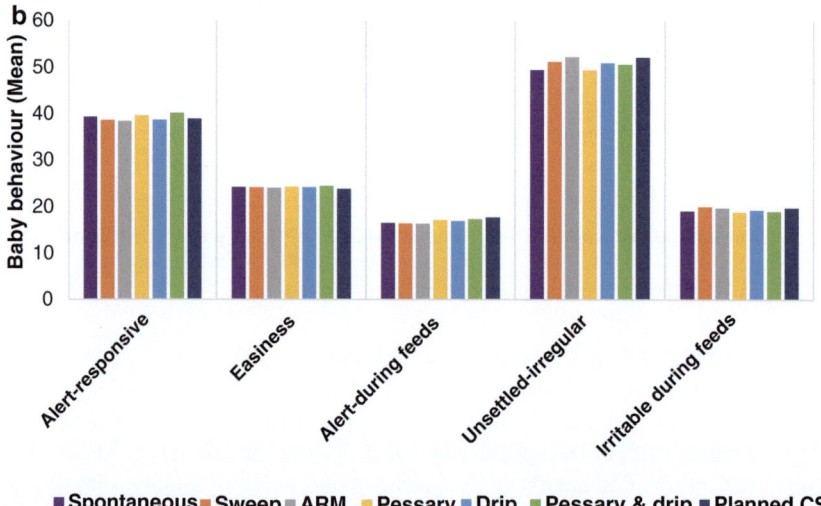

Fig. 7.10 Baby behaviour (0–6 months) according to start of labour

7.3 The Findings: Relationships Between Childbirth Experiences and Baby Behaviour 173

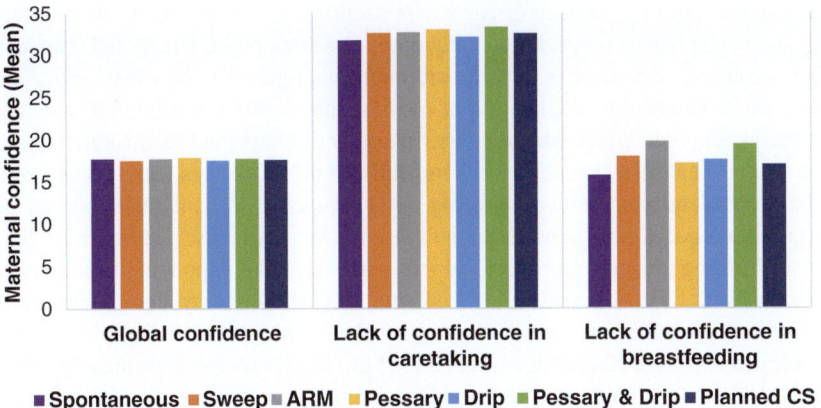

Fig. 7.11 Maternal confidence according to start of labour

several hours or even days. Mothers sometimes struggle to have their "pre-labour" pains taken seriously during this stage, although they can be experienced as extremely challenging, especially if they quickly escalate to full-blown labour [39]. The first stage also includes the "active stage" [25], which describes the progression from diagnosis or 4 cm (the point at which midwife-led units and hospitals generally encourage parents to come in and begin offering pain relief). This stage continues until the cervix reaches 10 cm (full dilation)—the width required for the baby to pass through the birth canal and be born. Then, comes a brief "transition" period where the intense pain caused by powerful contractions, together with a strong urge to push, might feel overwhelmingly difficult for the mother. The second ('pushing') stage of labour begins, where the mother voluntarily (or occasionally involuntarily via the oxytocin-induced foetal ejection reflex) pushes her baby out into the world. The "third stage" describes the womb contracting as it expels the placenta, although this final stage was not included in the survey.

As we saw in Chap. 3, the length of labour may affect the baby's health and wellbeing, particularly if it becomes prolonged during the active first stage or the pushing second stage. In the survey, mothers reported more cry-fuss behaviours after an extended labour [37]. Moreover, babies aged 0–6 months were reported as significantly *less* alert-responsive after a longer latent stage and *more* unsettled-irregular after longer first and second stages. Longer labours were also associated with *lower* maternal confidence [38].

Labour Interventions
Obstetric interventions are sometimes necessary; yet, they are not always available when needed, especially in low-resource settings. For this and other reasons, many regions of sub-Saharan Africa experience far higher perinatal mortality and morbidity rates than elsewhere in the world. In contrast to this potentially desperate situation, in better-resourced countries, medical interventions (such as episiotomy,

continuous foetal monitoring or caesarean sections) often become routine without adequate evidence to support their frequent use. At one point, Brazil had drastically high caesarean section rates of 90%, although this figure has now been reduced to under 60%. The routine application of medical interventions designed to save lives in emergencies can affect the birth experience for mothers (and their future physical and mental health) while negatively impacting birth outcomes [55]. For instance, continuous electronic foetal monitoring, used in place of intermittent handheld auscultation methods, lacks substantial evidence for its routine use. However, by limiting the birthing person's mobility—which is an essential component of spontaneous physiological birth—it denies low-risk mothers without any complications the opportunity to make informed choices about their birth [21]. The National Institute for Health and Care Excellence (NICE) [34] guidelines on foetal monitoring therefore emphasise the mother as decision-maker [35].

Given the potential impacts of unnecessary interventions on mothers and babies, mothers participating in the survey were asked a series of questions about which interventions they had experienced during labour and birth (note that some of these were the same as the induction methods discussed above). Mothers who experienced the artificial rupture of their membranes (ARM) during labour, continuous electronic foetal monitoring (restricting mobility), or labour acceleration through synthetic oxytocin tended to report more cry-fuss and fewer alert-content newborn behaviours. Newborns who underwent a foetal scalp electrode or a foetal blood sample exhibited similar behavioural patterns. Notably, the foetal blood sample, which involves scraping the surface of the baby's scalp to test for hypoxia (lack of oxygen), was associated with the highest scores for cry-fuss behaviours (Fig. 7.12), indicating that this could be the most stressful intervention for the unborn child.

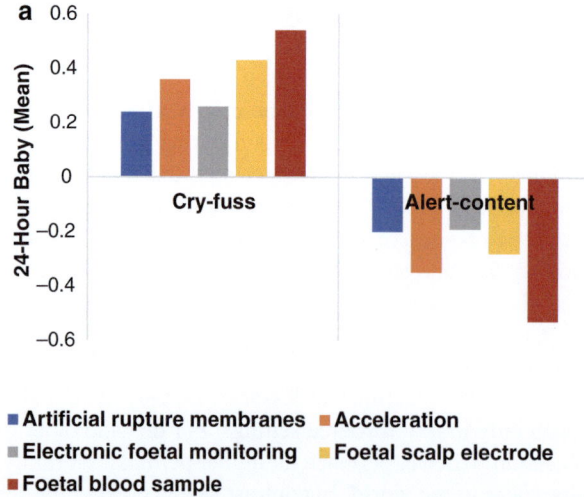

Fig. 7.12 Labour interventions and 24-Hour Baby

7.3 The Findings: Relationships Between Childbirth Experiences and Baby Behaviour

Indeed, due to insufficient evidence regarding its benefits and some evidence suggesting it could be harmful (as it is linked to reduced 5-minute Apgar scores), NICE guidelines no longer recommend foetal blood samples as a routine method for testing hypoxia [35].

Babies past this initial newborn stage tended to be more unsettled-irregular and irritable during feeds following the artificial rupture of membranes during labour, acceleration of labour or continuous foetal monitoring. There were no significant differences in baby behaviour (aged 0–6 months) following a foetal blood sample, although babies were significantly *more* unsettled and irregular after a foetal scalp electrode (Fig. 7.13). The pictorial representations of these results are slightly confusing as the tower for unsettled baby behaviour is higher for the foetal blood sample than for the foetal scalp electrode. However, fewer mothers responded to the question about foetal blood samples, meaning it failed to gain statistical significance, even though it was associated with higher scores for unsettled and irregular baby behaviours than any other intervention (scoring 53.26 compared to 49.67 for *no* foetal blood sample). As the data are too extensive to fit into one graph here, please refer to Power et al. [38] for numerical comparisons between each in-labour intervention compared to *no* intervention.

Mothers felt significantly less confident in caring for and breastfeeding their babies after experiencing artificial rupture of membranes, acceleration of labour or continuous foetal monitoring (Fig. 7.14). Once again, foetal blood sampling seemed to exert the most influence over scores, although it didn't gain significance as fewer mothers responded to this question.

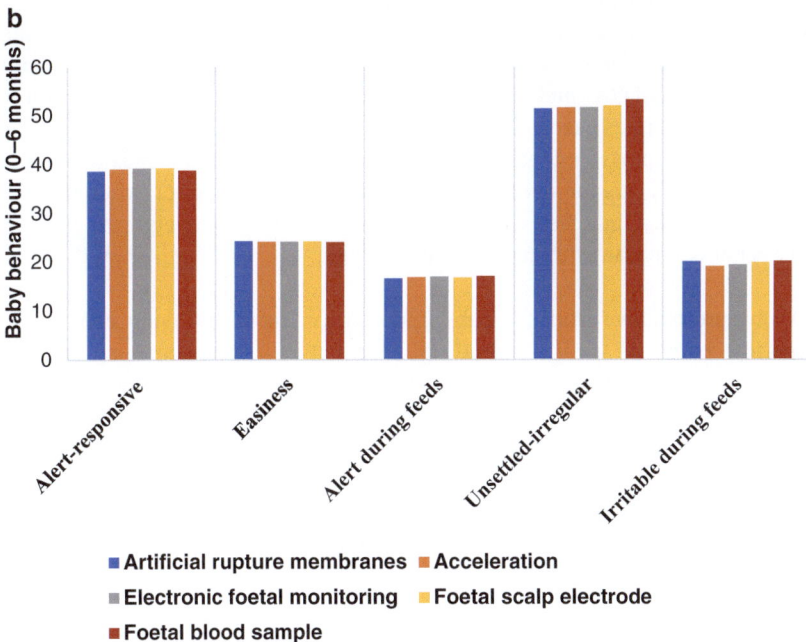

Fig. 7.13 Labour interventions and Baby Behaviour (0–6 months)

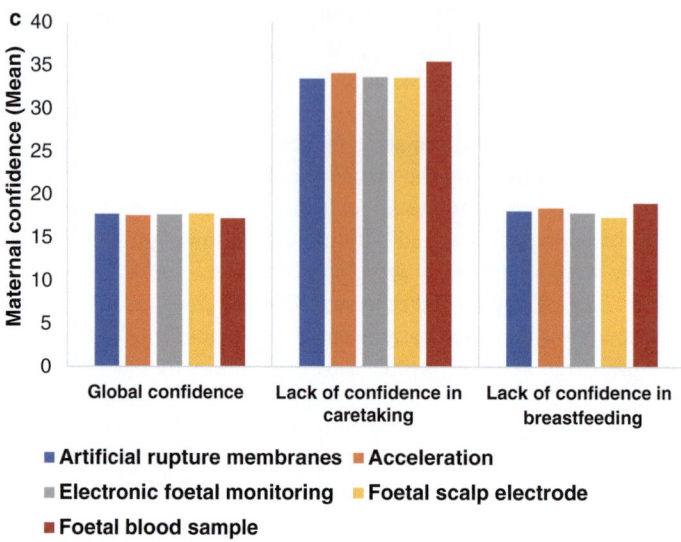

Fig. 7.14 Labour interventions and maternal confidence

Birth Mode

The way a baby is born may affect the mother and baby both physically and emotionally. These effects can last a long time and change the mother's and baby's lives for better or worse. Outcomes depend both on the nature of the birth and how it was experienced (see Chaps. 3 and 4). However, this topic is currently the subject of many contentious debates, with some believing that only the *physical* outcomes, rather than any *emotional* outcomes, significantly affect the mother's and baby's future health, happiness and wellbeing. Therefore, extremely high induction and caesarean section rates have become acceptable, no matter whether the physical and possibly long-term psychological harm caused to mothers and babies by unnecessary interventions (i.e. the over-use of some types of intervention when they have not been clinically indicated or fully consented to) may outweigh the presumed safety benefits for many mothers and their babies.

As a representative from the baby loss charity "Sands" (Saving babies' lives; Supporting bereaved families) gently pointed out in a recent meeting at Oxford University about the polarisation of maternity care issues, it's incredibly challenging, if not wholly impossible, to think past the first step (a live, healthy baby) when you're a bereaved parent. However, with birth trauma on the rise in parallel to the rising rates of what are at times *unnecessary* obstetric interventions [55], it is also essential that we understand the potentially life-long negative impacts for many mother and baby pairs of a one-size-fits-all approach to interventions, rather than a personalised assessment of each case according to that particular mother and baby's needs.

Consequently, as discussed in previous chapters, the World Health Organisation [55] has placed a strong emphasis on the importance of providing a "positive" and *psychologically safe* birth experience, as well as a *physically safe* one, for all mothers and babies. In fact, the body's natural physiology and psychology, when functioning properly, actively work together to promote *positive physical outcomes* for both mother and baby. Therefore, providing nothing is wrong with the mother and baby during a healthy pregnancy, supporting the woman's natural physiology is more likely to result in the outcome that everyone involved is aiming for: *a healthy, happy mother and baby.*

Modern medical textbooks, such as Obstetrics by Ten Teachers [25], encourage trainee obstetricians to remain aware that *thousands* of births may require unnecessary interventions (with all the negative repercussions these can entail) in order to save *one* life. Previous editions provided active warnings about unnecessary interventions, in particular the rising induction rates. In the 21st edition, similar cautions are presented about the blanket use of antibiotics after caesarean section, where thousands of women (and therefore also breastfeeding babies) must be treated to prevent one neonatal death. This kind of overuse could entail multiple risks to the long-term health and wellbeing of both mother and baby. We can't possibly cover all these risks here, but a growing body of research highlights negative impacts on the baby's developing microbiome [18, 42, 44]. For this reason, parents deserve to be fully informed about the risks associated with each intervention and, wherever possible, to be given the time and opportunity to discuss their individual situation with a health professional they know and trust before making potentially life-changing decisions. Instead, NICE guidelines are often misinterpreted and used to create different policies and protocols depending on the area, and a woman's childbirth experience can become a postcode lottery. While all mothers officially have the *right* to make informed choices suitable for themselves and their families and not be coerced into unnecessary or unwanted interventions, this autonomy is much more difficult to achieve in some parts of the UK than in others [8].

Given this background on birth mode, the way a baby is born might influence how they respond to their parents and the world around them. As shown in Fig. 7.15, the newborns in this study cried and fussed *most* after assisted births (see the high yellow tower for cry-fuss baby).

Older babies (aged 0–6 months) were also significantly more likely to be unsettled and irregular in their basic routines following an assisted birth or emergency caesarean section (Fig. 7.16). This aligns with previous research on the effects of birth mode on babies, indicating that these two modes of birth can be particularly stressful for mother and baby, especially if the mother isn't fully involved in the decision-making process, lacks effective pain relief or doesn't have adequate support throughout labour and birth (see Chaps. 3 and 4 for more details on this). In the column for unsettled-irregular baby behaviours, the yellow tower representing *assisted birth* is the highest, highlighting this as the most stressful way to be born for the baby.

Fig. 7.15 24-Hour Baby according to birth mode

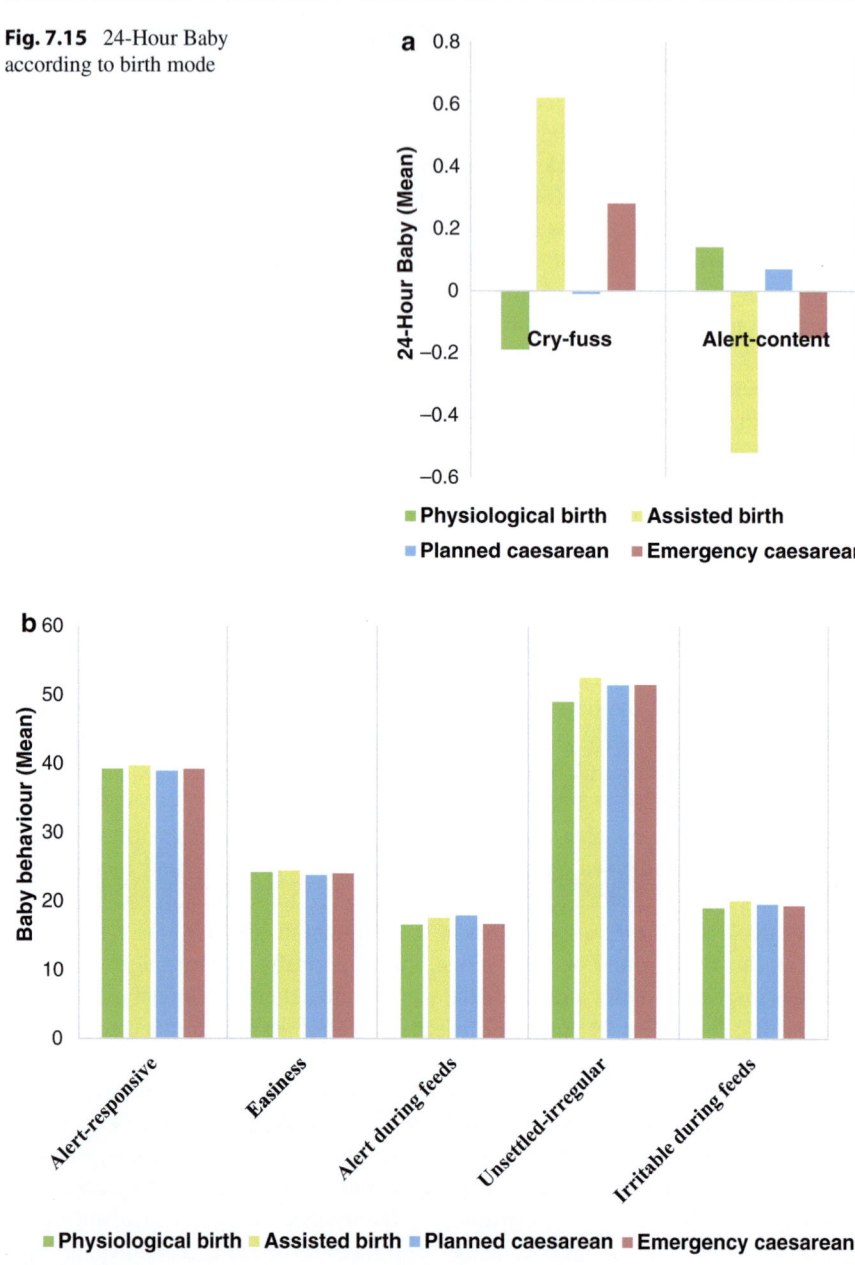

Fig. 7.16 Baby behaviour (0–6 months) according to mode of birth

7.3 The Findings: Relationships Between Childbirth Experiences and Baby Behaviour

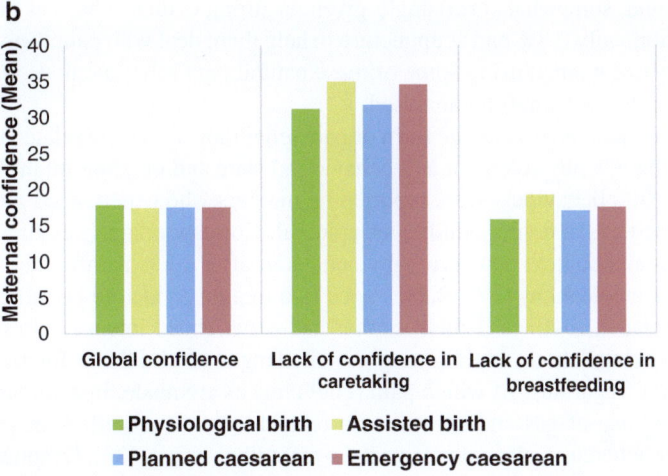

Fig. 7.17 Maternal confidence according to mode of birth

Mothers felt less confident in caring for and breastfeeding their babies after an assisted birth or emergency caesarean section. Planned caesarean sections were also linked to significantly *lower* breastfeeding confidence than for spontaneous births, although they did not seem to affect mothers' confidence in caring for their babies (Fig. 7.17).

Pain Ratings and Pain Relief

Pain relief is another contentious issue in current maternity care. While some believe pharmacological methods should be avoided at all costs, others argue that alleviating pain and fear during childbirth is crucial for the mother's and baby's wellbeing. The latter approach aims to lower the mother's cortisol (stress) levels, which helps protect her mental health (Chap. 3). Ultimately, as with any intervention, mothers must be fully informed about the pros and cons of each method and trusted to make their own decisions based on unbiased scientific evidence. If encouraged to maintain an open mind, they may also consider how they feel during labour. In theory, open-minded mothers (those with the personality trait of openness to new experiences) should be less likely to think they have "failed" at childbirth if they succumb to needing pain relief, even if it was not part of their original birth plan.

In this sample, approximately 8% of mothers used no pharmacological pain relief methods, 70% used Entonox, 14% used pethidine or an equivalent analgesic, 11% received a spinal block, 22.5% had an epidural and just over 1% underwent general anaesthesia. Some mothers used more than one form of pain relief or combined pharmacological medication with alternative methods. Approximately 26% used relaxation techniques during labour, 45% used breathing techniques, 24% used visualisations, 33% engaged in water therapy, 24% practised hypnobirthing and 22% used a TENS machine. Between 1 and 2% tried homoeopathy, reflexology or massage and, somewhat surprisingly given its strong evidence base as an effective intervention, only 0.8% had acupuncture to help them deal with pain. Consequently, the number of women using some of these natural pain relief methods was too low for them to be meaningfully analysed.

Mothers' pain levels and the form of pain relief they used were related to both the newborn baby's physiological and behavioural state and ongoing infant behaviour. More cry-fuss behaviours were reported by mothers who experienced greater pain, or who used gas and air, pethidine or epidural. Correspondingly, mothers reported more alert and content newborn baby behaviour after a *less* painful labour with *no* pain relief medications [37]. Babies aged 0–6 months tended to be more unsettled and irregular in routines if their mother had experienced intense pain or used an epidural during labour, highlighting the challenges of childbirth for mothers and their babies, regardless of which pain relief choices are made. In contrast to expectations, the use of gas and air was also related to more unsettled-irregular infant behaviour, whereas—also unexpectedly—pethidine was *not* [38]. Despite these surprising results, pethidine *did* seem to affect mother and baby in other ways, as it was linked to more irritable baby behaviour when feeding (possibly indicating an unsettled digestive system after pethidine) as well as to *lower* levels of maternal confidence and self-efficacy. Epidural use was associated with more unsettled-irregular baby behaviours, a less easy baby overall, and lower maternal confidence. The number of women who had a general anaesthetic was too low to assess the possible impacts of this in any meaningful way.

Relaxation exercises, breathing techniques, water immersion, hypnobirthing or positive visualisations during labour were all linked to *more* alert and content newborn behaviours and fewer cry-fuss behaviours [37]. In this sample, using a TEN machine, homoeopathy, reflexology and massage were not significantly related to outcomes, perhaps because there were so few mothers in most of these groups (with the exception of TENS, which was used quite frequently). Although water immersion seemed to help a little, hypnobirthing was the only natural method of pain relief that *significantly* correlated with ongoing baby behaviour (0–6 months). It was associated with *lower* unsettled-irregular scores, indicating that mothers who used hypnobirthing methods during pregnancy and childbirth tend to have calmer babies. However, mothers' reports on their confidence and self-efficacy didn't seem to be affected by whether they used any natural pain relief methods [38].

Figure 7.18 illustrates the significant relationships between pain ratings, pain relief medications, hypnobirthing and baby behaviour. The black arrows indicate *positive* correlations (where more of one thing implies more of the other). In this sample, the more severe the mother's perceptions of pain, and the more pharmacological pain relief she used, the more unsettled and irregular the baby's behaviour tended to be. The yellow arrow indicates a *negative* correlation (where more of one thing means *less* of the other). This negative relationship was between hypnobirthing and unsettled baby behaviour, meaning that babies were *less* unsettled if their

7.3 The Findings: Relationships Between Childbirth Experiences and Baby Behaviour

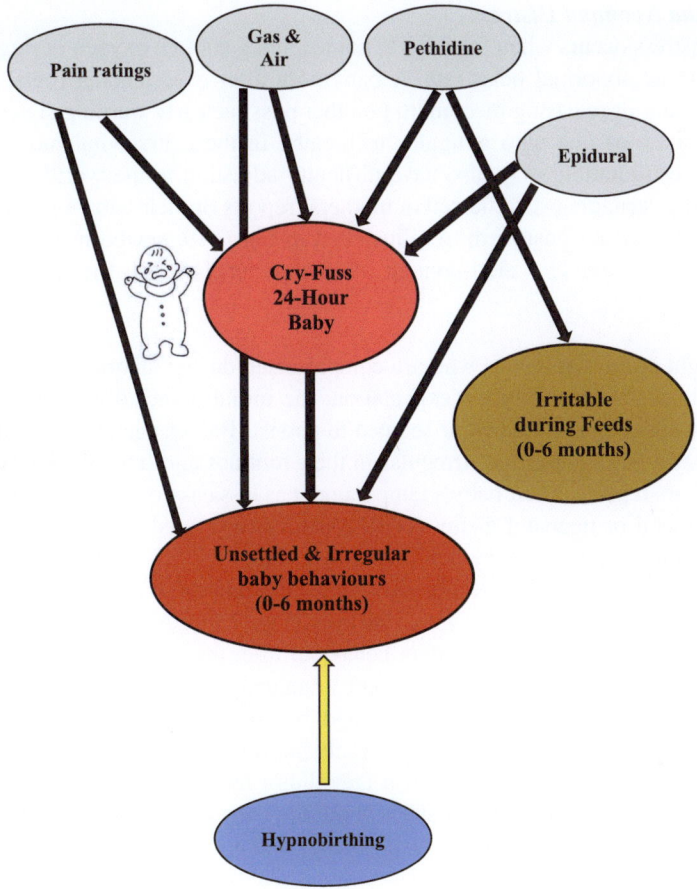

Fig. 7.18 Pain Ratings, Pain Relief and Baby Behaviour

Figure key

➡️ Positive correlations (more of one thing means more of the other)

➡️ Negative correlations (more of one thing means *less* of the other)

mothers had used hypnobirthing methods during childbirth. It's important to remember here that correlations are not causal. In other words, they neither show whether mothers' higher pain ratings led to negative baby behaviour nor the other way round. However, when one thing (maternal perceptions of labour pain) precedes the other (baby behaviour post-birth), we can *conjecture* the nature of the correlation, even though we don't have any objective scientific evidence of this until we get to the multiple linear regression models in Chap. 8.

Foetal and Neonatal Distress

Foetal distress occurs when the baby is not receiving enough oxygen during labour, leading to an abnormal heart rate. A baby born after experiencing foetal distress during labour or releasing meconium (another possible early warning sign of foetal compromise), or one who struggles to breathe in those first vital moments and requires resuscitation, may also have difficulty adjusting to the world outside the womb. This struggle was reflected in mothers' reports of their baby's physiological state and behaviour post-birth. As illustrated in Fig. 7.19, newborns were rated as *more* cry-fuss and *less* alert-content after experiencing any foetal or neonatal distress.

It might seem that babies who are compromised during labour would naturally bounce back. Contrary to this expectation, the initial associations with newborn babies' wellbeing and behaviour seemed to persist: Babies aged 0–6 months were significantly more Unsettled, Irregular in their routines and Irritable during Feeds, and mothers reported their baby's temperament as less easy overall after experiencing any foetal or neonatal distress. Foetal distress appeared to have the strongest influence on challenging baby behaviours (Fig. 7.20).

In addition, mothers had significantly *lower* confidence in caring for and breastfeeding their babies following foetal distress (Fig. 7.21). Although there were no significant differences in early infant behaviour after the presence of meconium in the waters (amniotic fluid), mothers more frequently experienced a lack of confidence in both caretaking (caring for) and breastfeeding their babies after this occurred. Mothers also reported significantly lower global (overall) confidence if their baby needed resuscitation than if they didn't require help to breathe, demonstrating that experiencing fear or stress about the baby during childbirth could seriously impact mothers' confidence, self-efficacy and postnatal wellbeing (Fig. 7.21).

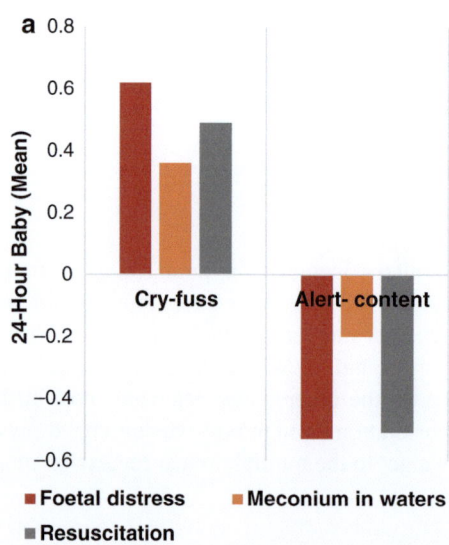

Fig. 7.19 Baby distress signals and 24-Hour Baby

7.3 The Findings: Relationships Between Childbirth Experiences and Baby Behaviour 183

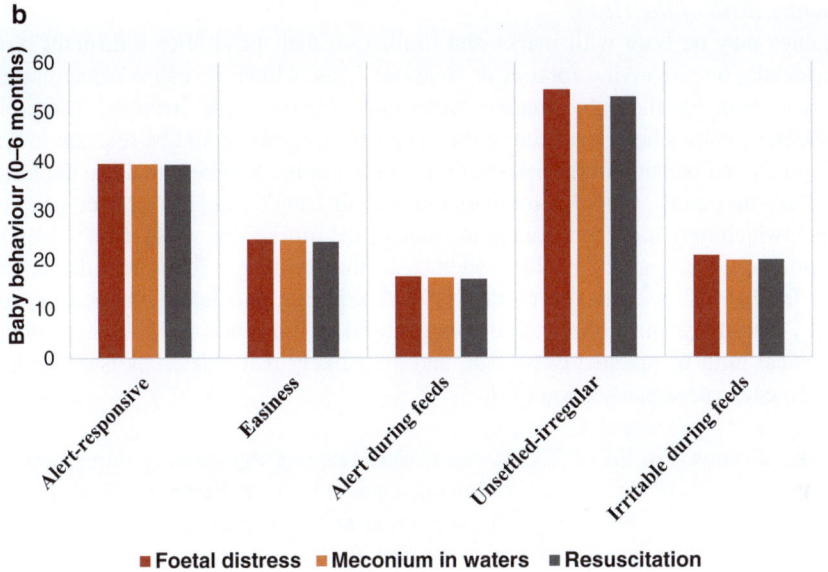

Fig. 7.20 Baby distress signals and baby behaviour (0–6 months)

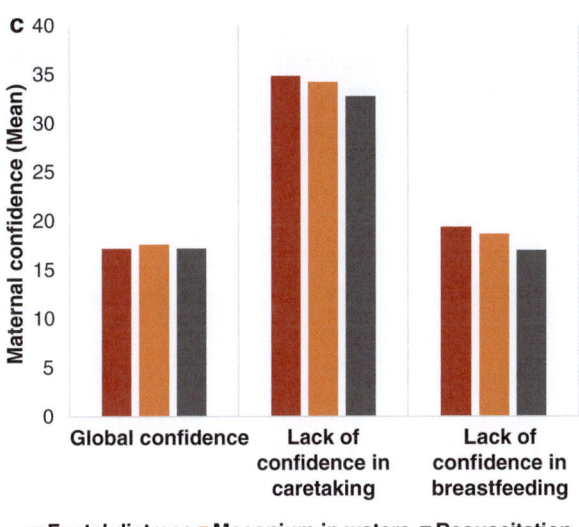

Fig. 7.21 Baby distress signals and maternal confidence

Gentle Birth of the Head

Babies may be born with marks and bruises on their head after a difficult birth, especially one involving forceps or ventouse. This is likely to cause some discomfort or pain for the baby, making them more fractious and irritable. Therefore, whether a baby's head has been birthed gently or *un*gently could be relevant to how they respond behaviourally post-birth. I should remind you here that the definition of "cry-fuss baby" included mothers rating their baby's head as "bruised or swollen", which may have contributed to some of the differences in cry-fuss scores for gentle versus non-gentle births. Nonetheless, this bruising is likely to indicate pain for the baby as well as the mother [19]. A separate calculation showed that the baby's head was most likely to be born gently if the birth was a spontaneous physiological birth or planned caesarean, and least likely if it was an assisted birth or emergency caesarean section [37].

As illustrated in Fig. 7.22, newborns were rated as significantly more alert and content (+0.26) in the 24 hours following a gentle birth of their head compared to a *non*-gentle birth (−0.15). Equally, they cried and fussed more after a *non*-gentle birth (+0.19) than they did after a gentle birth (−0.32).

Following this, babies aged 0–6 months were perceived as significantly more alert and responsive, *less* unsettled or irregular in their routines and easier overall after experiencing a gentle birth of their head (Fig. 7.23). While these differences in alert-responsive and easy baby behaviour were very small, they all contribute to the bigger picture. The difference in scores for unsettled-irregular baby behaviours was more substantial—babies scored a lower average of 47.51 points for unsettled-irregular behaviours after a gentle birth compared to the higher average of 51.44 points after a *non*-gentle birth.

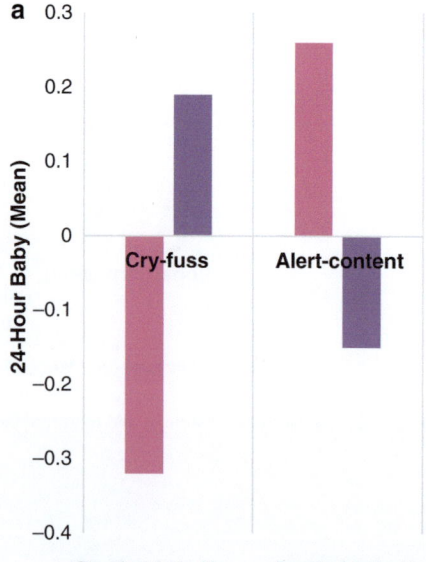

Fig. 7.22 Gentle birth and 24-Hour Baby

7.3 The Findings: Relationships Between Childbirth Experiences and Baby Behaviour

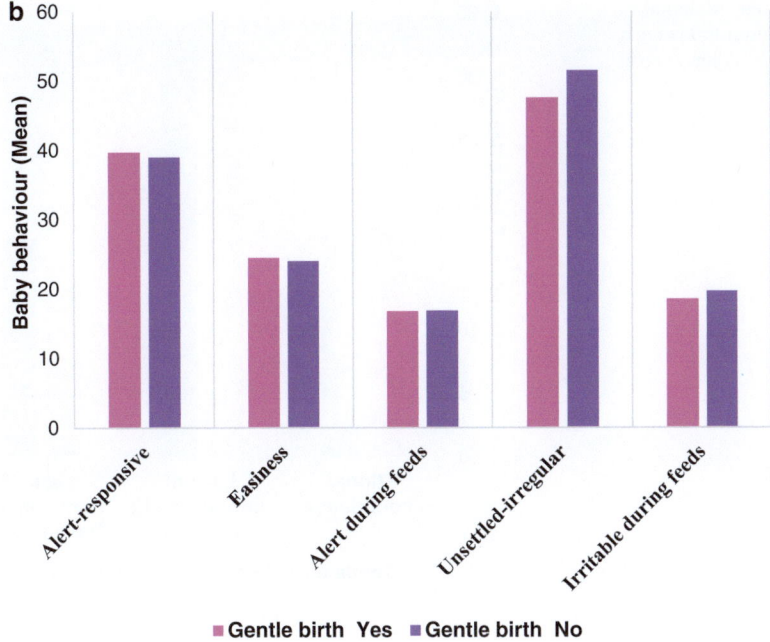

Fig. 7.23 Baby behaviour (0–6 months) following a gentle/non-gentle birth

Having a gentle birth of the baby's head also seemed to benefit mothers' confidence and self-efficacy (Fig. 7.24). On average, mothers experienced *less* lack of confidence in caretaking or breastfeeding—and therefore, *more* confidence in both these areas—following a gentle birth.

Skin-to-Skin Care

Skin-to-skin ("kangaroo") care is crucial for a newborn baby's immediate and ongoing health and physiological wellbeing as it keeps them warm and close, promoting the regulation of their temperature and heartbeat [51]. Importantly, kangaroo care reduces neonatal mortality and morbidity in low birthweight or preterm babies [27]. It also serves as a significant aspect of childbirth for new parents, alleviating symptoms of stress and depression while enabling them to release oxytocin, which facilitates breastfeeding and bonding [26]. It was therefore expected that immediate skin-to-skin contact between mother and baby would be associated with greater newborn and infant wellbeing and behaviour. As predicted, newborn babies receiving immediate skin-to-skin contact with their mother showed fewer cry-fuss behaviours during the first 24 hours post-birth. Corresponding with this, newborns were rated as more alert and content when they had immediate skin-to-skin contact with their mothers than when the mother-baby pair was separated (Fig. 7.25).

Fig. 7.24 Maternal confidence following a gentle/non-gentle birth

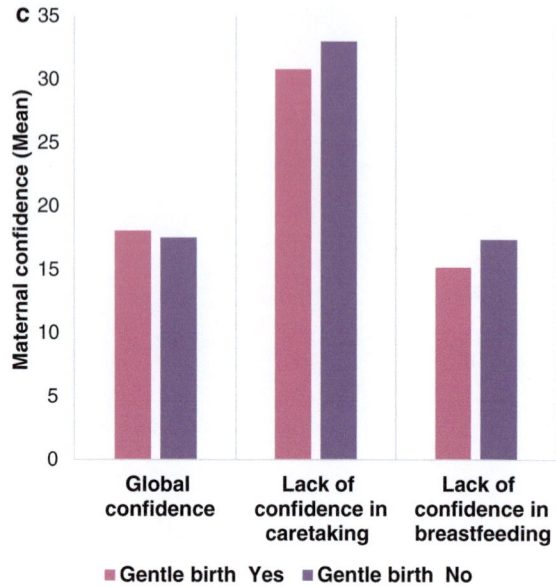

Fig. 7.25 24-Hour Baby following to skin to skin

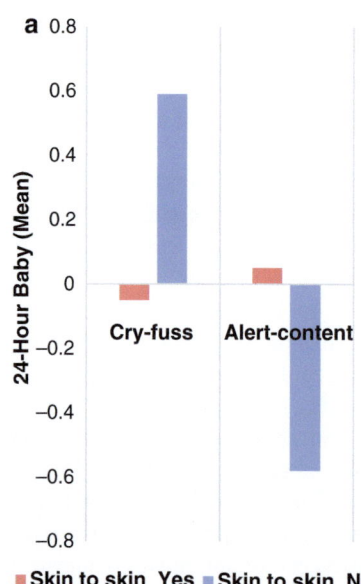

7.3 The Findings: Relationships Between Childbirth Experiences and Baby Behaviour   187

Looking beyond these initial 24 hours, 0–6-month-old babies who had immediate skin-to-skin contact with their mothers were seen as having a slightly easier overall temperament. More significantly, if they *didn't* have this close time with a parent immediately post-birth, babies aged 0-6 months tended to be more unsettled and irregular in their routines (Fig. 7.26).

Mothers who had immediate skin-to-skin time with their babies reported greater confidence in caring for and breastfeeding the baby and therefore had *lower* Lack of confidence scores in these areas after experiencing immediate skin-to-skin time with their babies (Fig. 7.27).

Initial and Current Feeding Practices

Finally, for the "physical" variables, the method used to feed the baby from birth to 6 months was explored. It's worth noting here that the MABS [53] were developed several decades ago. Since then, breastfeeding has become less popular, possibly more difficult to fit into our busy lives, known to be challenging to initiate successfully after major obstetric interventions, and therefore often replaced with other modes of feeding. Despite all these potentially intervening factors, 882 (88.3%) mothers in the survey initiated breastfeeding, while only 117 (11.7%) began feeding their baby using another method, such as formula or expressed milk. The sample was therefore initially skewed towards breastfeeding. Moreover, 850 mothers were still breastfeeding at the time of completing the survey, which is a much higher number than breastfeeding rates in the general population of British mothers.

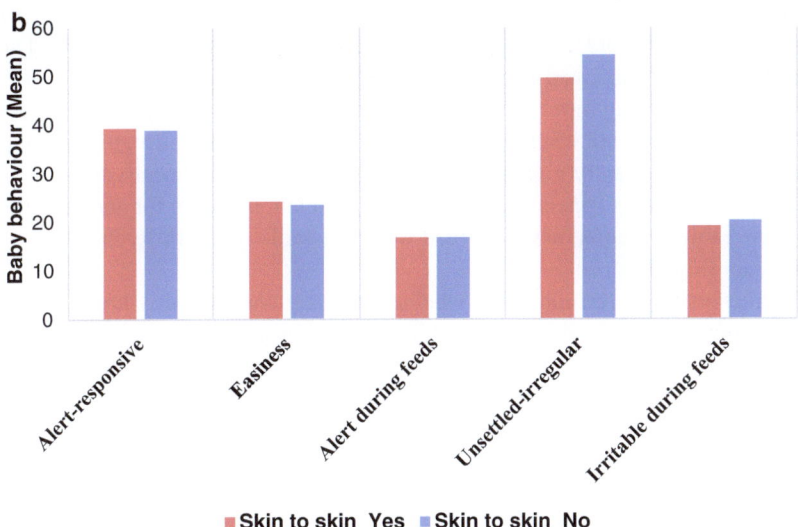

Fig. 7.26 Baby behaviour (0–6 months) following skin to skin

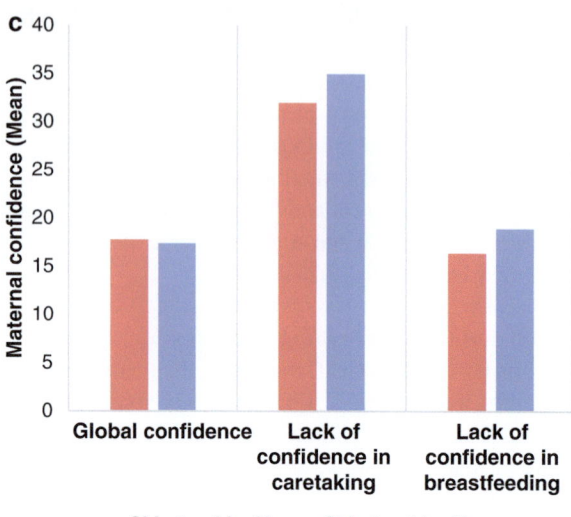

Fig. 7.27 Maternal confidence following skin to skin

Newborns were rated as being *less* cry-fuss and *more* alert-content if their first feed was breastfeeding (Fig. 7.28). This link between breastfeeding and alert-content baby wellbeing and behaviour is probably at least partially explained by one of the statements comprising the variable alert-content baby being directly related to breastfeeding: "My baby latched onto the breast easily". However, babies who found it easier to latch onto the breast straight away may have been more alert and content in their behaviour as well, and this seems likely if we look at the corresponding results for older babies' behaviour in Fig. 7.29, where non-breastfed newborn babies were perceived as more unsettled later.

Overall, exhibiting more crying and fussing behaviours appeared to be ongoing in babies who were not initially breastfed post-birth: unsettled-irregular behaviour scores were significantly higher for babies *first fed* by "other" means (Fig. 7.29).

Although mothers appeared slightly more confident in caring for and breastfeeding their babies when babies' first feed was breastmilk, these differences were not significant (Fig. 7.30).

While naturally presuming that whether the baby was currently breastfed at the time of completing the survey wouldn't be at all connected to 24-Hour Baby behaviour (unless the mother completed the survey within a day of giving birth), Currently breastfed *was* slightly (although not significantly) related to newborn baby behaviour (Fig. 7.31).

Babies who were still breastfeeding at the time their mother completed the survey were *less* alert during feeds, which could be due to the way breastfeeding babies often fall asleep or doze sleepily on the breast while feeding. Although, on average, older babies were rated as slightly *more* unsettled-irregular if currently breastfed, this difference in scores was *not* significant (Fig. 7.32). Nonetheless, the fact that breastfed babies were slightly more unsettled could be due to their need to feed more frequently. Breast milk is designed for the newborn baby's delicate system and is therefore more readily digestible than formula milk. It also contains enzymes

7.3 The Findings: Relationships Between Childbirth Experiences and Baby Behaviour 189

Fig. 7.28 24-Hour Baby according to first feed

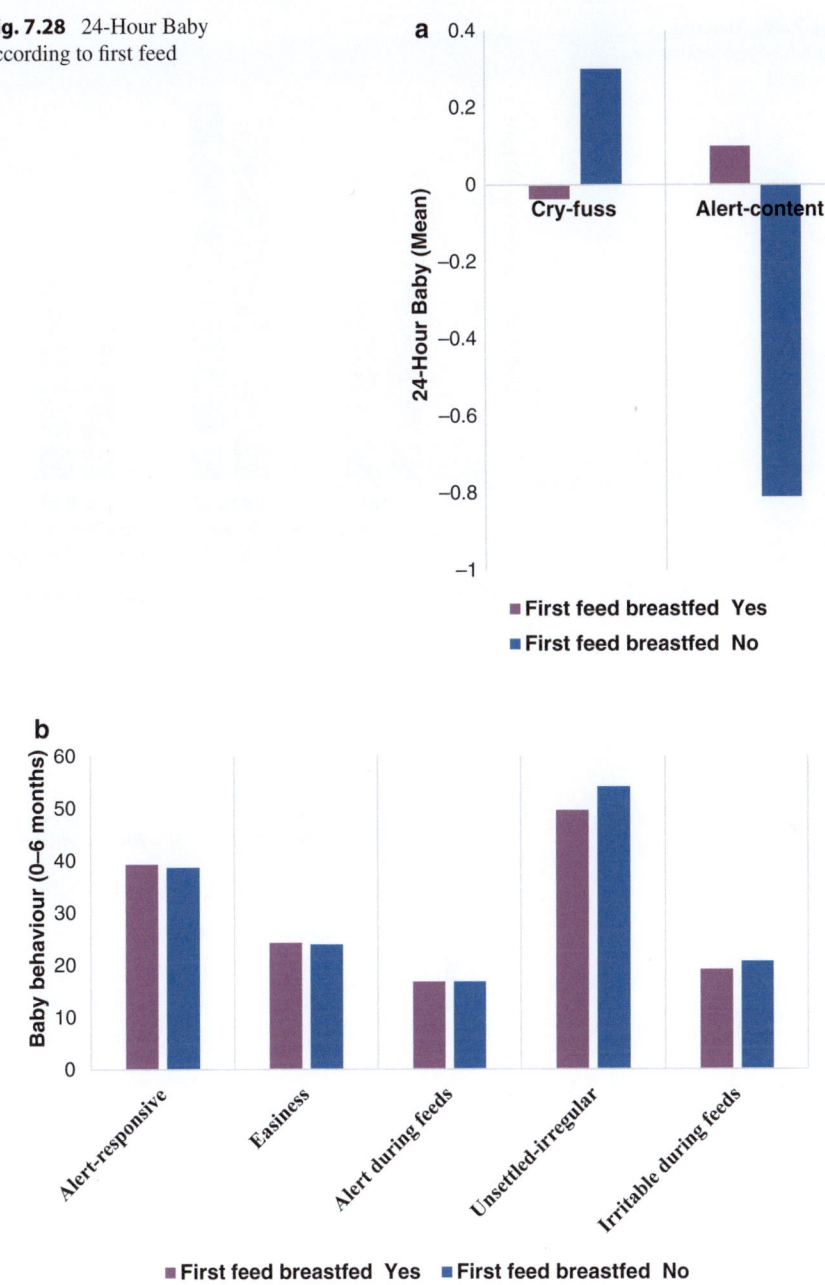

Fig. 7.29 Baby behaviour (0–6 months) according to first feed

Fig. 7.30 Maternal confidence according to first feed

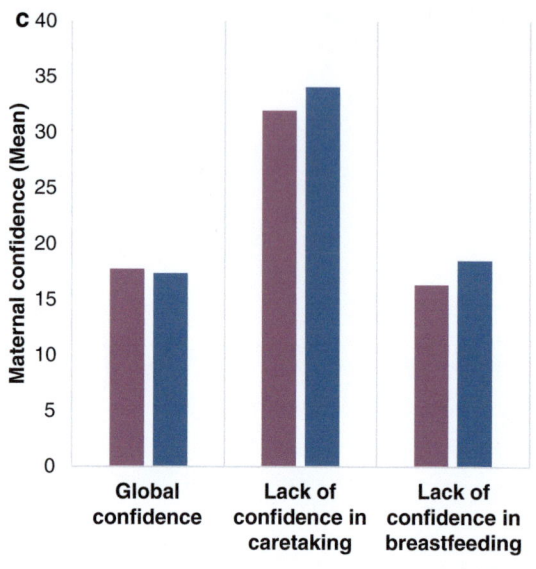

Fig. 7.31 24-Hour Baby according to current feeding method

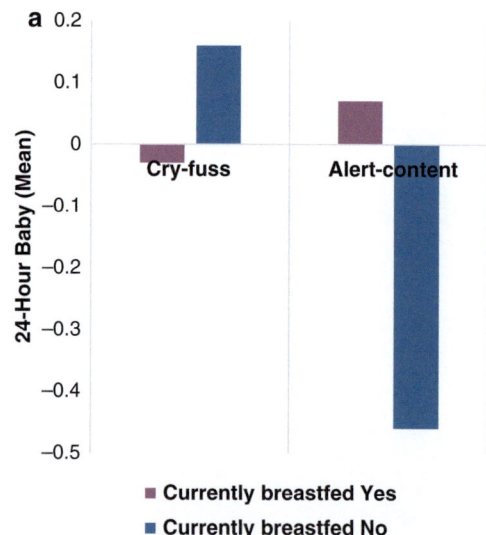

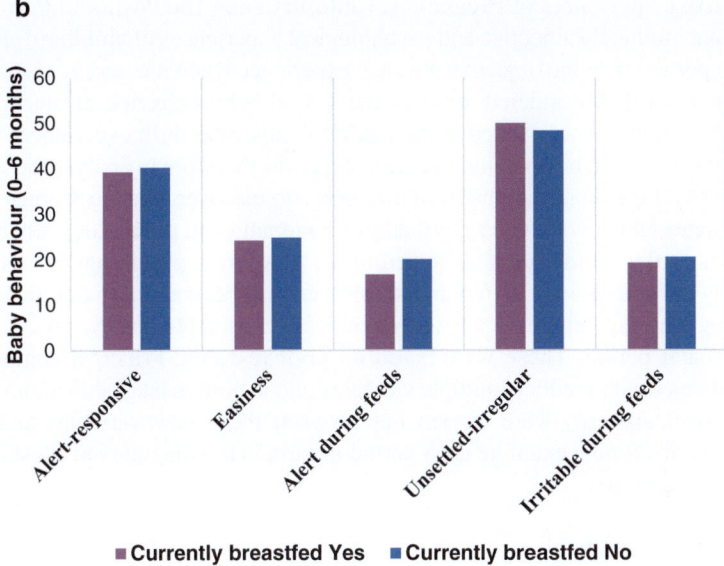

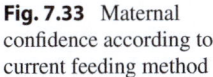

Fig. 7.32 Baby behaviour (0–6 months) according to current feeding method

Fig. 7.33 Maternal confidence according to current feeding method

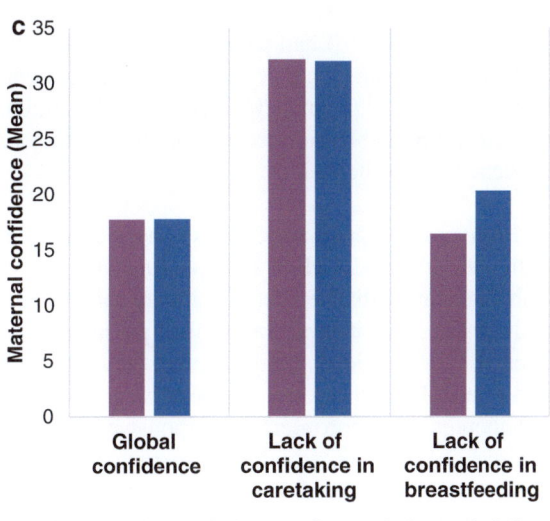

that aid digestion, which are likely to accelerate the digestion process, meaning the baby becomes hungry again more quickly.

As expected, mothers who were still breastfeeding at the time of completing the questionnaire felt more confident about breastfeeding than mothers who'd stopped (Fig. 7.33).

Subjective Experiences of Pregnancy, Childbirth and the Postnatal Period

Given that mothers' subjective and psychological experiences of childbirth are even more important than the objective physical experience when it comes to the issue of birth trauma [2], I wondered whether the key to baby behavioural outcomes of childbirth might *also* be related to the mother's subjective birth experience and her response to the birth postnatally. The next stage was therefore to analyse the subjective and psychological findings from the survey to discover whether women's subjective states and how they *felt* physically, emotionally and psychologically before, during and after childbirth were linked to the newborn's physiological wellbeing and early baby behaviour (0–6 months). Mothers had been asked to rate statements regarding how they felt physically and emotionally during pregnancy, childbirth and the postnatal period. These were based on prior research. Principal components analysis was used to reduce multiple variables into a more manageable number, and correlational analyses were carried out between these new variables and baby behaviour. We'll now examine each period in turn, using diagrams to illustrate the most notable results.

Pregnancy Experiences

Subjective pregnancy statements, including "I felt happy and excited" or "anxious and fearful about the birth", were named "positive pregnancy emotions". Negative items were inverse (or reverse) scored, meaning that higher scores indicated a more positive experience. The same treatment was given to the more *physical* subjective statements, such as "I had plenty of energy" or "felt tired", "drained" or "in pain", and these (including the inverse-scored negative items) were collectively labelled as "positive physical pregnancy". Physical and emotional pregnancy states were interrelated and probably bidirectional in the way they affected one another, as well as influencing baby behaviour.

Both positive pregnancy states (physical and emotional) positively correlated with alert-content 24-Hour Baby and *negatively* correlated with cry-fuss 24-Hour Baby, indicating that newborn babies appeared happier and more alert, while crying and fussing *less*, if their mother had *positive* physical and emotional pregnancy experiences. It follows, therefore, that they cried and fussed more if their mothers had physically and emotionally negative pregnancy experiences [37]. Babies aged 0–6 months were more alert and responsive with an overall easier temperament after positive physical and emotional experiences during pregnancy, and these mothers tended to feel more confident. Conversely, babies were more unsettled and irregular if their mothers had *not* experienced a positive pregnancy. Figure 7.34 illustrates the relationships between the two subjective positive pregnancy states, 24-Hour Baby and baby behaviour from 0 to 6 months [37].

Birth Emotions

A principal components analysis reduced multiple statements about mothers' feelings during labour and birth to four new variables describing different "birth emotions". Positive birth emotions described mothers feeling "strong", "happy",

7.3 The Findings: Relationships Between Childbirth Experiences and Baby Behaviour

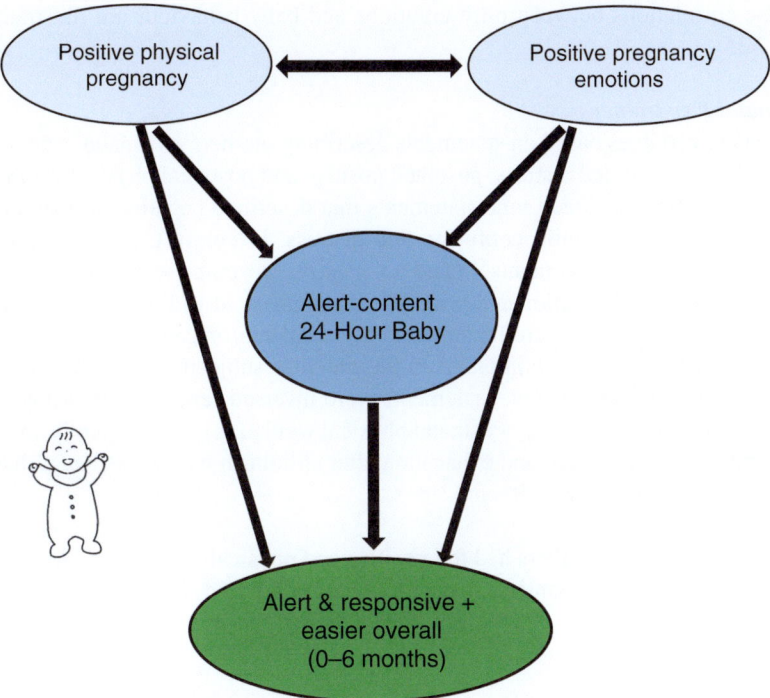

Fig. 7.34 Subjective pregnancy states and baby behaviour

Figure key

➡️ Positive correlations (more of one thing means more of the other)

⬅️➡️ Probable bi-directional associations, with each affecting the other

"energised" and "focused" during childbirth; neglected birth emotions described mothers who had felt "abandoned" or "ignored"; aware-alert birth emotions described mothers feeling "aware" and "alert"; and anxious-afraid birth emotions were based on feeling "anxious, afraid, vulnerable and overwhelmed". Feeling positive or aware and alert during childbirth was related to more alert and content newborn behaviours. In contrast, mothers who felt "neglected" or "anxious-afraid" during the birth were more likely to report their newborn baby as crying and fussing during the first 24 hours [37].

Following a similar pattern, babies whose mothers felt positive during childbirth were more alert, responsive and temperamentally easier overall, as well as significantly *less* unsettled-irregular or irritable during feeds than babies whose mothers had experienced more negative emotions during childbirth. As might be expected, mothers had significantly more confidence and self-efficacy in caring for their babies and greater global (overall) confidence following positive birth emotions (and therefore a positive birth experience) [38].

The correlations between birth emotions and baby behaviour are illustrated in Fig. 7.35.

Postnatal Experiences

Three new variables based on statements describing mothers' postnatal experiences were labelled postnatal distress, postnatal positive and postnatal physical wellbeing. Postnatal distress included nine statements that described negative postnatal emotions, such as anger, guilt, confusion and distress. In contrast, postnatal positive encompassed eight statements linked to positive postnatal emotions, including relief, euphoria, exhilaration and pride. Postnatal physical wellbeing was informed by negative statements regarding mothers' postnatal neurophysiological states, such as *feeling exhausted* and *in pain*. As in the previous subjective states during pregnancy and childbirth, negative statements were inversed scored when contributing to a named positive state (e.g. Postnatal physical wellbeing). Consequently, mothers who experienced *less* pain and exhaustion after childbirth were classified as having *better* postnatal physical wellbeing.

Newborns whose mothers had felt positive and physically well post-birth tended to exhibit *more* alert-content behaviour and cried and fussed *less* often. In

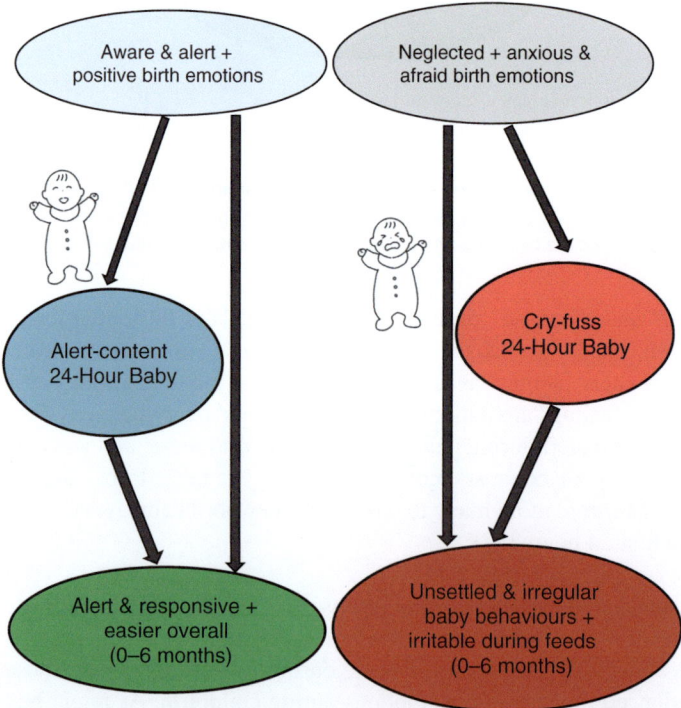

Fig. 7.35 Birth emotions and baby behaviour

Figure key

➤ Positive correlations (more of one thing means more of the other)

7.3 The Findings: Relationships Between Childbirth Experiences and Baby Behaviour

comparison, mothers who experienced postnatal distress reported more cry-fuss newborn behaviours [37].

The associations between postnatal states and baby behaviour continued along a similar line to the birthing states. Infants aged 0–6 months were easier and more alert and responsive if their mother felt physically and mentally well postnatally. Conversely, they tended to be *more* unsettled-irregular and irritable during feeds and *less* alert-responsive and have a more *difficult* temperament overall if their mother experienced postnatal distress, possibly linked to a traumatic birth experience. Mothers felt *more* confident in all areas (including looking after and breastfeeding their baby) if they had felt emotionally and physically well after childbirth. They reported themselves as *less* confident if they'd felt distressed postnatally [38].

The patterns of baby behaviour here were very similar to those of the subjective pregnancy states (Fig. 7.34) and birth emotions (Fig. 7.35). Therefore, positive *postnatal* physical and emotional states were linked to (or positively correlated with) positive baby behaviours and vice versa. Most notably, postnatal distress was linked to negative baby behaviours.

These correlations, which are likely to be bidirectional, are illustrated in Fig. 7.36.

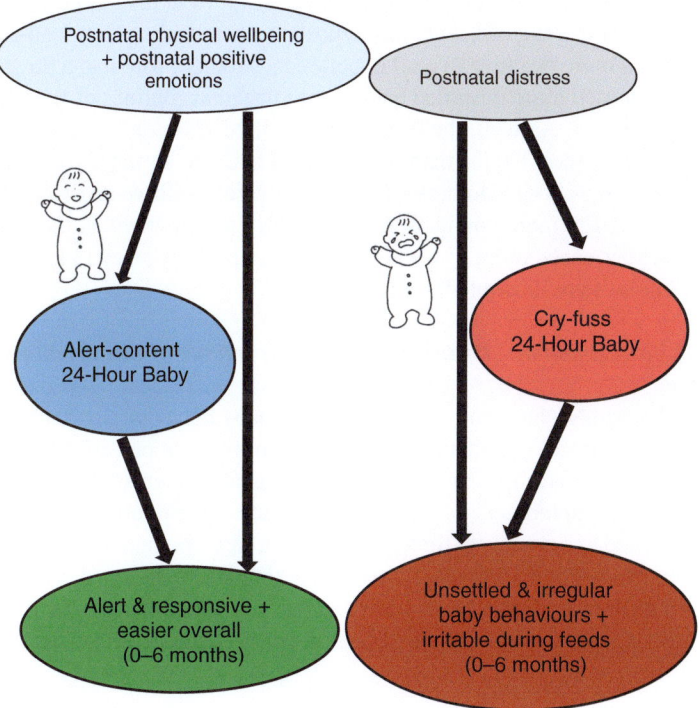

Fig. 7.36 Subjective postnatal states and baby behaviour

Figure key

➡ Positive correlations (more of one thing means more of the other)

Overall Perceptions of Childbirth

Lastly, mothers responded to statements about their *overall* birth experience. An overall "positive birth experience" involved mothers feeling positive, comfortable and in control and experiencing a gentle birth of their infant's head. A supported birth experience was characterised by helpful, informative and emotionally supportive birth attendants. A directed birth experience was characterised by a more directive approach, including being encouraged to remain on the bed, feeling unable to move about freely during labour (possibly due to the constraints of medical equipment such as continuous electronic foetal monitoring) and experiencing guided ("Valsalva") pushing techniques, as described in Chap. 3 [22].

As with all the other subjective variables discussed so far, mothers' overall postnatal perceptions of their birth experience were related to their baby's behaviour in the expected directions. "Positive" and 'supported" birth experiences were related to more alert-content newborn behaviour, including babies finding it easier to latch on and breastfeed. In contrast, having a more directed birth experience predicted more crying and fussing during the first 24 hours [37].

Beyond these first 24 hours, positive and well-supported birth experiences were positively associated with happier mothers and babies aged 0–6 months. These babies tended to be more alert and responsive. They were also rated as having an Easier overall temperament than babies whose mothers had *not* felt well-supported or who'd had a more negative overall experience. Mothers who had a directed birth experience reported more unsettled babies with irregular routines of feeding, sleeping and elimination. As well, these mothers reported less confidence in caring for and breastfeeding their babies than those who'd been given more freedom to give birth however they chose. Mothers who had an overall positive and well-supported birth experience felt more confident in their ability to breastfeed and care for their babies and experienced more overall confidence and self-efficacy [38].

These findings are illustrated in Fig. 7.37.

Maternal Birth Emotions, Postnatal Period, Perceptions of Childbirth and Birth Mode

Although the primary outcome of this study was baby behaviour, and the secondary outcome was maternal confidence (as this was an intrinsic part of the Mother and Baby Scales that relates to baby behaviour), I was also interested in how the *birth mode* might relate to mothers' subjective experiences of childbirth and the postnatal period. I decided to run a few extra tests to find out. The findings were clear: Mothers reported more positive birth emotions when they'd experienced a spontaneous labour and birth or a *planned* caesarean section, and more negative birth emotions if they had experienced an *assisted* birth or *emergency* caesarean section. These

7.3 The Findings: Relationships Between Childbirth Experiences and Baby Behaviour

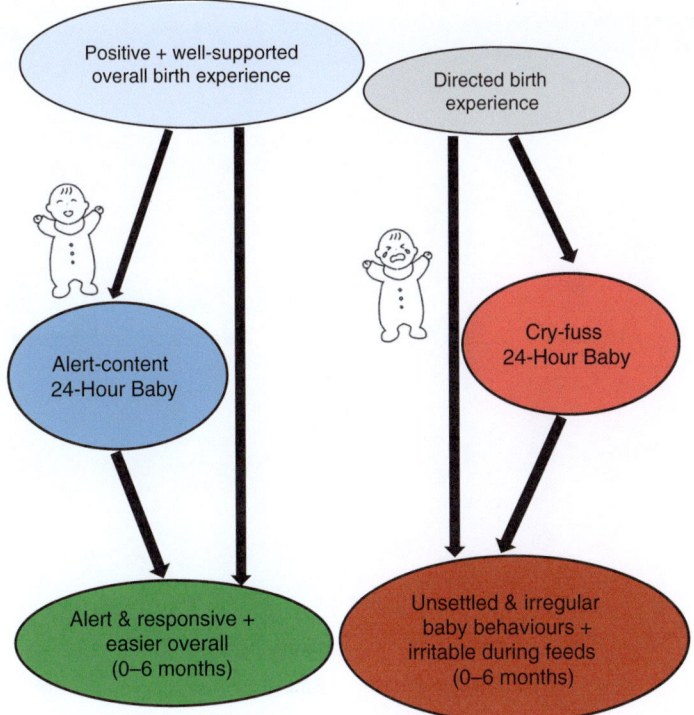

Fig. 7.37 Overall perceptions of childbirth and baby behaviour

Figure key

➡ Positive correlations (more of one thing means more of the other)

effects could be bidirectional, meaning that the physical birth experience may have triggered certain emotional states, and mothers' emotional states may have contributed to their physical birth experiences. Mothers were more likely to feel anxious and afraid during an assisted birth, and the relationship between emergency caesarean sections and anxious-afraid birth emotions was even stronger, highlighting how stressful both types of emergency birth can be for the mother and baby (Fig. 7.38).

Understandably, postnatal distress was significantly higher after an emergency caesarean section than after any other mode of birth, while mothers reported better physical and psychological outcomes following a spontaneous birth or a planned caesarean section. As you can see in Fig. 7.39, spontaneous birth was the only mode of birth that was *not* related to postnatal distress.

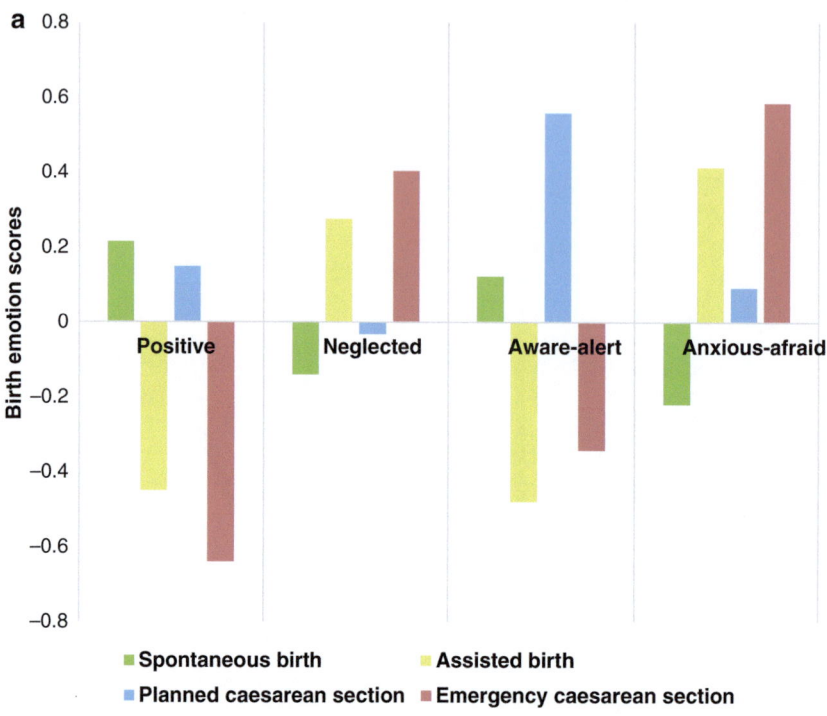

Fig. 7.38 Birth emotions according to birth mode

Mothers were more likely to rate their *overall* birth experience as positive after a spontaneous birth than after any other type of birth. However, a calm, planned caesarean could also be a positive experience. Spontaneous birth was the least likely to feel "directed" and, overall, mothers reported feeling less supported with a caesarean section compared to vaginal birth Fig. 7.40).

7.3 The Findings: Relationships Between Childbirth Experiences and Baby Behaviour 199

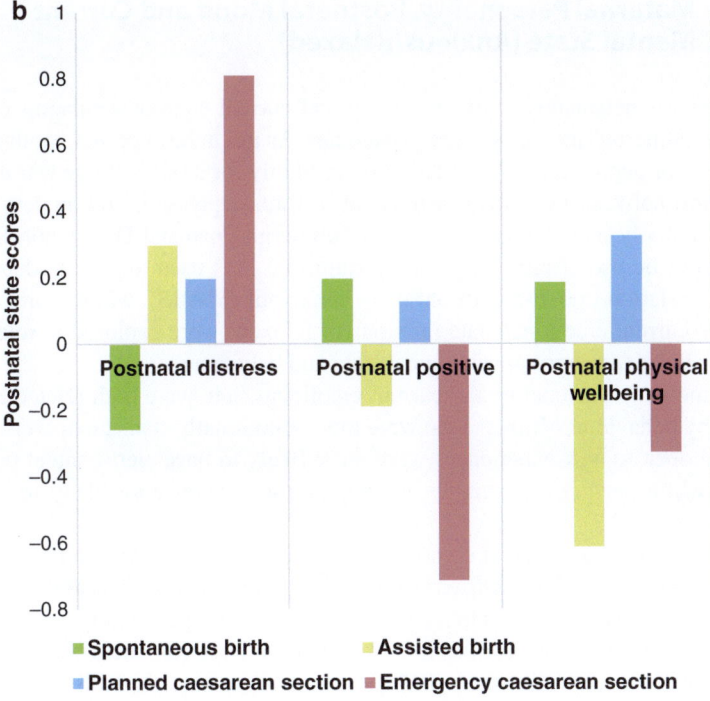

Fig. 7.39 Subjective postnatal states according to birth mode

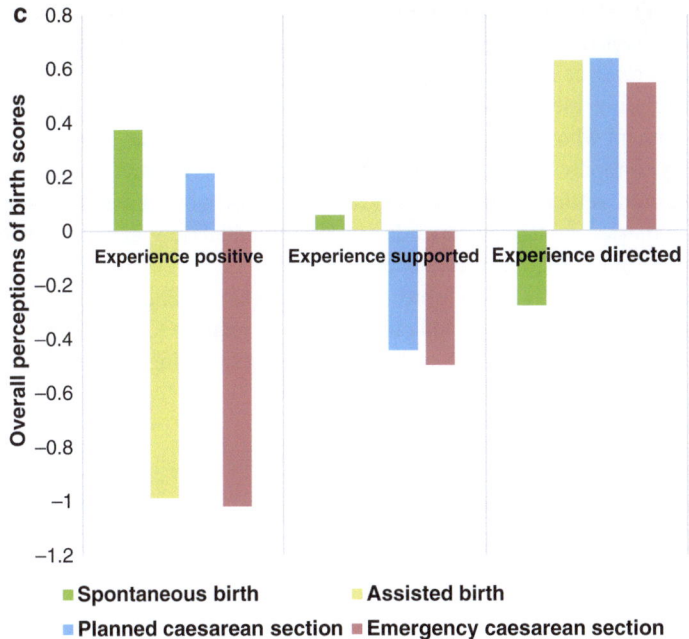

Fig. 7.40 Perceptions of childbirth according to birth mode

7.4 Maternal Personality, Postnatal Mood and Current Mental State (Anxious/Relaxed)

The mother's personality, postnatal mood and current state of wellbeing were all linked to numerous mother and baby outcomes. As might be expected, mothers with symptoms of depression also tended to score highly for anxiety (there was a strong correlation between the two measures); therefore, depression and anxiety scores were essentially interchangeable. As the Edinburgh Postnatal Depression Scale is designed to be used from 7 days postpartum, this was used to look at depression scores in relation to 0–6-month-old baby behaviour (MABS), while scores for the mother's current emotional state (anxious or relaxed) were explored in relation to 24-Hour Baby (newborn physiological state and behaviour).

The mother's personality and current emotional state were both related to newborn baby behaviour: Mothers who were more emotionally stable, extrovert, agreeable and open to new experiences were more likely to have alert-content newborn babies, while newborns of highly anxious mothers were more likely to cry and fuss [37].

Positive postnatal mood (i.e. mothers experiencing *fewer* symptoms of depression) and *feeling calm and relaxed* (scoring *lower* on the anxiety scale) at the time of completing the questionnaire, together with positive personality traits such as emotional stability, conscientiousness, openness and agreeableness were related to a more alert and responsive baby (0–6 months) with an easier overall temperament. Notably, the more emotionally stable mothers were, the *less* likely they were to feel anxious or depressed. Mothers with these personality traits were also more likely to feel confident. In contrast, babies tended to be more unsettled-irregular and irritable during feeds if their mothers were inclined towards being *introverted* or if they felt *anxious and depressed*. These mothers also tended to feel less confident about caring for and breastfeeding their babies [38].

When relating these results to mothers' childbirth and perinatal experiences, overall, mothers who had *positive* pregnancy, birth and postnatal experiences were more likely to report feeling *emotionally stable* and had happier, easier, more alert, responsive and settled babies. In contrast, mothers who had *negative* birth and perinatal experiences tended towards symptoms of anxiety and depression while reporting more unsettled, irritable babies [37].

Figure 7.41 is a pictorial representation of the findings regarding mothers' personalities, postnatal moods and current state in relation to baby behaviour.

The numerous physical and psychological factors relating to baby behaviour are summarised in Fig. 7.42.

7.4 Maternal Personality, Postnatal Mood and Current Mental State (Anxious/Relaxed)

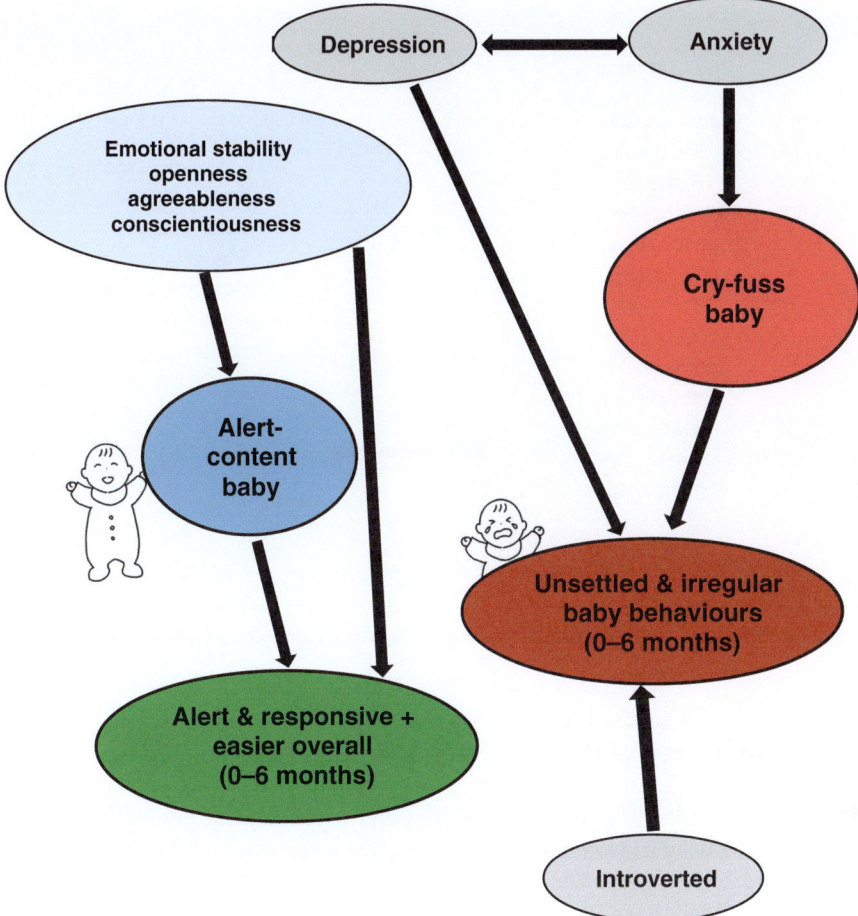

Fig. 7.41 Maternal personality, mental health and baby behaviour

Figure key

➡️ Positive correlations (more of one thing means more of the other)

⬅️➡️ Probable bidirectional associations, with each affecting the other

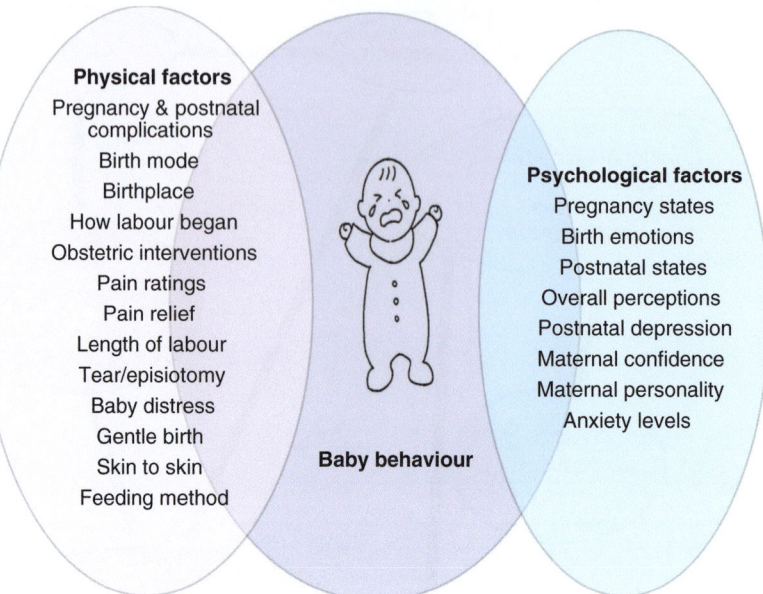

Fig. 7.42 Summary of physical and psychological factors relating to baby behaviour

7.5 Summary of the Survey Findings So Far

This chapter outlined the multiple physical and psychological perinatal variables relating to the baby's physiological wellbeing and behaviour and the mother's confidence and self-efficacy. The findings suggest that the baby's behaviour and the mother's confidence are likely to be influenced by the mother's personality, pregnancy, birth and postnatal experiences and emotional states. These findings are consistent with previous evidence that baby behaviour is shaped by both genetic and environmental influences, as discussed in Chap. 2. The next chapter will further explore this relationship by examining the *predictive* impacts of childbirth and other perinatal factors on mother and baby.

References

1. Apgar V. A proposal for a new method of evaluation of the newborn infant. Curr Res Anasth Analg. 1952;32(4):260–7.
2. Ayers S, Bond R, Bertullies S, Wijma K. The aetiology of post-traumatic stress following childbirth: a meta-analysis and theoretical framework. Psychol Med. 2016;46(6):1121–34.
3. Ayers S, Wright DB, Thornton A. Development of a measure of postpartum PTSD: the city birth trauma scale. Front Psychiatry. 2018;9:409.

4. Brazelton TB, Nugent JK. Neonatal behavioral assessment scale. 3rd ed. New York: Cambridge University Press; 1995.
5. British Psychological Society. BPS code of human research ethics. 2021. Available at: https://explore.bps.org.uk/binary/bpsworks/06096a55b82ca73a/9787a5959b2bfdff7ed2a43ad5b3f333a5278925cfd667b1b2e64b5387c91b92/inf180_2021.pdf. Accessed 15 Dec 2024.
6. Britton JR. Infant temperament and maternal anxiety and depressed mood in the early postpartum period. Women Health. 2011;51(1):55–71.
7. Brocklehurst P, Puddicombe D, Hollowell J, Stewart M, Linsell L, Macfarlane AJ, McCourt C. Perinatal and maternal outcomes by planned place of birth for healthy women with low risk pregnancies: the birthplace in England national prospective cohort study. Br Med J. 2011;343:d7400.
8. Coates D, Donnolley N, Foureur M, Spear V, Henry A. Exploring unwarranted clinical variation: the attitudes of midwives and obstetric medical staff regarding induction of labour and planned caesarean section. Women Birth. 2021;34(4):352–61.
9. Cox JL, Holden JM, Sagovsky R. Detection of postnatal depression: development of the 10-item Edinburgh postnatal depression scale. Br J Psychiatry. 1987;150(6):782–6.
10. Dahlen HG, Kennedy HP, Anderson CM, Bell AF, Clark A, Foureur M, Ohm JE, Shearman AM, Taylor JY, Wright ML, Downe S. The EPIIC hypothesis: intrapartum effects on the neonatal epigenome and consequent health outcomes. Med Hypotheses. 2013;80(5):656–62.
11. Denis A, Ponsin M, Callahan S. The relationship between maternal self-esteem, maternal competence, infant temperament and post-partum blues. J Reprod Infant Psychol. 2012;30:388–97.
12. Douglas PS, Hill PS. A neurobiological model for cry-fuss problems in the first three to four months of life. Med Hypotheses. 2013;81(5):816–22.
13. Feldman R. The neurobiology of human attachments. Trends Cogn Sci. 2017;21:80–99.
14. Fox H, Callander E, Lindsay D, Topp S. Evidence of overuse? Patterns of obstetric interventions during labour and birth among Australian mothers. BMC Pregnancy Childbirth. 2019;19:1–8.
15. Glover V, O'Donnell KJ, O'Connor TG, Fisher J. Prenatal maternal stress, fetal programming, and mechanisms underlying later psychopathology—a global perspective. Dev Psychopathol. 2018;30(3):843–54.
16. Goldberg LR. The development of markers for the big-five factor structure. Psychol Assess. 1992;4(1):26.
17. Gosling SD, Rentfrow PJ, Swann WB Jr. A very brief measure of the big-five personality domains. J Res Pers. 2003;37(6):504–28.
18. Grech A, Collins CE, Holmes A, Lal R, Duncanson K, Taylor R, Gordon A. Maternal exposures and the infant gut microbiome: a systematic review with meta-analysis. Gut Microbes. 2021;13(1):1897210.
19. Grunau RV, Craig KD. Pain expression in neonates: facial action and cry. Pain. 1987;28(3):395–410.
20. Gu S, Pei J, Zhou C, Zhao X, Wan S, Zhang J, Hua X. Selective versus routine use of episiotomy for vaginal births in Shanghai hospitals, China: a comparison of policies. BMC Pregnancy Childbirth. 2022;22(1):475.
21. Heelan L. Fetal monitoring: creating a culture of safety with informed choice. J Perinat Educ. 2013;22(3):156.
22. Hollins Martin CJ. Effects of valsalva manoeuvre on maternal and fetal wellbeing. Br J Midwifery. 2009;17(5):279–85.
23. Horsch A, Garthus-Niegel S. Posttraumatic stress disorder following childbirth. Vulnerability and Law: Childbirth; 2019. p. 49–66.
24. Jiang H, Qian X, Carroli G, Garner P. Selective versus routine use of episiotomy for vaginal birth. Cochrane Database Syst Rev. 2017;2(2):CD000081. https://doi.org/10.1002/14651858.CD000081.pub3.
25. Kenny LC, McCarthy F, editors. Obstetrics by ten teachers. Boca Raton: CRC Press; 2024.

26. Kulkarni A, Manerkar S, Paul N, Gupta A, Mondkar J. Impact of kangaroo mother care on mother-infant bonding in very low birth weight infants. J Neonatal Nurs. 2025;31:206–9.
27. Maguire L, Male F, Clarke H, Ndlovu B, Harris J, Chintende JM, Claudine BU. Skin-to-skin contact. Are we doing enough? J Neonatal Nurs. 2025;31:125–8.
28. Marteau TM, Bekker H. The development of a six-item short-form of the state scale of the Spielberger state—trait anxiety inventory (STAI). Br J Clin Psychol. 1992;31(3):301–6.
29. Martin CJH, Martin CR. Development and psychometric properties of the birth satisfaction scale-revised (BSS-R). Midwifery. 2014;30(6):610–9.
30. Matthies LM, Wallwiener S, Müller M, Doster A, Plewniok K, Feller S, Sohn C, Wallweiner M, Reck C. Maternal self-confidence during the first four months postpartum and its association with anxiety and early infant regulatory problems. Infant Behav Dev. 2017;49:228–37.
31. McAdams DP, Olson BD. Personality development: continuity and change over the life course. Annu Rev Psychol. 2010;61:517–42.
32. Mohammadi F, Kohan S, Farzi S, Khosravi M, Heidari Z. The effect of pregnancy training classes based on bandura self-efficacy theory on postpartum depression and anxiety and type of delivery. J Educ Health Promot. 2021;10:273.
33. Nakic Radoš S, Ayers S, Horsch A. From childbearing to childrearing: parental mental health and infant development. Front Psychol. 2023;13:1123241.
34. National Institute for Health and Care Excellence. Intrapartum care for healthy women and their babies (Clinical guideline CG190). 2017. Available at: https://www.nice.org.uk/guidance/cg190.
35. O'Heney J, McAllister S, Maresh M, Blott M. Fetal monitoring in labour: summary and update of NICE guidance. BMJ. 2022;379:o2854.
36. Pawlicka P, Wróbel W, Baranowska B, Macewicz D, Olech M, Hollins Martin CJ, Martin CR. Translation and validation of the Polish-language version of the Birth Satisfaction Scale-Revised (BSS-R) and its relationship to the type of delivery and the baby's Apgar score. 2024. https://napier-repository.worktribe.com/preview/3692200/%28131%29%20Health%20Psychology%20Report%20Polish-BSS-R.pdf.
37. Power C. The influence of maternal childbirth experience on early infant behavioural style. 2021. https://cronfa.swan.ac.uk/Record/cronfa57276/Details.
38. Power C, Williams C, Brown A. Physical and psychological childbirth experiences and early infant temperament. Front Psychol. 2022;13:792392.
39. Power C, Williams C, Brown A. Does a mother's childbirth experience influence her perceptions of her baby's behaviour? A qualitative interview study. PLoS One. 2023;18(4):e0284183.
40. Reck C, Noe D, Gerstenlauer J, Stehle E. Effects of postpartum anxiety disorders and depression on maternal self-confidence. Infant Behav Dev. 2012;35(2):264–72.
41. Renfrew M. Enabling Safe Quality Midwifery Services and Care In Northern Ireland. 2024. https://www.health-ni.gov.uk/publications/enabling-safe-quality-midwifery-services-and-care-northern-ireland. Accessed 25 Oct 2024.
42. Reyman M, Van Houten MA, Watson RL, Chu MLJ, Arp K, De Waal WJ, Bogaert D. Effects of early-life antibiotics on the developing infant gut microbiome and resistome: a randomized trial. Nat Commun. 2022;13(1):893.
43. Rosen NO, Dawson SJ, Leonhardt ND, Vannier SA, Impett EA. Trajectories of sexual Well-being among couples in the transition to parenthood. J Fam Psychol. 2021;35(4):523.
44. Schwartz DJ, Langdon AE, Dantas G. Understanding the impact of antibiotic perturbation on the human microbiome. Genome Med. 2020;12:1–12.
45. Spielberger CD. State-trait anxiety inventory. In: The Corsini encyclopedia of psychology. Hoboken: Wiley; 2010. p. 1.
46. Stuijfzand S, Garthus-Niegel S, Horsch A. Parental birth-related PTSD symptoms and bonding in the early postpartum period: a prospective population-based cohort study. Front Psychiatry. 2020;11:570727.
47. Taylor A, Fisk NM, Glover V. Mode of delivery and subsequent stress response. Lancet. 2000;355(9198):120.

48. UNICEF, & World Health Organization (2024). Levels and Trends Child Mortality-Report 2023: Estimates Developed by the United Nations Inter-agency Group for Child Mortality Estimation. https://data.unicef.org/resources/levels-and-trends-in-child-mortality-2024/.
49. Thomas K. Birth trauma inquiry report. Listen to mums: ending the postcode lottery on perinatal care. 2024. Available at: https://www.theo-clarke.org.uk/sites/www.theo-clarke.org.uk/files/2024-05/Birth%20Trauma%20Inquiry%20Report%20for%20Publication_May13_2024.pdf. Accessed 20 May 2024.
50. Uvnäs-Moberg K, Ekström-Bergström A, Berg M, Buckley S, Pajalic Z, Hadjigeorgiou E, Kotłowska A, Lengler L, Kielbratowska B, Leon-Larios F, Magistretti CM, Downe S, Lindström B, Dencker A. Maternal plasma levels of oxytocin during physiological childbirth– a systematic review with implications for uterine contractions and central actions of oxytocin. BMC Pregnancy Childbirth. 2019;19(1):285.
51. Widström AM, Brimdyr K, Svensson K, Cadwell K, Nissen E. Skin-to-skin contact the first hour after birth, underlying implications and clinical practice. Acta Paediatr. 2019;108(7):1192–204.
52. Wolke D. Parents' perceptions as guides for conducting NBAS clinical sessions. In: Brazelton TB, Nugent JK, editors. Neonatal Behavioral assessment scale. London: Mac Keith Press; 1995. p. 117–25.
53. Wolke D, James-Roberts I. Multi-method measurement of the early parent-infant system with easy and difficult newborns. Psychobiology and early development. 1987;46:49–70.
54. Wolke D, James-Roberts I. Mother and baby scales (MABS). Appendix 2. In: Brazelton TB, Nugent JK, editors. Neonatal Behavioral assessment scale. 3rd ed. London: Mac Keith Press; 1987. p. 135–7.
55. World Health Organization. World Health Organization recommendations: intrapartum care for a positive childbirth experience. 2018. Available at: https://www.who.int/reproductivehealth/intrapartum-care/en/. Accessed 7 Sept 2024.
56. World Medical Association. World Medical Association Declaration of Helsinki: ethical principles for medical research involving human subjects. JAMA. 2013;310(20):2191–4.

Physical and Psychological Experiences of Childbirth and Baby Behaviour

A Survey of a Thousand Mothers: Part Two

8.1 Introduction

In Chap. 7, we identified which childbirth and perinatal factors were linked to early infant behaviour and maternal confidence. Numerous physical (objective) and psychological (subjective) perinatal factors correlated with both the 24-Hour Baby Scale [12] and the Mother and Baby Scales (MABS, [16, 17]). Building on the significant variables identified in Part One of the survey analysis, this chapter explores what contributes *most* to outcomes. Thus, it investigates which variables best predict early infant physiological wellbeing and behaviour and maternal confidence, while holding all other significant variables (such as baby age or birth weight) constant (i.e. all other influencing variables are statistically controlled so as not to affect the variables under investigation).

The survey was a cross-sectional rather than a longitudinal study. Therefore, in the data analysis, overall comparisons were made between groups of mothers (e.g. those with high anxiety or depression scores) and groups of babies (e.g. those who were unsettled and irregular in their behavioural style) rather than following the same mother-infant pairs lengthwise across a period of time. For this reason, conducting multiple linear regressions was considered the most powerful and effective way to uncover the "predictors" of positive and negative mother and baby outcomes across a large data set. As might be expected given their well-known comorbidity, mothers' current state of anxiety on completing the questionnaire was strongly associated with their depression scores over the past 7 days. To avoid multicollinearity in the regression models (where two or more variables are highly interrelated, as indicated by a strong correlation over 0.7), and as the Edinburgh Postnatal Depression Scale (EPDS) is designed to be used from 7 days postnatally, this was used to look at depression scores in relation to early infant behaviour and maternal confidence (as measured by MABS), while the State and Trait Anxiety Inventory (STAI) scores for mothers' current emotional states (anxious or relaxed) were included in the equation when examining 24-Hour Baby outcomes.

8.2 Perinatal Factors Predicting 24-Hour Baby Outcomes

In Chap. 7, we learned that the 24-Hour Baby Scale included two variables (Cry-Fuss Baby and Alert-Content Baby) derived from seven statements about the newborn baby's initial appearance, physiological state, and behaviour: "My baby's head looked bruised and swollen", "My baby appeared calm and relaxed", "My baby seemed irritable", "My baby was very sleepy", "My baby cried a lot", "My baby smiled" and "My baby latched onto the breast easily". A Cry-Fuss Baby describes a newborn who may have a bruised or swollen head, cries excessively and appears irritable. In contrast, an alert-content baby describes a calm, relaxed, alert (*not* sleepy), smiling baby who latches onto the breast easily.

Cry-Fuss Baby

The results showed that certain birth events and emotional states during and after childbirth could negatively impact the newborn baby's appearance, physiological wellbeing and behaviour. The regression model for Cry-Fuss baby behaviour was highly significant [12]. Feelings of postnatal distress in the mother were the strongest predictor of Cry-Fuss 24-Hour Baby, followed by experiencing an assisted birth (Fig. 8.1). In addition, the emotions a mother experienced *during* childbirth contributed to the newborn baby's initial behavioural response to the world. Note that an *inverse* predictor (which works in a similar way to a negative correlation) means that *more* of the predictor variable leads to *less* of (or *lower scores* in) the outcome variable. Thus, positive birth emotions *inversely* predicted Cry-Fuss Baby (see yellow arrow), meaning the *more* positive emotions mothers experienced during childbirth, the *less* their babies tended to cry and fuss during the first 24 hours (and vice versa). Mothers' current anxiety levels when completing the questionnaire also played a small yet significant role in how mothers rated their baby's initial wellbeing and behaviour (Fig. 8.1).

Having reviewed previous research evidence regarding the potential bi-directionality of early infant behaviour and maternal distress (e.g. [15]), as well as the notion that stressed or depressed mothers may over-interpret their baby's cries, I decided it would be interesting to swap the roles of Cry-Fuss Baby and maternal postnatal distress, making postnatal distress the *outcome* variable and treating the baby's behaviour as a potential *predictor* by including it alongside the other significant variables illustrated in Fig. 8.1. Consequently, the *predictor* variables in the alternative regression model were Cry-Fuss Baby, assisted birth, positive birth emotions and current anxiety. This new regression model proved to be even more significant than the previous one [12]. Notably, while assisted birth had been a substantial factor for Cry-Fuss Baby (Fig. 8.1), it did *not* significantly predict maternal postnatal distress. Instead, experiencing *negative* emotions during the birth (positive birth emotions was an *inverse* predictor) and reporting a crying and fussing baby predicted postnatal distress for the mother. It's important to note that physical factors, such as birth mode, and psychological ones, like birth emotions, strongly correlated with one another throughout the study; therefore, the type of birth and the nature of the interventions experienced by the mother and baby continued to play a significant

8.2 Perinatal Factors Predicting 24-Hour Baby Outcomes

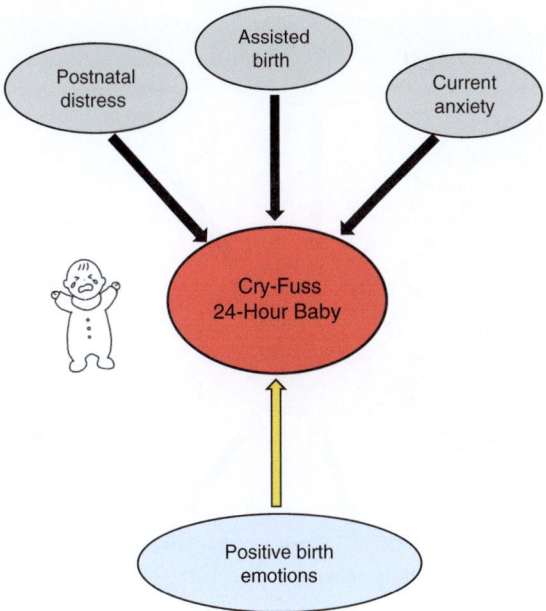

Fig. 8.1 Predictors of Cry-Fuss 24-Hour Baby

Figure key

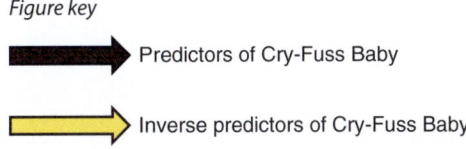

role in all outcomes, even though they didn't show up as "predictors" when standing alongside the more potent psychological variables.

Alert-Content 24-Hour Baby

The regression model for alert-content baby was also highly significant [12]. The strongest contributor to this positive physiological and behavioural state in newborns was the variable "Breastfed first". As noted in Chap. 7, it should be remembered that alert-content comprised several statements, including "My baby appeared calm and relaxed", "My baby smiled", "My baby was very sleepy" (inverse correlation) and "My baby latched onto the breast easily". This last statement may partially explain the statistical significance of the baby's breastfeeding behaviour in relation to the construct of alert-content baby.

Experiencing positive birth emotions and a sense of postnatal physical wellbeing also predicted alert and content newborns. Similarly, having more children, a female baby and the personality traits of extroversion and openness contributed to mothers reporting more alert and content baby behaviours. Mothers from lower-income households were more likely to perceive their newborn baby as alert and content, possibly due to lower expectations. Although there is no conclusive evidence to

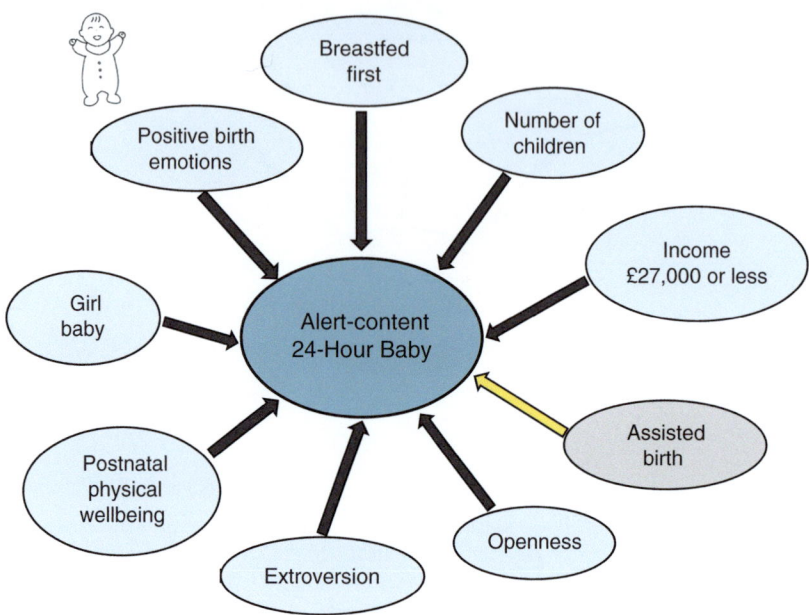

Fig. 8.2 Predictors of alert-content 24-Hour Baby

Figure key

▶ Predictors of Cry-Fuss Baby

▷ Inverse predictors of Cry-Fuss Baby

support this theory, a similar link has also been found in other research areas. Finally, as assisted birth was an *inverse* predictor of positive newborn physiological wellbeing and behaviour (note the yellow arrow), mothers perceived their newborn baby as *less* alert and content following an assisted birth (Fig. 8.2).

8.3 Perinatal Factors Predicting Mother and Baby Scale Outcomes (0–6 Months)

To explore which of the numerous correlating variables established in Chap. 7 most *effectively predicted* ongoing baby behaviour and maternal confidence during the first 6 months post-birth, a multiple linear regression was performed for each of the eight Mother and Baby Scales (MABS) outcome variables (please see Table 7.1 in Chap. 7 if you need to jog your memory on the definitions of the MABS items). The impacts of childbirth and perinatal experiences on positive, neutral and negative baby behaviours are illustrated here by Figs. 8.3, 8.4, and 8.5. For the numerical data underlying the diagrams, refer to Power et al. [13].

8.3 Perinatal Factors Predicting Mother and Baby Scale Outcomes (0–6 Months)

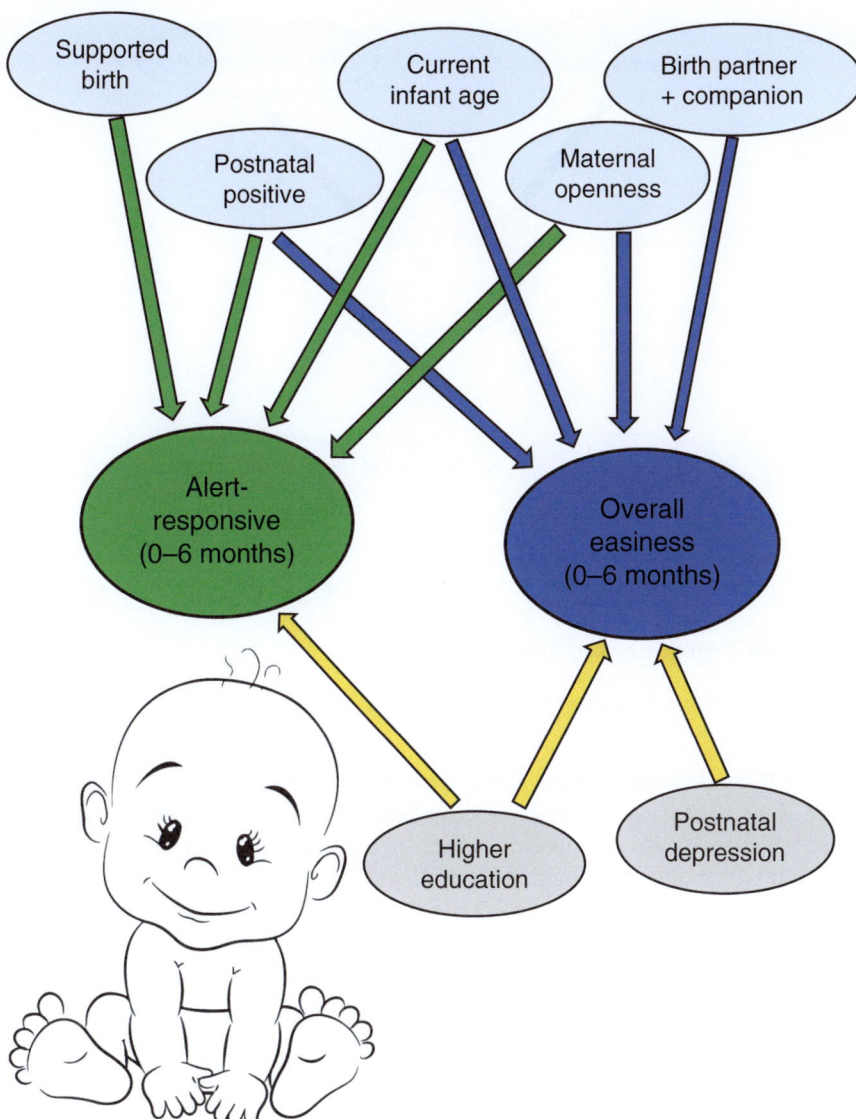

Fig. 8.3 Predictors of Positive Baby Behaviour

Figure key

➡ Predictors of overall infant Easiness

➡ Predictors of Alert-Responsive baby behaviour

➡ Inverse predictors of baby behaviour

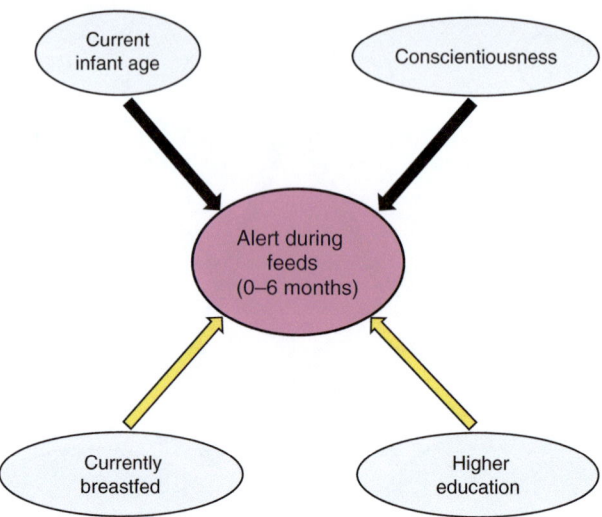

Fig. 8.4 Predictors of Neutral Behaviour (0–6 months)

Figure key

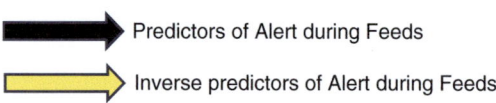   Predictors of Alert during Feeds

   Inverse predictors of Alert during Feeds

Positive Baby Behaviour: Alert-Responsive and Overall Easiness

There were several predictors of positive baby behaviours (Alert-responsive and overall Easiness). As described in Chap. 7, a Supported Birth Experience was one where the mother felt emotionally well-supported by her partner and midwife. "Postnatal positive" meant the mother had experienced positive emotions after childbirth, such as euphoria, exhilaration and pride. As illustrated in Fig. 8.3, older babies tended to be Easier overall as well as more alert and responsive. Mothers with the personality trait of openness to new experiences who felt positive postnatally perceived their babies as easier and more alert and responsive. Notably, mothers also reported more alert and responsive baby behaviour following a Supported Birth Experience, and Easier baby behaviours overall if they had received *two* sources of social support (in addition to professional support)—for example, their partner *and* a doula, relative or friend (labelled "birth companion").

Mothers reported *less* overall infant easiness if they experienced symptoms of postnatal depression. Interestingly, they reported more alert-responsive baby behaviours if they did *not* have higher education (see yellow arrows indicating *inverse* predictors). Similar to the connection shown in Fig. 8.2 between lower-income households and mothers reporting more Alert-Content newborn behaviours, it's possible that mothers who did *not* attend university perceive their babies as more alert and responsive because they have lower—and perhaps more realistic—expectations about birth and parenthood.

8.3 Perinatal Factors Predicting Mother and Baby Scale Outcomes (0–6 Months)

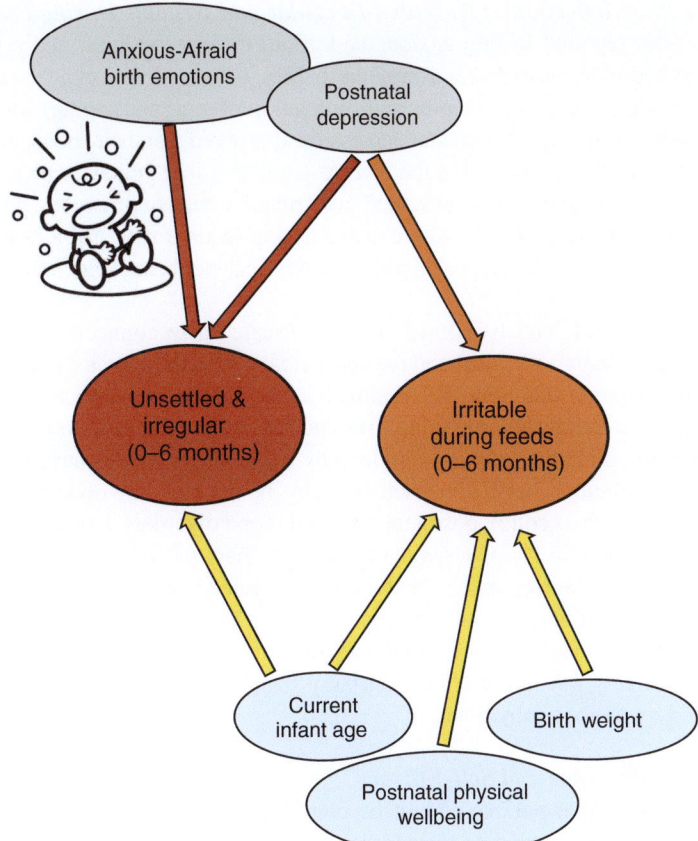

Fig. 8.5 Predictors of negative baby behaviours (0–6 months)

Figure key

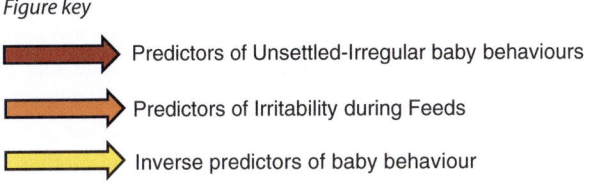

Neutral Baby Behaviour: Alert during Feeds

There's no right or wrong about whether young babies should be "alert during feeds" or sleepily dozing, often quite contentedly. It may depend on various factors such as their age and whether they're breastfeeding, as falling asleep at the breast is quite common. Consistent with this idea, mothers reported their babies as less alert during feeds if they were breastfeeding or had a higher education, possibly because these two factors are connected (educated mothers are more likely to breastfeed). Interestingly, "conscientious" mothers also reported that their babies were more alert during feeds, and — as expected — older babies were increasingly alert (Fig. 8.4).

Negative Baby Behaviours: Unsettled-Irregular and Irritable During Feeds

Mothers who reported feeling anxious and afraid during childbirth and postnatally depressed had more unsettled and irregular babies, who tended to cry, fuss and have irregular routines of feeding, sleeping and elimination (weeing and pooing). Meanwhile, mothers with symptoms of postnatal depression also noted that their babies were more irritable during feeds. Examining the *inverse* predictors (see yellow arrows), it's evident that babies displayed less unsettled and irregular behaviour as they grew older. Furthermore, they tended to be less irritable during feeds if they had a healthy birth weight and if their mothers reported postnatal physical wellbeing (Fig. 8.5).

Figures 8.3, 8.4, and 8.5 illustrate the intricate early connections between a mother and her baby's physical and psychological (or, in the baby's case, *physiological*) wellbeing and behaviour. The findings emphasise the importance of protecting the mother emotionally during childbirth and the perinatal period to achieve positive outcomes, including a happy and healthy baby. Other studies have found bidirectional correlations between unsettled baby behaviours (involving crying and tummy issues such as colic), postnatal maternal mood disorders and challenges with parent-infant bonding [6]. Consequently, how mothers *felt* and the amount of *support* they received during and after the birth impacted not only their own but also their baby's physiological wellbeing and behaviour. Moreover, based on the insights shared by mothers and health professionals in the two interview studies (Chapters 5 and 6), it's likely that these effects on baby behaviour both influenced and were influenced by mother-baby bonding.

Maternal Confidence and Self-Efficacy

It has been said that parents cannot be considered purely scientific observers of early infant behaviour due to the close emotional involvement that most parents have with their babies [2]. Although parents' perceptions are likely to be at least partially subjective, when asked for very specific, detailed elements of their baby's behaviour (e.g. how and when their baby cried over the past 7 days, as in the Mother and Baby Scales), the authors of the MABS found that parents made fairly trustworthy observations, comparable to trained observers. However, it's possible that a postnatal mood disorder, such as depression or post-traumatic stress (named "postnatal distress" here), could interfere with this process by affecting the mother's confidence and clouding her judgement of her baby [14]. Given that the mother's postnatal mood and confidence and the baby's behaviour are known to be interrelated, the Mother and Baby Scales [16, 17] were designed to assess mothers' confidence and self-efficacy alongside their perceptions of their baby's behaviour.

As might be expected, maternal confidence was connected to both postnatal depression scores and baby behaviour. The following two figures present the three

8.3 Perinatal Factors Predicting Mother and Baby Scale Outcomes (0–6 Months)

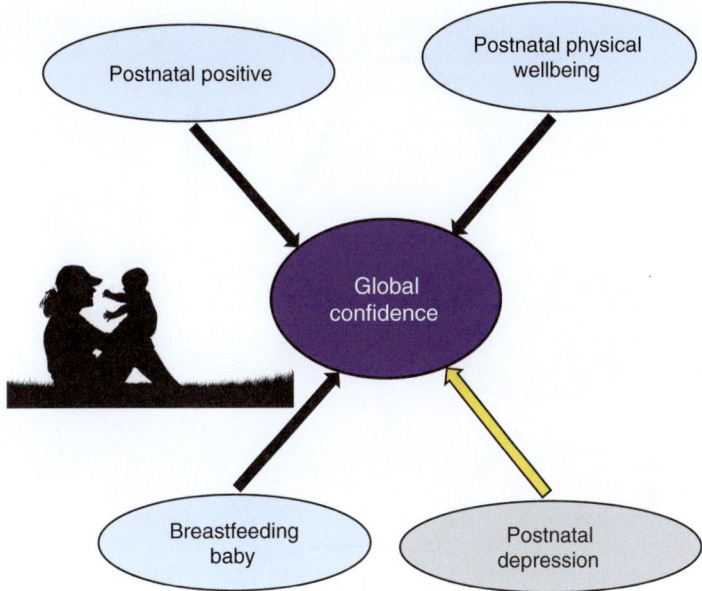

Fig. 8.6 Predictors of global confidence (during the first 6 months)

Figure key

➤ Positive predictors of global confidence

➤ Inverse predictors of global confidence

maternal confidence outcome variables: global (overall) confidence (Fig. 8.6) and lack of confidence in caretaking and breastfeeding (Fig. 8.7). As illustrated in Fig. 8.6, mothers' overall confidence and self-efficacy were predicted by their postnatal psychological wellbeing (Postnatal positive) and Postnatal physical wellbeing, as well as by whether they were currently breastfeeding their baby.

When analysing the results for mothers' lack of confidence in caretaking and breastfeeding (as depicted in Fig. 8.7), it was evident that the primary variable contributing to a *lack* of confidence was postnatal depression. Another factor influencing lack of confidence in breastfeeding was the presence of meconium in the waters, indicating that mothers may find this potential sign of foetal distress quite alarming and distressing. The number of children a mother had (known as "parity") emerged as an *inverse* predictor, suggesting that the more children a mother had, the more confident she tended to be about caring for and breastfeeding her baby.

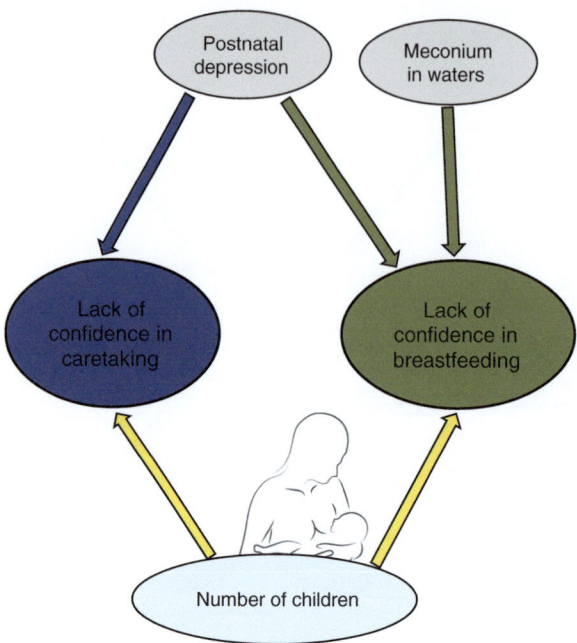

Fig. 8.7 Predictors of Lack of confidence in caretaking and breastfeeding (0–6 months)

Figure key

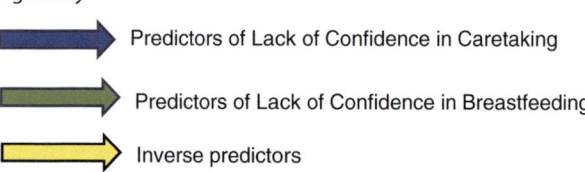

8.4 Summary of the Birth and Perinatal Factors Predicting Mother and Baby Outcomes

The key perinatal variables found to *predict* mother and baby outcomes of childbirth will now be summarised for clarity before presenting a diagram to illustrate the overall findings from this study.

Baby Behaviour Outcomes

The survey found that both *objective* physical variables (such as assisted birth) and the more *subjective* or psychological variables (including birth emotions, postnatal physical wellbeing and postnatal distress) affected baby behaviour during the first 24 hours after birth. However, alongside the mother's personality and certain mother and baby characteristics (such as age and education), subjective and psychological factors took precedence as the main predictors of baby behaviour during the first 6 months post-birth. It's important to remember here that objective and subjective childbirth factors are inherently intertwined [1]. This means that physical events and circumstances during childbirth (such as birth mode, birthplace, interventions or pain relief) undoubtedly influenced the outcomes of the birth experience for mother and baby, even when stronger subjective and psychological variables in the final regression models (such as positive or anxious-afraid birth emotions and postnatal physical wellbeing or distress) overrode them. The mother's personality traits of extroversion, openness and conscientiousness also featured prominently in baby behaviour outcomes, no doubt due to their dual influence on the baby's genetic makeup and early environment—as, in addition to passing on their genes, mothers feel, behave and arrange the home environment according to their personality. Consistent with other evidence about the adverse impacts of maternal mood disorders on infant wellbeing, behaviour and development, postnatal depression featured very strongly as a predictor too [11].

Maternal Confidence Outcomes
Multiple objective physical factors were related to maternal confidence (see Chap. 7). However, akin to baby behaviour, it was primarily subjective and psychological variables that *predicted* mothers' overall confidence and self-efficacy ("Global confidence"). For instance, feeling physically well and experiencing positive emotions post-birth ("Postnatal physical wellbeing" and "Postnatal positive") predicted higher levels of global confidence (Fig. 8.6). Although the multiple linear regression models weren't conducted in reverse after the experiment with the first one concerning postnatal distress and Cry-Fuss 24-Hour Baby (Sect. 8.2), it's highly likely that how babies behaved after childbirth influenced how confident mothers felt in their new role (and vice versa), particularly if it was their first child.

Predictably, mothers felt more confident if they had previously given birth and cared for a baby. Thus, the greater number of children a mother had *inversely* predicted Lack of confidence in caretaking and breastfeeding—meaning the more children she had, the more confident she felt (i.e. she had *less* lack of confidence). Notably, there was one physical factor that predicted mothers' lack of confidence in breastfeeding. This was meconium in waters, possibly because it induced lingering feelings of anxiety post-birth. Meanwhile, postnatal depression contributed to mothers' lack of confidence in all areas, as illustrated in Fig. 8.7.

As baby behaviour is our primary outcome of interest, Fig. 8.8 illustrates the childbirth and perinatal pathways leading to either settled or unsettled baby behaviours, highlighting which variables contributed most significantly to baby behaviour when all other influencing variables were held constant. This figure emphasises the significance of both physical *and* psychological experiences during childbirth and the perinatal period for mother and baby. It underscores the vital role that strong social and professional support play in positive outcomes, enhancing the wellbeing of both mother and baby while shielding them from some of the negative impacts associated with a challenging or distressing birth experience.

The figure consists of three main sections, each covering a key stage of the birth and perinatal journey. The first box illustrates the influential role that pregnancy

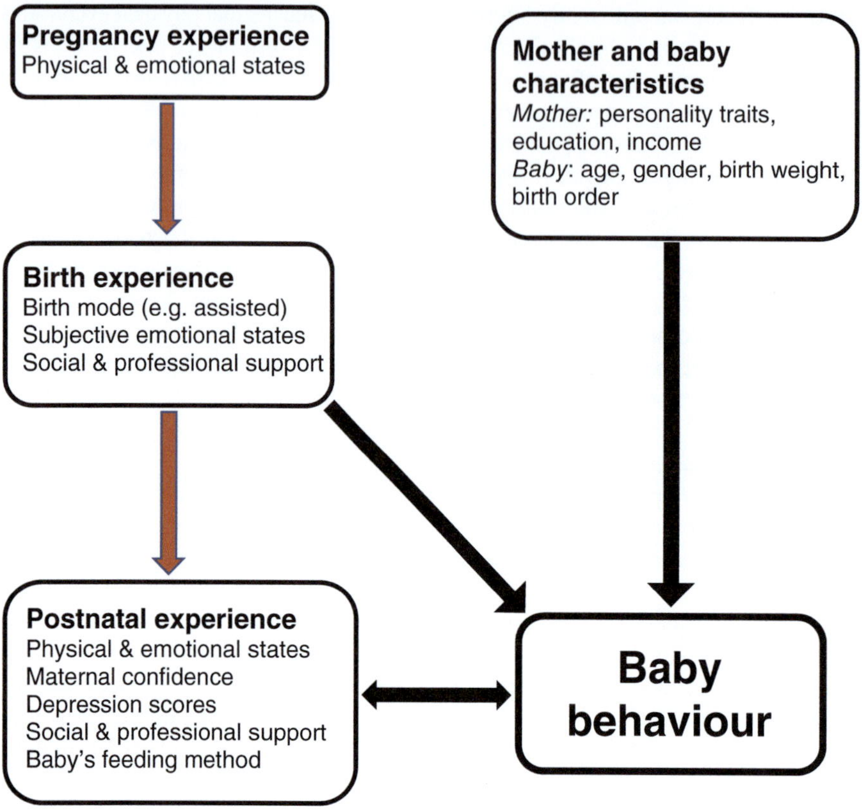

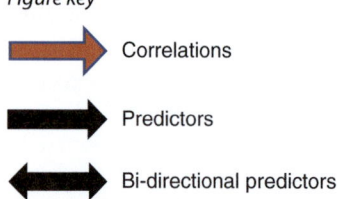

Fig. 8.8 Correlations and predictors of baby behaviour

Figure key

➡ Correlations

➡ Predictors

⬌ Bi-directional predictors

plays in the overall birth experience; however, pregnancy variables did *not* emerge as *predictors* of baby behaviour. The second box outlines the impacts of the mother's physical and psychological birth experiences on baby behaviour—both directly through birth events and intertwined mother-baby hormonal systems, and indirectly via the mother's postnatal mood. The third box illustrates how the mother's subjective postnatal state, encompassing both physical and emotional wellbeing (or distress), as well as her confidence and self-efficacy, predicts the baby's early behaviour. The additional right-hand box lists the sociodemographic variables and mother and baby characteristics also contributing to outcomes. Although other significantly

8.4 Summary of the Birth and Perinatal Factors Predicting Mother and Baby Outcomes

correlated variables (such as birth interventions or pain ratings) may have had an indirect influence on early baby behaviour, these are not included in Fig. 8.8, as they didn't feature in the final regression models. Therefore, they did *not* emerge as *predictors* when combined in one equation with the more powerful overriding factors, such as the mother's subjective birth and postnatal experiences, personality and postnatal mental health.

While Fig. 8.8 highlights potential adversities affecting baby behaviour, such as assisted birth, postnatal distress and depression, it also points to certain factors that appeared to benefit the mother-baby pair. As noted earlier, if mothers felt well-supported during their birth and had an additional birth companion (such as a friend or doula) alongside the health professional support (usually a midwife), they were more likely to report alert and responsive early baby behaviours and to perceive their baby as "easier" overall. This provides further evidence for the crucial role of providing strong emotional support during childbirth to prevent birth trauma and postnatal distress [4, 7]. Moreover, given the well-established links between baby behaviour and infant social-emotional development, it's highly likely that alert and responsive early baby behaviours directly influence the infant's developmental trajectory, potentially leading to long-term impacts on their happiness, wellbeing and educational success. Therefore, providing adequate social and professional support during childbirth is essential, not only for mothers and babies but also for families and the wider society.

This kind of intensive support, with its measurable benefits for mother and baby outcomes as demonstrated here, could also influence how their relationship with one another begins and develops (as represented by Fig. 8.9). Strong professional and social support helps to combat the adverse effects of a negative birth experience while further enhancing a positive birth, empowering the mother and baby for the best possible start to their lifelong journey together. In contrast, when a mother

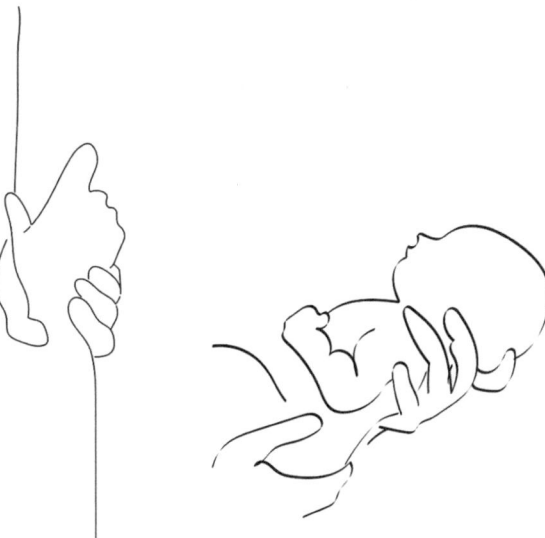

Fig. 8.9 Mother-infant bonding predicts the ongoing mother-child relationship

experiences a lack of support during childbirth and the transition to parenthood, this could lead to long-term negative consequences for her mental health. And as we have seen in previous chapters, poor postnatal mental health has a substantial adverse effect on mother-baby bonding and infant development [9, 10].

8.5 What Does This Study Show Us, and Where Do We Go from Here?

The study presented in the last two chapters investigated various physical and psychological variables that could affect mothers and babies during childbirth and throughout the perinatal period. It explored the potential pathways between mothers' physical and psychological birth experiences and how both mothers and babies may feel and respond after the birth. For the baby, this response was assessed through their earliest form of communication—*baby behaviour*. The mother's reaction to the birth was measured through her postnatal confidence, anxiety and depression scores, alongside responses to questions concerning her physical and psychological experiences of pregnancy, childbirth and the postnatal period.

The survey highlighted a range of influential factors contributing to baby behaviour and early infant temperament. These included the mode of birth, particularly assisted birth, the mother's subjective perceptions of the birth, and how she felt afterwards, both physically and emotionally. It also investigated how the mother's personality and postnatal mood contributed to her confidence as a new mother, as well as to her baby's behaviour post-birth. The birth experience and postnatal depression scores correlated with one another, both predicting baby behaviour and maternal confidence. Ultimately, depression scores emerged as the strongest contributor to unsettled, irregular and irritable baby behaviours, as well as to a lack of confidence, particularly in new mothers.

Notably, postnatal distress in mothers predicted increased crying and fussing behaviours in newborn babies, and vice versa—a crying baby also induced distress in the mother, confirming previous research, especially if the mother feels unable to soothe them [15]. These effects of birth and postnatal experiences on baby behaviour were ongoing, as the babies aged 0-6 months of postnatally distressed mothers tended to be more unsettled and irregular in their feeding, sleeping and elimination routines. Since the sample only included mothers with babies aged 0–30 weeks, these influencing factors may have impacted babies for even longer. Although older babies generally appeared more settled, this didn't seem to apply to babies whose mothers developed postnatal depression. Instead, babies of depressed mothers exhibited more challenging and negative behaviours, regardless of their age.

The findings from the survey advance previous research by investigating the potentially dire consequences of childbirth and early postnatal experiences for the baby's wellbeing, as reflected in their earliest behaviours and developing temperament. We know that early stressors can have devastating and sometimes enduring effects on the baby's regulatory stress response system [3, 5]. In turn, a crying,

8.5 What Does This Study Show Us, and Where Do We Go from Here?

unsettled baby could make life even more difficult for parents who are already struggling to cope after a challenging birth experience. Although pregnancy factors influence how the birth unfolds and play a direct role in infant temperament development through a combination of genetic influences and foetal programming, these results indicate that an ongoing negative cycle of reciprocal distress between mother and baby may begin at the time of birth. The finding that 24-Hour Baby (newborn baby wellbeing and behaviour) correlated with the Mother and Baby Scales (0–6 months) suggests that initial baby wellbeing and behaviour is linked to infant temperament development.

Giving birth to a baby in a calm environment (including when a caesarean section is required) not only positively affects the mother's subjective birth experience but also creates an optimal setting for the baby to receive the best possible start in life with a warm welcome to life outside the womb. Moreover, the mother's subjective birth and postnatal experiences seem to indirectly influence the baby's behavioural response, potentially through their interlinked neurohormonal systems (via the placenta, breastfeeding and other close contact) as well as through the mother's feelings and behaviour towards the baby after birth, which are influenced by her postnatal mood.

Although assisted birth remained a predictor of initial crying and fussing in newborn behaviours, and physical factors such as induction, pain relief and birth mode correlated with unsettled baby behaviour during the first 6 months, the most vital aspects of childbirth for ongoing infant behaviour, when all other variables were held constant, were the mother's subjective and psychological experiences. Experiencing negative birth emotions, such as feeling anxious, afraid, ignored, neglected or abandoned during childbirth and feeling distressed postnatally—or conversely, experiencing positive emotions during and after childbirth—significantly contributed to baby behaviour. Moreover, these birthing and postnatal emotional states greatly influenced the mother's (lack of) confidence and self-efficacy, as well as her postnatal depression scores. These were much healthier (i.e. *lower*) after a positive birth experience. They were significantly (and rather concerningly) higher after a negative, complex or medicalised birth—in other words, mothers experienced more postnatal depression and lack of confidence following a negative birth experience. The study therefore supports the idea that mothers' subjective perceptions of their birth experience are *at least* as important as the physical aspects [1].

The survey findings emphasise the essential need to protect mothers' psychological wellbeing during childbirth and the perinatal period, ensuring that all mothers and babies receive nurturing care from health professionals, as well as adequate emotional and practical support throughout their perinatal journey and transition into parenthood. It demonstrates that providing such support could help prevent the all-too-common extreme distress that arises in both mother and baby after traumatic birth and postnatal experiences. Emotional nurturing urgently needs to return to maternity and neonatal care to protect mother and child, not only from immediate distress but also from the longer-term consequences of a negative birth experience with inadequate care [8].

8.6 Summary

In this chapter, we discovered which specific childbirth and perinatal factors had the strongest impact on baby behaviour during the first few months of life. Although individual statistical relationships between each childbirth or perinatal factor and baby behaviour were not particularly large when considered as stand-alone items, the mother's experience of childbirth and the early postnatal period appeared to have a substantial influence on outcomes for both mother and baby when taken together. Notably, subjective and psychological factors such as a positive, well-supported birth experience—or, conversely, postnatal distress and postnatal depression—predicted baby behaviour even more than objective physical factors like pain ratings, pain relief, medical interventions and birth mode. These findings send a clear message to those who care for women during childbirth and seek the best overall outcomes for mother and baby: *the birth experience matters*. How mothers *perceive* their birth and postnatal experiences is significant, not just for the mother but also for the baby, as it may affect their wellbeing and behaviour following birth, with potentially long-term consequences for infant behaviour, temperament and development, as well as the child's future physical and mental health.

References

1. Ayers S, Bond R, Bertullies S, Wijma K. The aetiology of post-traumatic stress following childbirth: a meta-analysis and theoretical framework. Psychol Med. 2016;46(6):1121–34.
2. Brazelton TB, Nugent JK. Neonatal behavioral assessment scale. 3rd ed. New York: Cambridge University Press; 1995.
3. Dahlen HG, Kennedy HP, Anderson CM, Bell AF, Clark A, Foureur M, Ohm JE, Shearman AM, Taylor JY, Wright ML, Downe S. The EPIIC hypothesis: intrapartum effects on the neonatal epigenome and consequent health outcomes. Med Hypotheses. 2013;80(5):656–62.
4. Delicate A, Ayers S, McMullen S. Health-care practitioners' assessment and observations of birth trauma in mothers and partners. J Reprod Infant Psychol. 2022;40:34–46.
5. Douglas PS, Hill PS. A neurobiological model for cry-fuss problems in the first three to four months of life. Med Hypotheses. 2013;81(5):816–22.
6. Frankel LA, Umemura T, Pfeffer KA, Powell EM, Hughes KR. Maternal perceptions of infant behavior as a potential indicator of parents or infants in need of additional support and intervention. Front Public Health. 2021;9:630201.
7. Horsch A, Garthus-Niegel S. Posttraumatic stress disorder following childbirth. In: Pickles C, Herring J, editors. Childbirth, vulnerability and law. London: Routledge; 2019. p. 49–66.
8. Miyauchi A, Shishido E, Horiuchi S. Women's experiences and perceptions of women-centered care and respectful care during facility-based childbirth: a meta-synthesis. Jpn J Nurs Sci. 2022;19(3):e12475.
9. Murray L, Cooper P, Fearon P. Parenting difficulties and postnatal depression: implications for primary healthcare assessment and intervention. Community Pract. 2014;87(11):34–8.
10. Murray L, Halligan S, Cooper P. Postnatal depression and young children's development. New York: Guilford Press; 2018.
11. Oyetunji A, Chandra P. Postpartum stress and infant outcome: a review of current literature. Psychiatry Res. 2020;284:112769.

12. Power C. The influence of maternal childbirth experience on early infant behavioural style. 2021. Available at: https://www.researchgate.net/publication/353039432_The_Influence_of_Maternal_Childbirth_Experience_on_Early_Infant_Behavioural_Style. Accessed 20 Sept 2024.
13. Power C, Williams C, Brown A. Physical and psychological childbirth experiences and early infant temperament. Front Psychol. 2022;13:792392.
14. Power C, Williams C, Brown A. Does a mother's childbirth experience influence her perceptions of her baby's behaviour? A qualitative interview study. PLoS One. 2023;18(4):e0284183.
15. Radesky JS, Zuckerman B, Silverstein M, Rivara FP, Barr M, Taylor JA, Lengua LJ, Barr RG. Inconsolable infant crying and maternal postpartum depressive symptoms. Pediatrics. 2013;131(6):e1857–64.
16. Wolke D, James-Roberts I. Multi-method measurement of the early parent-infant system with easy and difficult newborns. Psychobiology and early development. Adv Psychol. 1987;46:49–70.
17. Wolke D, James-Roberts I. Mother and baby scales (MABS). Appendix 2. In: Brazelton TB, Nugent JK, editors. Neonatal behavioral assessment scale. 3rd ed. London: Mac Keith Press; 1987. p. 135–7). (1995).

9 Joining the Dots: *What Does This All Mean for the Future of Maternity Care?*

9.1 Placing the Findings in the Context of Other Research

In this final chapter of the Birth, Bonding and Baby Behaviour book, I attempt to "join the dots" and draw conclusions from all the evidence explored here, including my own and others' research. The chapter examines how these conclusions can be applied to improve maternity and neonatal care, ensuring that all babies receive the best possible start, enabling them to thrive and grow into physically and mentally healthy members of society. Bringing together the research findings from three studies on childbirth and baby behaviour, a key aspect of maternity care that often seems to be overlooked amid an increasingly medicalised system is the enormous value of sustaining emotionally supportive relationships during and after the momentous and life-changing event of childbirth. Positive interactions between mothers and midwives are recognised as one of the most effective ways to increase birth satisfaction and reduce trauma [29, 46]. Thus, ensuring that mothers receive appropriate social and professional support throughout their maternity care journey can significantly increase their confidence in mothering and has positive outcomes for breastfeeding, bonding and baby behaviour [49–51]. When mothers are well cared for, they become better equipped to care for their babies. In turn, warm, sensitive and responsive care from the mother nurtures and protects the baby's regulatory system, promoting easier baby behaviour and better cognitive growth, thereby optimising infant development [38].

We have seen how various childbirth and perinatal factors—including assisted birth, health professional authority and coercion, feeling anxious, afraid or neglected during the birth or suffering with postnatal distress and depression afterwards—can adversely impact the baby's wellbeing, as reflected in their behaviour and developing temperament. The survey showed that providing practical and emotional support during and after childbirth may go a long way towards lessening this link. Maternal distress or depression after the birth impairs the mother's ability to support the baby's regulation, increasing the risk for long-term social and emotional problems in the child [61]. On the other hand, enhancing social and professional support helps reduce this intergenerational transmission of stress-related vulnerabilities [22, 38]. Consistent with other research in this field [13, 30], the findings presented in this book reinforce how negative communications between health professionals and the mothers they care for promote trauma. They also demonstrate how continuous, personalised emotional support can reduce the impacts of a challenging birth or difficult postnatal experience on three very precious outcomes: breastfeeding, bonding and baby behaviour.

The survey results suggested that a negative baby behavioural style can substantially add to maternal distress. Therefore, connections between the birth experience, baby behaviour and the mother's postnatal mood seem to be two-way (bidirectional), and possibly cyclical. For instance, a baby who is crying and fussing after a difficult induction, emergency caesarean or forceps delivery will no doubt contribute to their mother's distress. As we saw across all three studies, when the mother is distressed, this is likely to make the baby even more unsettled, further adding to maternal distress.

The pandemic-related study I carried out in collaboration with a team of German scientists, based on their extensive dataset of mothers and fathers, identified strong correlations between parents' stress levels, symptoms of anxiety, depression, anger-hostility and parent-infant bonding, affecting both parents in varying degrees. High stress levels increased parents' mental health symptoms, influencing parent-infant bonding both directly (through the stress itself) and indirectly via the impact of stress on parents' mental health [52]. Considering these findings, along with the established links between postnatal depression, PTSD and infant development [25, 39], it seems likely that both depression *and* postnatal distress would disrupt mother-infant bonding as well as the outcome we were initially investigating—baby behaviour [50].

Taking on board the midwives' and health visitors' central concepts of "baby mirrors mother" in terms of mood and behaviour, and the mother's subjective birth experience influencing mother and baby bonding, these two factors could be the critical missing links in the association we discovered between a mother's emotional response to childbirth and the baby's temperament and behaviour [50]. If the mother feels distressed about the birth and this feeling continues postnatally, the baby will reflect this negative mood in his behaviour. Likewise, if a challenging birth experience, postnatal distress or depression and a fractious baby follow one another, it is perhaps not surprising that this combination of factors, at least to begin with, affects the mother's perceptions of the baby, making it more difficult to bond. Meanwhile, the baby will be affected by his mother's feelings and behaviour towards him and react accordingly, mirroring her behaviour. It is easy to see how these initial issues could establish an ongoing cycle of negative neurobehavioural patterns between mother and baby, rather than a positive cycle of reciprocal communication, intimacy and bonding.

Bringing the findings presented in this book together with the wider literature, I designed a theoretical model to illustrate this potential pathway between childbirth and baby behaviour (Fig. 9.1). While establishing predictive links between maternal

9.1 Placing the Findings in the Context of Other Research

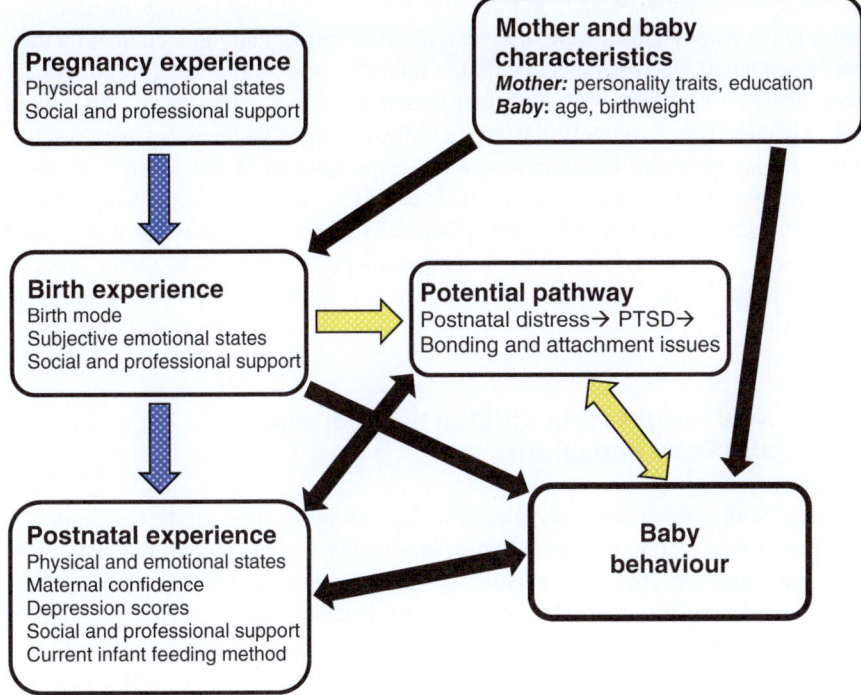

Fig. 9.1 Factors that most contribute to baby behaviour during the first 6 months

postnatal distress, symptoms of PTSD and bonding difficulties, Suzannah Stuijfzand and colleagues [64] found that professional and social support matter during pregnancy too. Therefore, although pregnancy did not feature as strongly as birth and postnatal experiences in my studies, support during pregnancy is included in the model to represent this broader evidence. As illustrated in Fig. 9.1, how a mother feels physically and emotionally during pregnancy can affect both the type of birth she has (birth mode) and her subjective birth experience. In turn, the birth experience influences how the mother feels physically and emotionally during the postnatal period; for example, whether she feels euphoric and empowered after a positive birth experience where she felt calm and in control or whether she feels depressed and distressed after a negative birth experience where she felt anxious, afraid and neglected. These physical and psychological birth experiences impact not only the mother's postnatal mental health but also how she perceives and interacts with her baby. The *Potential Pathway* box, therefore, illustrates the possible impacts of subjective birth and postnatal experiences and mothers' emotional states on mother-baby bonding, ultimately affecting baby behaviour.

This pathway between childbirth experience, maternal mental health, bonding and baby behaviour seems to be influenced by how the mother feels and how well she is cared for during and after childbirth: Emotional support was a key predictor of higher maternal confidence and more alert and responsive baby behaviour.

In some cases, baby behaviour may also be influenced by feeding methods, as breastfed newborn babies were often perceived as calmer and more content by their mothers. Genetic factors (specifically the mother's personality and level of education) played a significant role in infant temperament outcomes too, as did certain baby characteristics—namely, the baby's birthweight and their current age. Notably, while babies generally became more alert, responsive and easier overall, mothers who felt positive postnatally viewed their babies as having more of these positive traits. In contrast, mothers who were postnatally distressed or depressed perceived their babies as having more difficult temperaments and tended to report them as more unsettled and irritable with irregular routines in feeding, sleeping and elimination.

9.2 New Insights into Childbirth Experiences and Baby Behaviour

So, what findings and new insights can we take from the three studies presented in this book? This section summarises the main points arising from all the data. First, how much the subjective birth experience matters, not only to how the mother feels postnatally but also to the baby and how they behave—which is an expression of their physiological state and sensations (e.g. pain, hunger, wanting to be held and comforted). Second, it demonstrates how closely connected the physical experience is to the psychological one—we can't separate one from the other because if a mother has a more challenging or different physical birth experience than the one she was expecting, it's almost inevitable she will be at the very least disappointed. She may also experience distress, shame, guilt and even depression, because she couldn't give her baby the perfect start in life she had planned.

Providing regular and accessible antenatal classes to educate mothers about the physiology of childbirth and natural pain relief methods (as well as pharmacological ones) while explaining what happens during other childbirth methods that might be used if needed might help with this. However, when preparing parents better for the reality of childbearing and early parenting, a careful balance must be struck between disseminating the necessary information and scaring or overwhelming expectant parents by providing an overload of too many facts and unnecessary details. The potentially empowering knowledge provided by this type of childbirth education needs the support of partners and health professionals. However, a recent Australian study has demonstrated that antenatal education can be challenging to sustain in highly medicalised birth environments, which are often constrained by the limitations inherent in such maternity care systems [65].

Another important finding was that, just as there is a continuum between pregnancy, birth and postnatal states in the mother, babies who were born crying and fussing seemed to remain unsettled and irritable. At the same time, those who emerged from the womb as alert, content newborns were more likely to grow into alert, responsive babies with an easy behavioural style. This shows that, while babies may recover from their birth experience to some degree, they do not simply "bounce back". Therefore, it is essential to provide them with the best possible start in life.

These findings will now be discussed in more depth, and possible solutions offered.

The Subjective Birth Experience Matters
Although the survey indicated that the physical birth had an initial impact on the newborn baby, it was the mother's perceptions of her overall birth experience that accounted for the baby's longer-term temperament. How mothers *felt* both physically and emotionally during and after childbirth—especially if experiencing postnatal distress or depression—had a much stronger effect on how they perceived their babies' temperament during the first 6 months than the more objective aspects of childbirth, such as birth mode, pain level and pain relief. Although it's possible that depressed mothers perceive their babies differently, maternal reporting of baby behaviour is generally considered to be fairly consistent when compared to trained external observers. Therefore, the mother's subjective birth experience matters, not just to herself but also to her baby [50]. Moreover, when speaking with mothers, midwives, health visitors and other maternity care providers, I discovered that the subjective birth experience affects the mother-baby pair on multiple levels, impacting mothers' mental health, confidence, self-esteem, self-efficacy, and ability to bond with their baby [49, 51].

Connections Between the Physical and Psychological Birth Experience
Complications and unplanned interventions occurring during childbirth seemed to influence mothers' postnatal perceptions of both the birth experience and their babies' behaviour. We know that unnecessary (as opposed to necessary) medical interventions increase stress for the physiologically intertwined pair, disrupting the natural progression of labour while affecting the baby's ability to self-regulate [19, 24]. The survey data highlighted strong connections between the physical birth experience and the psychological birth experience, so mothers who had a challenging time physically tended to experience psychological consequences too. These mothers were more likely to feel anxious and afraid during their birth and distressed or depressed afterwards. Equally, those who had an easier physical ride during childbirth were more likely to feel positive about their birth and their baby postnatally.

Preventing postnatal depression or PTSD from developing requires intensive professional support during the early postnatal period [14]. Intervention strategies can also begin during pregnancy in the form of childbirth education classes, mindfulness training and cognitive behavioural therapy. These strategies help prevent postnatal depression, with benefits extending beyond the mother to the baby and wider family [6]. If a psychological distress response to childbirth is left untreated and a mother becomes even more distressed or depressed, withdrawn and emotionally unavailable, the midwives and health visitors interviewed in Chap. 5 emphasised how the mother may then struggle to respond appropriately to her baby's distress. This increases the risk of an insecure attachment developing, which is associated with higher cortisol levels in the baby and a greater risk of developing later mood disorders such as anxiety or depression. It may also affect the child's future social and emotional development [39].

Intervention treatments, such as psychological counselling, trauma-focused cognitive behavioural therapy or eye movement desensitisation and reprocessing (EMDR), are all potentially beneficial treatments for reducing symptoms after a traumatic event [12, 16, 70]. Sometimes though, mothers simply need to talk and debrief with a known and trusted midwife. A study testing a midwife-led follow-up counselling session 6 weeks after childbirth in a Swiss university hospital achieved positive results, reducing rates of postnatal depression and childbirth-related PTSD diagnosis [1]. Providing this time to talk and discuss their birth experience was found to be "extremely useful" by 87% of the women who took part in the study.

Newborn Behavioural State and Ongoing Temperament

The survey found that crying and fussing during the first 24 hours post-birth was linked to unsettled baby behaviours from 0 to 6 months. This finding has significant implications for maternity and neonatal care as it means that babies do not necessarily recover as easily and automatically as we once thought they did. Therefore, they need to be treated as gently as possible during their journey from the womb into the world, though unfortunately, this does not always happen. Babies are sentient beings who respond to the birth environment and to their mother's physiology and emotional states. The three original studies contained in this book, together with a wealth of other research evidence presented in Chaps. 1, 2, 3 and 4, highlight that babies are sensitive and social new human beings born programmed to interact with their parents, siblings, wider family and the world around them. This intrinsic need (and skill) can easily be thwarted by treating babies as physical objects rather than as small, non-vocal yet highly intelligent human beings who are acutely aware of their surroundings and fully capable of experiencing either calm and contentment or intense pain and distress.

Why All the Fuss About Oxytocin?

One of the mechanisms behind the impact of childbirth experience on baby behaviour is probably endogenous oxytocin—the hormone produced by mothers and babies during pregnancy, birth, bonding and breastfeeding. This essential hormone is effectively blocked during challenging birth situations where the mother requires an epidural or is releasing too much cortisol, the stress hormone [72]. Babies share and are therefore sensitive to their mother's physiological (hormonal) and emotional states and reflect these back through their own physiology and behaviour. Babies who lack endogenous oxytocin during childbirth may become stuck in a state of poor regulation that remains during toddlerdom and early childhood, potentially contributing to the development of psychiatric disorders such as autism or ADHD [37, 60]. Furthermore, the synthetic version of oxytocin so frequently used in inductions and accelerations of labour has been linked to an increased likelihood of the baby developing one of these challenging behavioural and developmental disorders [33]. Perhaps this is one of the reasons why autism and ADHD diagnoses in young children are on the rise. As we saw in Chap. 3, these effects worsen for babies exposed to epidural analgesia, as this may also affect the baby's brand-new and hyper-sensitive neurobiological system [53]. Although a recent study has shown promising results for reducing symptoms of postnatal depression and enhancing the mother's perceptions of her baby by administering intranasal oxytocin post-birth, this did *not* improve mothers' physiological arousal and sensitivity towards their babies [57]; so it seems oxytocin is a complex hormone that is not easy to fully replicate by artificial means.

An undisturbed, physiological birth experience without any complications or *unnecessary* interventions—in other words, one where the mother releases plenty of oxytocin and only limited amounts of cortisol—is more conducive to positive mother-and-baby behaviours. Mothers who have an empowering, joyful or positive experience without any significant distress find it easier to "tune in", as one health visitor put it, and develop "biobehavioural synchrony" with their baby. The Israeli scientist Ruth Feldman [20] coined this phrase to describe the mutual exchanges of gaze and touch between mother and baby, as well as how well the mother responds to her baby's needs while the baby mirrors her mood and behaviour. Feldman established that the first few days are the most sensitive time for developing mother-baby synchrony. She also discovered that newborn babies who had prolonged skin-to-skin contact behaved differently due to the close proximity they experienced with their mothers. This intimate exposure to their mother's natural release of oxytocin, which generally occurs when she's in close contact with her baby resulted in these babies being less reactive to stressors, sleeping better and exhibiting more biobehavioural synchrony with their mothers than babies who received "care as usual" without prolonged skin-to-skin contact [21].

Once the mother-baby pairs got off to a good start, the babies in Feldman's [21] longitudinal study had higher oxytocin levels and better biobehavioural synchrony with their mothers, not just during this early period but throughout the first year and beyond. Other research has found that this closeness is also beneficial to parents as the oxytocin exchange moderates their autonomic nervous and stress response systems alongside the baby's, shielding them against anxiety and postnatal depression [63]. In contrast, raised cortisol levels in mother and baby lead to disturbed mother-infant interactions and disrupted biobehavioural synchrony [23]. This may also be the first stage in the development of postnatal distress or depression, and—as we discovered in the survey (Chaps. 7 and 8)—these conditions are strong predictors of unsettled, irritable and irregular baby behaviours [50]. Thus, protecting mother and baby's reciprocal neurohormonal states during and after childbirth should be of paramount importance. High cortisol levels and consequently reduced oxytocin may affect the pair's burgeoning relationship, influencing bonding and attachment as well as the baby's future wellbeing, temperament and development.

What Can We Do About Difficult Infant Temperament?

Difficult infant temperaments are undoubtedly extremely challenging to manage, especially for parents experiencing depression. They may also place a significant strain on mother-baby interactions, leading to weaker mother-infant bonding during the first year [67]. Added to this is the risk of a "vicious cycle" of negative effects, with poorer parental functioning due to postnatal depression affecting the baby's temperament and vice versa. This could have negative long-term consequences for infant development [31].

Martha Gartstein—the infant temperament expert who, together with her close colleague Mary Rothbart, designed the widely used Infant Behaviour Questionnaire [26]—believes that early intervention is crucial as temperament is less stable (and therefore more malleable) during infancy than in later childhood [27]. One practical example of such an intervention is the 8-week *Mindful with Your Baby* programme, which has been found to benefit parental functioning, self-efficacy, stress levels and mental health, with positive effects on both the couple relationship and infant temperament. In this intervention study, educating parents in mindful parenting techniques improved infant smiling, laughter and soothability while reducing babies' negative emotional states, such as sadness or distress [48]. Consequently, if a birth has been very challenging and the mother and baby appear distressed, an intervention programme that encourages the mother to focus outwards on how her baby might be feeling and how she can help them feel better could be beneficial.

Applying the Findings to Practice

The findings from the three studies have significant implications for the mother and baby pair and their ongoing wellbeing and relationship with one another. How we manage maternity and neonatal care in our hospitals and midwife-led units is of vital importance. Regardless of which physical interventions occur, whether a mother has a positive or a distressing birth experience seems to affect mother-infant bonding and the baby's behaviour and developing temperament. Likewise, the baby's early behavioural style influences his mother's postnatal mood, mother-infant interactions, and whether the pair will manage to establish biobehavioural synchrony. In turn, these outcomes affect the baby's social engagement, fear regulation and stress reactivity [20–23].

The parent-infant relationship provides the foundation for infant development in all areas—behavioural, social-emotional, cognitive, and language and communication [22, 38, 39]. If the mother's stress response system (HPA axis) is dysregulated during or after childbirth, this could contribute to the development of emotional disorders such as postnatal depression. According to the midwives and health visitors in our maternity care providers' study [49], the baby will tend to reflect this response. Therefore, if the mother is stressed, the mother-baby pair is more likely to struggle with bonding and forming a secure attachment. Meanwhile, the research evidence clearly shows that, without positive interventions, early child attachment patterns may persist into adulthood [71]. Consequently, building positive mother-baby bonds and a secure attachment style lie at the centre of the baby's future stability. Any issues in this area could impact the child's future happiness and wellbeing, as well as their social and emotional development [34].

In the mothers' interview study, it was notable that those who had *unplanned* interventions perceived their birth and their baby's behaviour in a much more negative light than those who had taken an active part in the decision-making process, making *informed choices* about their care. Mothers who felt coerced, directed, bullied or neglected by health professionals could feel quite traumatised after the birth, and this seemed to affect their baby's behaviour and mother-infant bonding during the postnatal period. These findings emphasise the necessity of empowering mothers to feel in control of what is happening to them. Making informed decisions about their own care is key to a positive birth experience [11], and "genuine" choice involves carving out time and space for women to talk through all their options with an experienced health professional they know and trust [42]. Therefore, encouraging all pregnant women to attend antenatal classes where they learn about birthing physiology and all the complex, multidimensional decisions they may need to make could be very helpful. Incorporating the validating and empowering process of informed decision-making with a known and trusted midwife should help to keep women's psychological wellbeing at the centre of the birth process [46, 58].

Thanks to our current human rights laws, making space for "informed choice" is now a legal requirement in UK maternity care [9]; however, not all mothers in our study (or in subsequent studies) felt they were given the opportunity to do so [51]. Parents don't always realise they can request a different midwife if they feel their concerns are not being addressed—and this can be a very positive move for outcomes [46]. Unfortunately, in an urgent situation where there is no time for much discussion, experiencing some trauma can become almost inevitable. However, if the mother has established a trusting relationship with the midwives or doctors caring for her, making a swift decision about what to do in an emergency might be easier.

The main findings of this research—that the subjective birth experience affects the mother's mental health and ability to bond with her baby while also influencing the baby's behaviour and therefore their social and emotional development—mean that we need to begin taking the subjective birth experience much more seriously. Mothers should receive well-supported, one-to-one, continuous and personalised care throughout labour and childbirth, as this promotes the safest and most positive birth outcomes for both mother and baby [58, 59]. A lack of this essential support can profoundly affect the mother's mental health post-birth [30, 46]. As Dr. Emma Svanberg (clinical psychologist and co-founder of the charity *Make Birth* Better) noted poignantly in her discerning book on birth trauma, "Too often, a kind word or a loving touch would have made all the difference" [66, p. 14].

Ideally, there should be mandatory training for all maternity care health professionals about the subjective nature of the birth experience and its link to postnatal mental health, parent-infant bonding and baby behaviour. This training would aim to empower midwives and obstetricians to work together to create an atmosphere of physical and psychological safety and support, thereby reducing parents' fear and stress during childbirth, which are both key contributors to postpartum depression and PTSD [5, 30]. Prompt medical interventions can be absolutely vital and even life-saving when childbirth becomes complicated. Parents undergoing such interventions, especially where they occur in an emergency, need immediate access to postnatal care and mental health counselling to support their confidence, self-efficacy, parental functioning, mental health and parent-infant bonding alongside their baby's wellbeing, behaviour and development. In the meantime, when mother and baby are healthy, their birthing physiology is being well protected by creating a calm and compassionate birth environment, and labour is progressing smoothly, childbirth should be treated as a normal biological human event [35, 55]. In this scenario, the holistic physiological and psychological health and wellbeing of the mother and baby are paramount, and interfering with labour's natural course could result in a cascade of unnecessary, non-evidence-based medical interventions that might create more harm than good [75].

When analysing data and writing a report for the Parent Infant Foundation's Securing Healthy Lives project following the pandemic, one of the things that struck me most was parents' reluctance to disclose their current state of mental health or any parent-baby bonding issues for fear of their baby being "taken away" [3, 4]. This seems to be a very real fear and one that needs tackling urgently, as parents who are struggling postnatally often fail to reach out for the support they so desperately need. Mothers in the Parent Infant Foundation's study spoke about how their partners could also find it very difficult to talk about mental health, even when they seemed depressed. One recurring suggestion parents made was around the benefits of community and peer support groups, the general lack of them, and how it would be beneficial if health professionals could facilitate and promote them to provide much-needed contact with other parents at a similar stage or experiencing similar issues.

According to a survey conducted by the Care Quality Commission [8], although improvements have been made in some areas (e.g. women being asked more frequently about their mental health), the overall quality of maternity care has deteriorated over the past 5 years. This includes parents not feeling as though they are being listened to or properly consulted, a trend that needs to be reversed if we are to stand any chance of improving outcomes for mothers and babies. Meanwhile, an independent review of maternity services in Northern Ireland highlights the urgent need for high-quality maternity care to be provided everywhere [54]. It states that the outcomes and experiences of many mothers and babies are unacceptable and in conflict with the "best evidence" and "international benchmarking". According to the author, good maternity care must achieve two main objectives to ensure the safety and wellbeing of mothers and babies:

1. Help women to stay physically and psychologically healthy so they can enjoy the birth of a new life and the formation of positive new family relationships.
2. Offer timely and appropriate treatments or interventions if and when they are required.

The report emphasises the importance of evidence-based, relationship-based, physically and psychologically safe, personalised woman-centred maternity care delivered with kindness, continuity, compassion, trust, understanding and respect. Currently, this type of compassionate care is often forgotten in the name of "physical safety". Yet "if childbirth is treated like a high-pressure, high-risk environment, that is how staff will behave and women's physiology will respond accordingly, with high levels of stress hormones, fear and distress" [54].

Compassionate care is, of course, vitally important for health care in general, not just maternity care. However, there are growing concerns that it is lacking in areas where resources are overstretched, and these days, midwives have no time to sit and nurture the mothers and babies they are caring for. Compassionate care includes validating and being attuned to the mother's needs (including responding to simple requests for pain relief) and empowering her during and after the birth. "Small acts of kindness" may go a long way towards achieving these aims [74]. When compassionate care is lacking, this poses a major threat to positive physical and psychological outcomes, leading to difficulties in the transition to parenthood and an increase in symptoms of depression, anxiety or PTSD [5, 74].

The Northern Ireland report further emphasises how providing high-quality, compassionate, enabling and empowering care that encompasses the whole perinatal period leads to better physical and psychological outcomes for mothers and babies. The author, Professor Mary Renfrew (OBE), states: "What happens in pregnancy, birth, and following birth affects women, babies, and families for the rest of their lives. Improving maternity care must be a priority for the health services and for society. Investing in improvement will contribute to better physical and mental health for women, better health, well-being and development for babies, better attachment and family relationships, better population health and reduced inequalities, better health and well-being for staff with improved staff retention, and better use of health service resources" [15].

While the complexities of modern childbirth—including rising maternal age, poverty, diabetes, obesity and unhealthy sedentary lifestyles—also need to be considered, if we want to avoid trauma and distress, safe and compassionate continuous care delivered by knowledgeable, skilled midwives needs to be available to all women everywhere. Meanwhile, the current system in the UK and elsewhere suffers from a lack of resources, dangerous levels of staff shortages and "unsafe working conditions" [41]. This physically and psychologically unsafe working environment—where many midwives, nurses and doctors feel they cannot give the quality of care they know is needed and desperately want to provide—compromises the safety and quality of maternity care with detrimental and life-altering outcomes for some families. The current working environment in maternity care means that, alongside reports of consistently rising maternal and neonatal distress and trauma with their associated short and long-term physical and mental health problems for mother and baby [69], for the first time in decades the stillbirth, neonatal and extended perinatal death rates are rising too [36].

Maternal deaths are also rising, particularly among vulnerable ethnic groups, including Black, Brown and younger mothers as well as those from poorer sociodemographic backgrounds [36]. According to figures from the annual UK report on "Saving Lives, Improving Mothers' Care", suicide remains the most common cause of maternal death within the first year after having a baby. And it's not just in the UK where this is happening, but across Western countries, including Europe and North America. Neil Shah, a Harvard University obstetrician and professor who studies safety in pregnancy, has distilled the data and written about the "soaring maternal mortality rate" across the USA. According to him, women giving birth today are 50% more likely to die during the perinatal period than their mothers were, and the risk is "consistently 3–4 times higher" for Black mothers than white mothers [62]. He has worked out that, for every maternal childbirth or perinatal death, there are approximately 100 "severe injuries" due to undetected pregnancy-related conditions such as blood clots or high blood pressure, and for every severe injury, there are tens of thousands of "inadequately treated" physical and mental illnesses.

These stark figures are not due to hospital errors alone (which amount to approximately one in five maternal deaths). Rather, they tend to occur within our communities, where women's natural social support networks have rapidly diminished over the past few decades. Such networks are essential in offering a lifeline to otherwise isolated, overwhelmed and "disempowered" mothers who may be struggling with sleep deprivation, the transition to parenthood, depression or all three [62]. They may also help mothers to recognise the early warning signs of a physical issue that requires urgent medical attention, such as pre-eclampsia. In describing the extreme vulnerability of new and pregnant mothers during the perinatal period, Neil Shah [62] declares that it is *everybody's business*—we all need to "step up"—and that includes health professionals, birth partners, grandparents, friends and neighbours. Vulnerable parents and babies in particular need to receive appropriate levels of practical and emotional support during the extended perinatal period. This care may need to continue for longer and should cater for both parents if they have experienced a devastating perinatal loss. As Renfrew [54] noted, "One woman who lost her baby said, 'I have never felt so held by the health service'. Every woman deserves to experience this standard of care".

It's estimated that up to 60% of new mothers report a negative birth experience, with up to a third describing their birth as traumatic [66]. These figures are neither healthy nor sustainable. Mothers may seek alternative routes if the support they need during and after childbirth cannot be provided within their community or within a physically *and* psychologically safe maternity care system. Rather than risking the continuing growth of unattended "free births"—where the baby is born without a qualified accompanying midwife—it would be sensible to ensure that all options for planned homebirths and continuity of midwifery care models remain open. A homebirth typically ensures the presence of a known midwife and continuity of care throughout labour, with two birth attendants during the second stage, which provides a safe option for healthy, low-risk pregnancies, as discussed in Chap. 3 [7]. Waterbirths are also considered safe for healthy pregnancies [2]. In the mothers' interview study (Chap. 6), homebirths and waterbirths generally seemed to empower the mother, reducing pain and allowing her to remain in control of her birth experience, thereby benefitting the mother and baby's mutual wellbeing and reciprocal behaviour postnatally [51].

Approximately a fifth of all mothers experience some form of postnatal emotional disorder following childbirth. As we have firmly established, parental mood disorders can have significant negative impacts on infant behaviour and development. This 20% figure could be even higher, as many parents are thought to slip under the radar, avoiding confessing to mental health problems or possibly not even realising they could do with some help. Public Health England [28] has emphasised the need to integrate physical and psychological perinatal care, yet the focus is increasingly on physical health and life-or-death situations within the birth room. Meanwhile, the central importance of the mother and baby's physiological and psychological wellbeing to longer-term outcomes frequently gets discarded as an insignificant side issue. Consequently, thousands of women are subjected to blanket interventions they may not want or need—for example, blanket inductions at 40–41 weeks' gestation or antibiotic administration prior to caesarean sections, without fully knowing the risks these practices may entail for the baby. Rather than this potentially harmful approach, policymakers need to look at the first year as a whole and find ways to ensure that mother and baby thrive. They need to make it possible for midwives and health visitors to do everything in their power to facilitate physiological and psychological wellbeing, breastfeeding, bonding and settled baby behaviour.

Instead, women may see up to 10–20 different health professionals during their perinatal journey and are often denied what they have consistently asked for in surveys—continuous care from known midwives who can create an atmosphere of trust, safety and empowerment by getting to know the women they care for and providing personalised care [47]. In a systematic review of studies taking place across 19 different countries, Professor Soo Downe and colleagues [18] found that a positive birth experience truly matters to women. This includes giving birth to a live baby within a clinically *and* psychologically safe environment with kind, competent and reassuring health professionals while receiving both practical and emotional support from chosen birth companions. When a medical intervention is needed, women want to have a say in the decision-making around this so they can remain empowered and in control. This feeling of empowerment stays with women long after childbirth, contributing to positive mental health, successful breastfeeding and bonding, and subsequently easier and more settled baby behaviour.

9.3 Conclusion

Baby behaviour is affected both directly through the physiological impacts of medicalised interventions on the baby's stress response system [17, 68] and indirectly through the mother's subjective birth experience and postnatal emotional state, whether positive or negative [50]. Extensive research has shown that maternal postnatal distress and depression impact the baby's physiological wellbeing, behaviour and development by adversely affecting natural bonding and attachment processes. Therefore, the mother and newborn baby should be viewed as biologically *and* psychologically inseparable, interconnected by their mutual neurohormonal pathways throughout the perinatal period. Caring for mother and baby respectfully and compassionately during this time optimises physiological and psychological outcomes. When they are well cared for during the birth and postnatally, we maximise their chance of successful bonding and breastfeeding. These processes promote mutual wellbeing, positive baby behaviour and healthy infant development [22, 38].

To achieve the best long-term outcomes for mother and baby, we must therefore protect their naturally interwoven physiology during childbirth and postnatally as much as we can, given the circumstances of the birth [44, 73], and this should be engraved into maternity care policy and practice [43]. The concept of safety in maternity and neonatal care needs updating to incorporate all the latest research on the psychology of childbirth, so that the word "safety" means more than just the *physical* care of mother and baby. Defensive medical decision-making based on concerns about litigation must be carefully balanced against the very real possibility of inflicting lasting physical and psychological trauma on mother and baby. The notion of "safety" in childbirth should include physiological, psychological, social, emotional and cultural safety for everyone who gives birth, regardless of their background, gender, creed or colour.

Medical interventions can be life-saving and therefore "essential when used appropriately", and it is important for women to have the right to choose them [56]. In line with the National Institute for Health and Care Excellence [40] guidance, this should include granting mothers a "requested caesarean birth" if they have made an informed choice to have one and all other options have been discussed. Where a pain-inducing intervention such as an induction or caesarean section is needed, the pain needs to be carefully managed and the mother should be treated by trauma-informed health professionals (including the anaesthesiologist) throughout the process [32].

As we witnessed in several of the mothers' horrific birth stories in Chap. 6, women are not always involved in the decision-making [10], and interventions often occur without their informed choice or consent. For example: "And then everything I didn't want to happen happened, which was, I didn't want to have stirrups or anything like that, and the next thing was they took the gas and air away and said I wasn't pushing hard enough..." (Rachael: hospital induction, third-degree tear, postpartum haemorrhage—[51]). Experiences like these are highly likely to increase maternal stress, raising cortisol levels and decreasing oxytocin, disrupting healthy birthing physiology and causing trauma to mother and baby. In contrast, when the mother is well-supported, listened to, respected and involved in the decision-making process, she is more likely to have a positive birth experience, free from fear, anxiety or stress. Moreover, breastfeeding, bonding and positive baby behaviours are all optimised. In this scenario, the mother and baby pair are set up not only to survive but to thrive.

Childbirth affects us all. We have all been born, and most of us become parents. Therefore, it is time to re-humanise the childbirth experience. It is time to listen to women and hear what they want for themselves and their babies. We also need to listen to the wisdom of highly experienced practising or academic midwives and obstetricians. In the words of Page and Wardhaugh [45], "Childbirth (the period around pregnancy, labour and birth and the early weeks of life) is a time of promise and potential. It is a time of infinite possibilities, with the potential for love and social thriving, as well as for optimal health and wellbeing. The consequences can resonate beyond the short term, over a lifetime and into the next generation".

In a similar vein, Renfrew [54] states: "This is formative time for the baby. It is the start of life, and what happens to the baby in pregnancy, birth, and in the early days and weeks will affect the rest of their life; it is well known that the first 1000 days of life influence lifelong health and wellbeing. This time offers a unique opportunity not only to avoid harm, but to positively enhance the baby's health, wellbeing and development". In an urgent plea for evidence-based changes to the current maternity care system, midwifery professor Mary Renfrew goes on to explain: "It is the beginning of a whole new human being… It is the beginning of the population over time. Every person goes through this system … and we forget that at our peril" [54][1].

References

1. Avignon V, Annen V, Baud D, Bourdin J, Horsch A. Evaluating a midwife-led consultation for women after a traumatic birth experience: preliminary results. Midwifery. 2025;144:104358.
2. Barry PL, McMahon LE, Banks RA, Fergus AM, Murphy DJ. Prospective cohort study of water immersion for labour and birth compared with standard care in an Irish maternity setting. BMJ Open. 2020;10(12):e038080.
3. Bateson K, Power C. Building strong infant bonds: what support do parents want? Community Pract. 2023;2023:40–3. https://www.researchgate.net/publication/375381093_httpswwwcommunitypractitionercoukparents-perceptions-and-experiences-of-support-to-develop-a-secure-parent-infant-relationship
4. Bateson K, et al. The parent-infant foundation. Securing health lives: an extended summary of research about parent-infant relationship help and support across Cwm Taf Morgannwg. 2021. https://parentinfantfoundation.org.uk/publications/resources-for-professionals/.
5. Bell AF, Andersson E. The birth experience and women's postnatal depression: a systematic review. Midwifery. 2016;39:112–23.
6. Bjertrup AJ, Rasmussen KH, Miskowiak KW. Psychological prevention of postpartum depression for expectant parents. J Affect Disord. 2025;378:58–73.
7. Brocklehurst P, Puddicombe D, Hollowell J, Stewart M, Linsell L, Macfarlane AJ, McCourt C. Perinatal and maternal outcomes by planned place of birth for healthy women with low risk pregnancies: the birthplace in England national prospective cohort study. BMJ. 2011;343:d7400.
8. Care Quality Commission. Maternity survey. 2024. https://www.cqc.org.uk/publications/surveys/maternity-survey.
9. Chan SW, Tulloch E, Cooper ES, Smith A, Wojcik W, Norman JE. Montgomery and informed consent: where are we now? BMJ. 2017;357:j2224.
10. Coates R, Cupples G, Scamell A, McCourt C. Women's experiences of induction of labour: qualitative systematic review and thematic synthesis. Midwifery. 2019;69:17–28.
11. De Schepper S, Vercauteren T, Tersago J, Jacquemyn Y, Raes F, Franck E. Post-traumatic stress disorder after childbirth and the influence of maternity team care during labour and birth: a cohort study. Midwifery. 2016;32:87–92.
12. Dekel S, Papadakis JE, Quagliarini B, Jagodnik KM, Nandru R. A systematic review of interventions for prevention and treatment of post-traumatic stress disorder following childbirth. medRxiv. 2023; https://doi.org/10.1101/2023.08.17.23294230.
13. Delicate A, Ayers S, McMullen S. Health-care practitioners' assessment and observations of birth trauma in mothers and partners. J Reprod Infant Psychol. 2020;40:1–13.
14. Dennis CL, Dowswell T. Psychosocial and psychological interventions for preventing postpartum depression. Cochrane Database Syst Rev. 2013;2013(2):CD001134.
15. Department of Health. Radical system-wide change needed in maternity services. 2024. https://www.health-ni.gov.uk/news/radical-system-wide-change-needed-maternity-services.

---

[1] Professor Mary Renfrew discussing her recent maternity care in Northern Ireland report on the Maternity and Midwifery Hour, 15th February 2025.

16. Doherty A, Nagle U, Doyle J, Duffy RM. Eye movement desensitisation and reprocessing for childbirth-related post-traumatic stress symptoms: effectiveness, duration and completion. Front Glob Womens Health. 2025;6:1487799.
17. Douglas PS, Hill PS. A neurobiological model for cry-fuss problems in the first three to four months of life. Med Hypotheses. 2013;81(5):816–22.
18. Downe S, Finlayson K, Oladapo O, Bonet M, Gülmezoglu AM. What matters to women during childbirth: a systematic qualitative review. PLoS One. 2018;13(4):e0194906.
19. Downe S, Calleja Agius J, Balaam MC, Frith L. Understanding childbirth as a complex salutogenic phenomenon: The EU COST BIRTH Action Special Collection. PLoS One. 2020;15(8):e0236722.
20. Feldman R. Parent–infant synchrony: a biobehavioral model of mutual influences in the formation of affiliative bonds. Monogr Soc Res Child Dev. 2012;77(2):42–51.
21. Feldman R. Sensitive periods in human social development: new insights from research on oxytocin, synchrony, and high-risk parenting. Dev Psychopathol. 2015;27(2):369–95.
22. Feldman R. The neurobiology of human attachments. Trends Cogn Sci. 2017;21:80–99.
23. Feldman R, Granat A, Pariente C, Kanety H, Kuint J, Gilboa-Schechtman E. Maternal depression and anxiety across the postpartum year and infant social engagement, fear regulation, and stress reactivity. J Am Acad Child Adolesc Psychiatry. 2009;48(9):919–27.
24. Fuemmeler BF, Lee CT, Soubry A, Iversen ES, Huang Z, Murtha AP, Schildkraut JM, Jirtle RL, Murphy SK, Hoyo C. DNA methylation of regulatory regions of imprinted genes at birth and its relation to infant temperament. Genet Epigenet. 2016;8:59–67.
25. Garthus-Niegel S, Ayers S, Martini J, von Soest T, Eberhard-Gran M. The impact of postpartum post-traumatic stress disorder symptoms on child development: a population-based, 2-year follow-up study. Psychol Med. 2017;47(1):161–70.
26. Gartstein MA, Rothbart MK. Studying infant temperament via the revised infant behavior questionnaire. Infant Behav Dev. 2003;26(1):64–86.
27. Gartstein MA, Putnam SP, Aron EN, Rothbart MK. Temperament and personality. In: Oxford handbook of treatment processes and outcomes in counseling psychology. New York: Oxford University Press; 2016. p. 11–41.
28. Gov.uk. Public Health England guidance. 4. Perinatal mental health. 2019. Retrieved from https://www.gov.uk/government/publications/better-mental-health-jsna-toolkit/4-perinatal-mental-health#fn:2.
29. Harris R, Ayers S. What makes labour and birth traumatic? A survey of intrapartum 'hotspots'. Psychol Health. 2012;27(10):1166–77.
30. Horsch A, Garthus-Niegel S. Posttraumatic stress disorder following childbirth. In: Childbirth, vulnerability and law. Oxford: Routledge; 2019. p. 49–66.
31. Ortiz RMR, Barnes J. Temperament, parental personality and parenting stress in relation to socio-emotional development at 51 months. Early Child Dev Care. 2019; ISSN 0300-4430. https://core.ac.uk/download/pdf/146458523.pdf.
32. Kountanis JA, Vogel TM. Unveiling the anesthesiologist's impact on childbirth-related post-traumatic stress disorder. Anesth Analg. 2024;139(6):1156–8.
33. Kurth L, O'Shea TM, Burd I, Dunlop AL, Croen L, Wilkening G, et al. Intrapartum exposure to synthetic oxytocin, maternal BMI, and neurodevelopmental outcomes in children within the ECHO consortium. J Neurodev Disord. 2024;16(1):26.
34. Le Bas G, Youssef G, Macdonald JA, Teague S, Mattick R, Honan I, et al. The role of antenatal and postnatal maternal bonding in infant development. J Am Acad Child Adolesc Psychiatry. 2022;61(6):820–9.
35. Maga G, Magon A, Caruso R, Brigante L, Daniele MAS, Belloni S, Arrigoni C. Development and validation of the midwifery interventions classification for a salutogenic approach to maternity care: a Delphi study. Healthcare. 2024;12(22):2228. MDPI.
36. MBRRACE. Saving lives, improving mothers' care 2024 – lessons learned to inform maternity care from the UK and Ireland confidential enquiries into maternal deaths. 2024. https://www.npeu.ox.ac.uk/mbrrace-uk/reports/maternal-reports/maternal-report-2020-2022.

References

37. Moerkerke M, Peeters M, de Vries L, Daniels N, Steyaert J, Alaerts K, Boets B. Endogenous oxytocin levels in autism—a meta-analysis. Brain Sci. 2021;11(11):1545.
38. Murray L, Cooper P, Fearon P. Parenting difficulties and postnatal depression: implications for primary healthcare assessment and intervention. Community Pract. 2014;87(11):34–8.
39. Murray L, Halligan S, Cooper P. Postnatal depression and young children's development. New York: Guilford Press; 2018.
40. National Institute for Health and Care Excellence. Caesarean birth. 2024. https://www.nice.org.uk/guidance/ng192/documents/draft-guideline.
41. Nursing and Midwifery Council. NMC responds to independent review of midwifery services in Northern Ireland. 2024. https://www.nmc.org.uk/news/news-and-updates/nmc-responds-to-independent-review-of-midwifery-services-in-northern-ireland/.
42. O'Brien D, Butler MM, Casey M. A participatory action research study exploring women's understandings of the concept of informed choice during pregnancy and childbirth in Ireland. Midwifery. 2017;46:1–7.
43. Page L. Women and babies need protection from the dangers of normal birth ideology: AGAINST: support for normal birth is crucial to safe high-quality maternity care. BJOG Int J Obstet Gynaecol. 2017;124(9):1385.
44. Page L, Newnham E. Humanisation of childbirth 8: where do we go from here? Pract Midwife. 2020;23(4):1–6. https://www.all4maternity.com/humanisation-of-childbirth-8-where-do-we-go-from-here-2/
45. Page L, Wardhaugh C. Love and the humanisation of childbirth. In: Love and midwifery. Abingdon: Routledge; 2025. p. 24–37.
46. Patterson J, Hollins Martin C, Karatzias T. PTSD post-childbirth: a systematic review of women's and midwives' subjective experiences of care provider interaction. J Reprod Infant Psychol. 2019;37(1):56–83.
47. Perriman N, Davis DL, Ferguson S. What women value in the midwifery continuity of care model: a systematic review with meta-synthesis. Midwifery. 2018;62:220–9.
48. Potharst ES, Kraakman R, Bögels SM, Colonnesi C. Effect of mindful with your baby training on infant temperament: what parental factors are at play? Personal Individ Differ. 2025;238:113084.
49. Power C, Williams C, Brown A. Does childbirth experience affect infant behaviour? Exploring the perceptions of maternity care providers. Midwifery. 2019;78:131–9.
50. Power C, Williams C, Brown A. Physical and psychological childbirth experiences and early infant temperament. Front Psychol. 2022;13:792392.
51. Power C, Williams C, Brown A. Does a mother's childbirth experience influence her perceptions of her baby's behaviour? A qualitative interview study. PLoS One. 2023;18(4):e0284183.
52. Power C, Weise V, Mack JT, Karl M, Garthus-Niegel S. Does parental mental health mediate the association between parents' perceived stress and parent-infant bonding during the early COVID-19 pandemic? Early Hum Dev. 2024;189:105931.
53. Qiu C, Carter SA, Lin JC, Shi JM, Chow T, Desai VN, et al. Association of labor epidural analgesia, oxytocin exposure, and risk of autism spectrum disorders in children. JAMA Netw Open. 2023;6(7):e2324630.
54. Renfrew M. Enabling safe quality midwifery services and care in Northern Ireland. 2024. https://www.health-ni.gov.uk/sites/default/files/publications/health/doh-midwifery-renfrew-report-oct-2024_0.pdf.
55. Renfrew MJ, McFadden A, Bastos MH, Campbell J, Channon AA, Cheung NF, et al. Midwifery and quality care: findings from a new evidence-informed framework for maternal and newborn care. Lancet. 2014;384(9948):1129–45.
56. Renfrew MJ, Cheyne H, Burnett A, Crozier K, Downe S, Heazell A, et al. Responding to the Ockenden review: safe care for all needs evidence-based system change-and strengthened midwifery. Midwifery. 2022;112:103391.
57. Riem MM, Loheide-Niesmann L, Beijers R, Tendolkar I, Mulders PC. Boosting oxytocin in postpartum depression: intranasal oxytocin enhances maternal positive affect and regard for the infant. Psychoneuroendocrinology. 2025;179:107530.

58. Sandall J, Soltani H, Gates S, Shennan A, Devane D. Midwife-led continuity models of care compared with other models of care for women during pregnancy, birth and early parenting. Cochrane Database Syst Rev. 2016;4(4):CD004667.
59. Sandall J, Turienzo CF, Devane D, Soltani H, Gillespie P, Gates S, et al. Midwife continuity of care models versus other models of care for childbearing women. Cochrane Database Syst Rev. 2024;4(4):CD004667.
60. Sasaki T, Hashimoto K, Oda Y, Ishima T, Kurata T, Takahashi J, et al. Decreased levels of serum oxytocin in pediatric patients with attention deficit/hyperactivity disorder. Psychiatry Res. 2015;228(3):746–51.
61. Schechter DS, Willheim E, Hinojosa C, Scholfield-Kleinman K, Turner JB, McCaw J, Zeanah CH, Myers MM. Subjective and objective measures of parent-child relationship dysfunction, child separation distress, and joint attention. Psychiatry Interpers Biolog Processes. 2010;73(2):130–44.
62. Shah N. A soaring maternal mortality rate: what does it mean for you? vol. 16. Harvard Health Blog; 2018.
63. Stuebe AM, Grewen K, Meltzer-Brody S. Association between maternal mood and oxytocin response to breastfeeding. J Women's Health. 2013;22(4):352–61.
64. Stuijfzand S, Garthus-Niegel S, Horsch A. Parental birth-related PTSD symptoms and bonding in the early postpartum period: a prospective population-based cohort study. Front Psych. 2020;11:941.
65. Sutcliffe K, Dahlen H, Newnham E, Mackay L, Levett K. Pulled in different directions–the experiences of birth partners and care-providers when supporting women to implement what they learn in childbirth education classes. Midwifery. 2025;145:104372.
66. Svanberg E. Why birth trauma matters. London: Pinter & Martin; 2019.
67. Takács L, Smolík F, Kaźmierczak M, Putnam SP. Early infant temperament shapes the nature of mother-infant bonding in the first postpartum year. Infant Behav Dev. 2020;58:101428.
68. Taylor A, Fisk NM, Glover V. Mode of delivery and subsequent stress response. Lancet. 2000;355(9198):120.
69. Thomas K. Birth trauma inquiry report. Listen to Mums: ending the postcode lottery on perinatal care. 2024. https://www.theo-clarke.org.uk/sites/www.theo-clarke.org.uk/files/2024-05/Birth%20Trauma%20Inquiry%20Report%20for%20Publication_May13_2024.pdf.
70. Torres-Giménez A, Garcia-Gibert C, Gelabert E, Mallorquí A, Segu X, Roca-Lecumberri A, et al. Efficacy of EMDR for early intervention after a traumatic event: a systematic review and meta-analysis. J Psychiatr Res. 2024;174:73–83.
71. Ulmer-Yaniv A, Waidergoren S, Shaked A, Salomon R, Feldman R. Neural representation of the parent–child attachment from infancy to adulthood. Soc Cogn Affect Neurosci. 2022;17(7):609–24.
72. Uvnäs-Moberg K. Why oxytocin matters, vol. 16. London: Pinter & Martin Ltd.; 2019.
73. Uvnäs-Moberg K, Ekström-Bergström A, Berg M, Buckley S, Pajalic Z, Hadjigeorgiou E, Kotłowska A, Lengler L, Kielbratowska B, Leon-Larios F, Magistretti CM, Downe S, Lindström B, Dencker A. Maternal plasma levels of oxytocin during physiological childbirth–a systematic review with implications for uterine contractions and central actions of oxytocin. BMC Pregnancy Childbirth. 2019;19(1):285.
74. Vedeler C, Nilsen ABV, Downe S, Eri TS. The "doing" of compassionate care in the context of childbirth from a women's perspective. Qual Health Res. 2024;35(10–11):1177–90. https://doi.org/10.1177/10497323241280370.
75. WHO. World Health Organization recommendations: intrapartum care for a positive childbirth experience. 2018. https://www.who.int/publications/i/item/9789241550215.

MIX
Papier aus verantwortungsvollen Quellen
Paper from responsible sources
FSC® C105338

If you have any concerns about our products,
you can contact us on
ProductSafety@springernature.com

In case Publisher is established outside the EU,
the EU authorized representative is:
**Springer Nature Customer Service Center GmbH
Europaplatz 3, 69115 Heidelberg, Germany**

Printed by Libri Plureos GmbH
in Hamburg, Germany